THERAPEUTIC
CHANGE
WITH
DIFFICULT
CLIENTS

Even the most experienced and skilled therapists encounter challenges with clients that can stifle progress and bring frustration into the therapeutic relationship. In this volume, Wilkinson and Hanna explore a compassionate approach to working with these challenges that considers the unique individual client. It is an excellent resource for any therapist.

—Louis Hoffman, PhD, Editor, *APA Handbook of Humanistic and Existential Psychology* and coeditor, *The Evidence-Based Foundations of Existential–Humanistic Therapy*

If I could only grab one book to give to psychotherapists in training at any level it would be *Therapeutic Change With Difficult Clients*. It has enough theory, so it hangs together well, but the real treasure is the host of tools and techniques that are wonderfully explained and exemplified. No therapist, even experienced ones, should miss this valuable volume. This old dog learned lots of new tricks!

—David M. Young, PhD, Professor Emeritus, Psychology, Purdue University Fort Wayne, Fort Wayne, IN; coauthor of *The Silent Language of Psychotherapy, Third Edition*

Drs. Wilkinson and Hanna are percipient thinkers who have put together a truly invaluable book on how to work with some of the most challenging clients. Filled with keen insights and practical wisdom for practice, I am confident that this second edition will be widely read and cited for years to come.

—Matthew E. Lemberger-Truelove, PhD, American Counseling Association Fellow; Professor of Counseling at the University of North Texas, Denton, TX

Finally, a book about how to support people in their change process! This book's focus on facilitating and enhancing people's change process is a must-read for all mental health providers. Too often it is assumed our clients want to change, when in reality, most people have ambivalence about change. The authors guide readers, step-by-step, with practical tools they can use to help encourage change. The case examples and applications bring to life the most important thing we do as helpers—support others in their change process.

—**Victoria Kress, PhD,** Distinguished Professor, Youngstown State University, Youngstown, OH

THERAPEUTIC CHANGE
WITH
DIFFICULT CLIENTS

Second Edition

Precursors and Techniques
in the CHANGES Model

BRETT D. WILKINSON | FRED J. HANNA

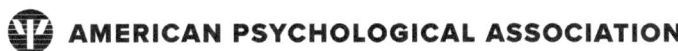 AMERICAN PSYCHOLOGICAL ASSOCIATION

The opinions and statements published are those of the Authors, and do not necessarily represent the policies of the American Psychological Association. The information contained in this work does not constitute personalized therapeutic advice. Users seeking medical advice, diagnoses, or treatment should consult a medical professional or health care provider. The Authors have worked to ensure that all information in this book is accurate at the time of publication and consistent with general mental health care standards.

Published by
American Psychological Association
750 First Street, NE
Washington, DC 20002
https://www.apa.org

Order Department
https://www.apa.org/pubs/books
order@apa.org

Typeset in Meridien and Ortodoxa by Lumina Datamatics, India

Printer: Sheridan Books, Chelsea, MI
Cover Designer: Anthony Paular Design, Newbury Park, CA

Library of Congress Cataloging-in-Publication Data

Names: Wilkinson, Brett D. author | Hanna, Fred J. author
Title: Therapeutic change with difficult clients : precursors and
 techniques in the CHANGES model / by Brett D. Wilkinson and Fred J.
 Hanna.
Other titles: Therapy with difficult clients
Description: Second edition. | Washington, DC : American Psychological
 Association, [2025] | Revised edition of: Therapy with difficult clients :
 using the precursors model to awaken change / Fred J. Hanna.
 Washington, DC : American Psychological Association, c2002. | Includes
 bibliographical references and index.
Identifiers: LCCN 2024061452 (print) | LCCN 2024061453 (ebook) | ISBN
 9781433843167 paperback | ISBN 9781433843174 ebook
Subjects: LCSH: Impasse (Psychotherapy) | Attitude change
Classification: LCC RC489.I45 H36 2025 (print) | LCC RC489.I45 (ebook) |
 DDC 616.8914—dc23/eng/20250307
LC record available at https://lccn.loc.gov/2024061452
LC ebook record available at https://lccn.loc.gov/2024061453

https://doi.org/10.1037/0000451-000

Printed in the United States of America

10 9 8 7 6 5 4 3 2 1

CONTENTS

PREFACE

We have spent our careers seeing clients in therapy, training and supervising graduate students, providing consultations in the community, and conducting research on therapy processes. Across these avenues, our study of therapeutic change has been a persistent theme. We consider the subject of therapeutic change to be one of the most intriguing and extraordinary topics among the vast range of phenomena that constitute human life. Change remains ever at the heart of our work as therapists and, indeed, at the root of our personal experiences in navigating a fulfilling life.

Well-established techniques quite often hit the mark with relative ease among those clients who are willing and able to intentionally engage in the therapeutic change process. However, one of the most challenging aspects of therapy is working with clients who have little interest in change, or who think that change is a waste of time, or who somehow have come to believe that change is a threat to their personal freedom or sense of being. The limits of psychotherapy effectiveness become starkly evident when we look steadfastly at the difficulty of creating change for such clients, making it one of the most important areas of consideration for ongoing research efforts.

The many theories of psychotherapy, from behavioral to psychodynamic and from existential to family systems, are remarkably instructive and descriptive of the subtleties and complexities of human thought, feeling, behavior, and relationships. There is no substitute for the study of the great insights these theories catalog and represent. Add to those the integrative and eclectic approaches to psychotherapy, and one has a rich and wide spectrum of perspectives on human problems. Nevertheless, classic theories and innovative integrative approaches do not go far enough in capturing the essential structures and dynamics of change. We remain in need of the knowledge of what makes people change. We also believe there is a need for more techniques and approaches to help such clients and the therapists who work with them.

Our investigations of therapeutic change with difficult clients have revealed a host of subtle processes that affect change. Such subtle processes often go unacknowledged in routine psychotherapy, not because they are hidden but because they are pervasive. Such pervasiveness often makes them difficult to identify and articulate. For example, what are the subtle processes that move a callous, cruel man from nearly exclusive self-centeredness toward opening up to the feelings and views of others? What are the dynamics that make an involuntary, defiant, court-ordered client wake up to become aware of a problem and involved in therapy? What brings a helplessly depressed person to the point of realizing that depression is something that can be influenced and relieved? Similarly, when a client is sitting on the fence between taking responsibility and blaming others, what nudges the person toward responsibility? These are difficult questions and certainly require further research, but we now know that such changes result not from a single process but a combination of many.

A major purpose of this book is to identify seven of these processes and move them from the vague to the defined. We have called the processes precursors because they herald the arrival of change. When the precursors dawn, change is on the horizon. We hope to outline the intricate and variable manner in which the precursors act interdependently to produce change. To help therapists use the CHANGES model, we propose a clinical assessment tool that reveals which of the precursors is missing in the client who is not achieving change. Finally, we provide techniques for implementing each precursor in accordance with the assessment. This is the essence of the precursors approach to therapeutic change. The precursors are offered as an aid to clients for whom therapy is a painful and fruitless struggle.

From the outset, we want to make it clear that the precursors are neither our invention nor our discovery. They were recognized long before the dawn of psychotherapy. We have only shown how they interact and described an array of techniques that stimulate the precursors in clients who may not otherwise achieve positive change. We share these techniques and approaches in the hope they will help therapists work with difficult clients to achieve change sooner rather than later.

ACKNOWLEDGMENTS

I (Brett) have had the privilege of learning from and connecting with so many inspiring figures, wise friends, and good colleagues over the years. I would like to first thank Fred Hanna, who has been an inspirational mentor and good friend. The opportunity to collaborate on this important work has been a pleasure, and I am grateful for the chance to contribute to the field in this way.

To my wife, Katherine, whose insightfulness as a therapist, patience as my life partner, and boundless love as a mother, has been my lodestar. To our children, Elianora and Rowan, whose earnestness and curiosity are a welcomed reminder of what matters most in life. To my father, stepmother, and sister, for their unwavering love and support, I am forever grateful. And to my late mother, of course, whose heart endures.

I would also like to share my gratitude for the mentorships of the late counselor Tim Robertson, the evolutionary psychologist Harmon Holcomb, and the Husserlian scholar Ronald Bruzina, all of whom fostered my curiosity and lent compassionate guidance at critical stages in my journey. Appreciation also extends to my friend of 30 years, Kusha Sefat, whose intellectual virtuosity is equaled only by his humor, adaptability, and brilliance at the piano. And to my many colleagues, graduate students, and former clients: I have gained so much from my relations with each of you, and I am thankful for the chance to have played a small part in your big life story.

I (Fred) have been inspired by many people in this field. Some I have met in person, and others I have not. I am grateful to them all for providing insights that have helped me find my path in this fascinating and gratifying work. First, I want to thank my wife, Constance Hanna, a wonderfully effective and empathic therapist. Her wisdom and advice have kept me practical and concrete.

I also thank two professional philosophers from whom I benefited enormously. Ramakrishna Puligandla taught me the subtleties and liberating potential of dialectical philosophy from the viewpoints of both Kant and Nagarjuna. James Daley, friend and mentor, validated my ideas and taught me the insider's perspective on phenomenology as a philosophical discipline and its implications for psychology. Studying with him brought Husserl and Heidegger to life, especially in terms of consciousness, dialectics, and ontology. My study with both of these men afforded great insight into the nature and goals of psychotherapy from a philosophical perspective.

My collaboration with Kaisa Puhakka has been nothing less than extraordinary. I am deeply thankful to her for teaching me the subtleties of object relations therapy. Most of all, she has always been willing to take part in a vital interchange of ideas on Asian philosophy and psychology that was part of our perennial quest to understand the human predicament.

The pioneering insights of Jerome Frank are now legendary, and I am deeply grateful to him for the extraordinarily helpful conversations we had during my time at Johns Hopkins. I thank George Howard for his wisdom, innovative research, and progressive ideas concerning psychotherapy. When I was a graduate student, he took me under his wing and patiently answered dozens of questions. He helped shed light on a path that would have taken me many years to find on my own.

I also thank Hal Arkowitz, who encouraged me to write the original article on which this book is based. Michael Mahoney's comments on my work have been of great value. His deep and global view of psychotherapy and therapeutic change has been a rich source of insight for me for many years. I extend my heartfelt thanks to him for his invaluable suggestions concerning the original draft of this book. I have also found the work of Arnold Lazarus to be a source of instruction and learning. I have greatly admired his teachings, bold thinking, and commentary on psychotherapy as well as his therapeutic wisdom. I owe a debt of gratitude to Al Ottens, who has always been there for perceptive comments, support, and reassurance. I also thank Martin Ritchie, Chris Aanstoos, and Lorean Roberts for their professional and personal support. Finally, I want to acknowledge and extend deep thanks to my friend and coauthor, Brett Wilkinson. He is a person of great insight, creativity, and vision. Our nearly 15-year association has been most rewarding, supportive, and fortuitous.

In terms of the manuscript itself, we would like to thank Susan Reynolds, Senior Acquisitions Editor at American Psychological Association Books, for her patience and encouragement in this long process. We thank Molly Gage for her guidance in development.

THERAPEUTIC CHANGE
WITH
DIFFICULT CLIENTS

Introduction

In this book, we endeavor to clarify that which brings about beneficial change in human beings. Its promise lies in the fact that it concentrates on within-individual catalysts that bring therapeutic change into being. Psychotherapy has grown and evolved immensely in the intervening 140 years since Sigmund Freud studied hypnosis under Jean-Martin Charcot at the Pitié-Salpêtrière Hospital in Paris. Nowhere is this more evident than in the area of theory-into-practice, as more than 500 theories of, and approaches to, psychotherapy have been proposed as an efficacious means to facilitate change with clients (Goldfried, 2019). Yet we still know relatively little about the intricacies of therapeutic change itself; much of this essential knowledge remains to be discovered.

Psychotherapy researchers have expended considerable effort demonstrating that psychotherapy facilitates change, whereas mechanisms or processes by which such change is produced remain a bit of a mystery, which is not to say that valuable inroads have not been made. Outcome research does not always present a sufficiently detailed or accurate picture of therapeutic change in practice, which led Gendlin (1986) to promote the value of microprocess moments in therapy. Such change process research has long been a valuable route to "identifying, describing, explaining, and predicting the effects of the processes that bring about therapeutic change" (Greenberg, 1986, p. 4) that complements process-outcome research, randomized control trials, and experimental designs.

Yet, even within the tighter sphere of change process research, the primary methods of analysis tend to emphasize change only within the context of therapeutic practice. As outlined by Elliott (2010), qualitative helpful factors design asks clients to identify what in the therapeutic process helped facilitate

https://doi.org/10.1037/0000451-001

Therapeutic Change With Difficult Clients: Precursors and Techniques in the CHANGES Model, Second Edition, by B. D. Wilkinson and F. J. Hanna

change, microanalytic sequential process design tends to closely scrutinize coded therapist–client interactions to identify change catalysts, and the significant events approach examines major transition points in the therapeutic process. Taking a closer look at research that employs such designs, the focal points of analysis tend to be therapist behaviors, attitudes, and dispositions; therapist-led interventions, techniques, and methods; and therapist–client relationship factors.

The CHANGES model is an outgrowth of qualitative research in the spirit of a significant events approach but without the within-session task analysis features often associated with such designs (Pascual-Leone et al., 2009). Instead, Hanna and Ritchie (1995) compiled 32 variables cited in the psychotherapy literature as having the capacity for producing change. Participants were screened for having undergone a major, significant moment of therapeutic change and were then asked to rate those 32 variables on a "perceived potency scale" to gauge perceived causal relationships between variables and events. Ratings on the 5-point scale included: 0 = *not present*; 1 = *present but not a factor in change*; 2 = *somewhat of a factor*; 3 = *a definite factor*; 4 = *a necessary condition for change*; and 5 = *a sufficient condition for change*. The study concluded that several of the 32 variables may regulate both the rate and magnitude of therapeutic change, seven of which have been identified as fundamental precursors of therapeutic change in the CHANGES model.

FUNDAMENTAL QUESTIONS

A more thorough understanding of the intricacies of therapeutic change may be the most important step toward improving the effectiveness of psychotherapy. Procedures can then be developed that derive from that new and vital knowledge. When it comes to using techniques, therapists still rely, for the most part, on those that have been cataloged in alignment with the various theories, such as behavioral, Adlerian, gestalt, or cognitive. Are there undiscovered change principles that can lead to the development of more effective techniques and more efficient use of the techniques we have?

There are some fundamental questions about change that need to be addressed in this regard. Why is it that some clients change relatively quickly in therapy while others make little, if any, progress? Why is change painfully difficult for some clients and comparatively easy for others? Why do some clients welcome change, but others resist and struggle against it every inch of the way? Why do some clients achieve core personality changes, whereas others make relatively minor, linear adjustments? Why do some clients recognize that therapeutic change is important, but others see it as threatening? And how can the most beneficial change be produced in the shortest amount of time, especially in this age of managed care?

Each of these questions emphasizes client-specific, within-individual factors for which we have an incomplete understanding. We hope to persuade therapists that a better understanding of within-individual change factors is crucial to fostering change, particularly for difficult clients. The latter point is of universal concern in psychotherapy as we continue to wrangle with how to help clients who are disinterested in change. Tried and true techniques, rigorous treatment methods, and every bit of efficacy evidence born of research are of little use to the therapist who sits across from a client who has no interest in changing. As the American journalist Sydney J. Harris (1986) wrote, "Our dilemma is that we hate change and love it at the same time. What we really want is for things to remain the same but get better" (p. 36). As a principle, this is perhaps what makes therapy one of the most difficult professions there is. Like chess, it is relatively easy to learn principles and maneuvers, but it is incredibly difficult to master and more difficult still when working with a disengaged client.

PRECURSORS OF CHANGE

This book offers one approach to these fundamental questions by suggesting a set of seven critical variables called "precursors" that are conducive to psycho-therapeutic change. A *precursor* is generally defined as that which precedes and, so to speak, "announces" the arrival of something else. We refer to these seven variables as precursors because their presence indicates the imminent manifestation of change. The seven precursors are not focused on the therapist, theories, or techniques. Each has to do with client-specific factors, that is, what the client brings to the session.

The seven precursors are concerned with pivotal within-individual processes upon which change depends. Each has empirical validation. The precursors are not arranged in terms of potency or order of implementation, but rather to produce the acronym *CHANGES* as a mnemonic device:

- **C**onfronting the problem
- **H**ope for change
- **A**wareness of the problem
- **N**ecessity for change
- **G**rit, or a willingness or readiness to experience anxiety or difficulty
- **E**ffort or will toward change
- **S**ocial support for change

Each precursor is a transient and conditional state that may be present, or not, within a person at any given time for a particular problem or issue. They are not dispositions, personality traits, or characteristics, such as ego strength or hardiness. Confronting the problem, one of the most powerful of the precursors, is something that a person does, or not, in real time. It is not a part of a person's personality makeup. Even if a person is particularly skilled or attentive to the process of confronting many of their life problems, there may still be problems about which they are unaware, or are aware but would rather not be, or are aware and would simply prefer to put off considering until some later date or set of conditions. Anyone with any kind of personality, disordered or not, can activate precursors, assuming there are no neurophysiological impediments.

The seven precursors are a set of interdependent, necessary conditions for therapeutic change. When precursors are not activated in a client, change is unlikely to occur regardless of how great the therapist is, how potent the theory is, how close the relationship is, or how capable the person is. These client-specific ingredients, working in various combinations, seem to regulate the speed, intensity, and magnitude of change and can be considered regulators of the change process (see Hanna & Ritchie, 1995). In other words, the more they are present in a person, the more quickly change will occur and, in some cases, the deeper that change will be in the person's psyche.

Each precursor can be formulated in different ways and with different terms and jargon, but we have tried to keep them as theory-free as possible. In fact, they are assumed by all the theories and techniques of counseling and therapy. The precursors are pervasive; one can pick up virtually any book on therapy that contains successful case examples, and the precursors will be very much in evidence in each case. In unsuccessful cases, the precursors will be absent. There may be more precursors than those discussed in this book, but these seven seem to be key ingredients of change.

UNIQUE ASPECTS OF THE CHANGES MODEL

Several aspects of the CHANGES model are rather unique. One unique aspect of the CHANGES model is that it concentrates solely on a set of within-individual change factors without focusing on stages, theories, or personality traits. Additionally, the CHANGES model is a taxonomy of client-specific processes with corollary interventions and techniques developed across virtually all the schools of psychotherapy. The activation of precursors can be brought about by myriad, well-established therapy practices regardless of whether or not the therapist or client is aware that the activation of an underlying precursor was responsible for the change. Finally, focusing on client-specific change factors means that therapeutic change can occur outside of therapy, as maintained by Gendlin (1986). As such, therapeutic change does not require therapy; techniques to activate precursors abound, and the CHANGES model addresses the common factors of change itself.

Therapeutic Change as a Metacognitive Skill

The CHANGES model is also unique in its consideration of metacognitive aspects of change. Rather than addressing first-order thought processes, metacognition has to do with thinking about thinking, intentional psychological acts, or what were once called "acts of consciousness" (Husserl, 1913/1982), those inner decisions about where to direct awareness, the act of regulating one's thoughts and behaviors, or degree of awareness of awareness (Hanna et al., 1995). Barring a few exceptions, metacognition has seldom been considered in relation to change processes.

Most research tends to focus on the role that metacognition plays in mal-adaptive behaviors and associated beliefs; for instance, in how worrying arises from a metacognitive belief that worry is an effective means of coping, while the idea that "people are dangerous" is an instance of cognitive belief that feeds into that metacognitive style (Wells, 2007). However, when therapeutic change itself is examined from a metacognitive perspective, it begins to look more and more like a skill.

Behavior therapists have long emphasized the importance of skill building. In the metacognitive context, change itself is a skill, and mastery of the precursors is tantamount to mastery of therapeutic change itself (Hanna, 1996). As noted earlier, precursors are not traits or dispositions. Each precursor is a transient, conditional state that may or may not be present in a person at a given time for a given problem. However, having an awareness of the role that the precursors play in the change process can profoundly impact one's relationship to, and understanding of, change itself. If one understands that grit, confronting, and a sense of necessity are required catalysts for change to take place, then it becomes possible to orient oneself toward the activation of these core states. In this respect, the intentional, metacognitive activation of precursors is a skill that can be learned.

The Role of Interpersonal Savvy in Facilitating Change

Although therapeutic change is a metacognitive skill that can be learned and engaged without the need for therapy, therapists obviously play a central role in the activation of precursors and, thus, the facilitation of therapeutic change for clients. While the value of using various techniques and strategies to facilitate precursor activation and client change is a founding premise of this book, the pivotal role of interpersonal dynamics must also be underscored, particularly in therapy with difficult clients. Insofar as the CHANGES model broadly aligns with the common factors model, a therapist's ability to successfully activate precursors is oft contingent upon a strong therapeutic relationship. As such, Chapter 3 is dedicated to techniques for both building the relationship and building the therapeutic encounter around the principle of therapeutic change itself.

However, a considerable portion of the content within this book implicitly—and in some cases, explicitly—suggests that therapists with a degree of interpersonal savvy may be particularly well suited to the task of activating precursors in work with difficult clients. It is basically understood that it takes a certain degree of interpersonal skill, ability, or savvy to convince someone that the challenge of change is a worthwhile endeavor. If change were mundane or simple, then everyone would do it whenever necessary, and there would be absolutely no need for psychotherapists.

The truth is, change is hard. When a client shows up for therapy and makes immediate progress toward their goals, that client likely already had many, if not all, established precursors in place. Difficult clients are, as discussed in Chapter 2, only "difficult" insofar as they do not have activated precursors in place. The task of establishing those precursors is often not an easy one, and the barriers presented by a client to their activation are often complex. In the end, it often takes a certain degree of interpersonal savvy, and perhaps perspicacity (see Chapter 14), to break through with such difficult clients, making relational contact and getting the client onboard with the idea that therapy is about change and that change itself is worthwhile.

Techniques Oriented Around Change Principles

Perhaps the most unique aspect of this book is the vast array of techniques that have been compiled and described for activating each of the precursors. It is unusual for techniques to be cataloged in terms of change principles. In Part II, each chapter includes a subsection that lists and describes various techniques to activate each particular precursor. Many of the techniques have not been previously described, while others are more familiar and well-established techniques that have been adapted specifically for bringing about the presence of precursors among difficult clients.

Precursors in Group and Family Therapies

The CHANGES model is not limited to work with individuals. It also applies to group and family therapy. The precursors can be assessed and identified not only with each individual member of the group or family but also with the group or family as a whole. A group will display a configuration of precursors of its own. Whitaker held that a family has its own character as an entity in its own right (Simon, 1985). Therapy groups can be seen in the same way. Thus, the CHANGES model and assessment can help a therapist working with difficult groups and families.

Human Being as Active Agent

The CHANGES model makes great use of the concept of *active agency*, the view that human beings function as agents, actively influencing both their own minds and their environments (see Avdi et al., 2015; Gorlin & Békés, 2021; Harré, 1984). The behaviorist view of human beings leaned more toward a mechanistic or deterministic conception of human beings as merely effects of and responses to environmental forces. The latter perspective did not allow for the idea that human beings actually determined or shaped events in their lives, only that their environments and events determined and shaped them. This perspective, albeit useful, is obviously limited and has steadily diminished in popularity across decades of advancement in the cognitive sciences.

In parallel with the decline of this behaviorist view, the active agency conception that was central to the approaches of Rogers and Adler has gained considerable attention and widespread acceptance (Hoener et al., 2012). Led by deepening philosophical and neuroscientific discussions on the mind–body problem, the rise of influential research based on principles of embodied cognition and enactivism reflects a significant advancement in phenomenological discourse on the relation between self and world (Chemero, 2013; Gallagher, 2017; Wilkinson & Wilkinson, 2024). People are indeed influenced by the world just as much as they are agents influencing that same world in return (Zahavi, 2008).

In truth, the idea of active agency in psychology has been around for over a century. It was the basis of the psychology of William James, for example, and is assumed in almost all the major schools of psychotherapy today. In fact, many historians of psychology believe that contemporary psychology in general is now returning to the approaches and conceptions found in James's (1890/1981) classic *Principles of Psychology* (Hergenhahn, 1996). Metacognition also rests comfortably within the active agency conception, especially with regard to the realms of awareness, making decisions, consciously changing thoughts, exerting effort, forming and reforming mental images, and deliberately acting on the body and its impulses to enact new behaviors. Nowhere are such processes better described than in James's classic book. The CHANGES model shows how research confirms active agency and how therapeutic change depends to a large degree on it.

DEGREE OF CHANGE: FIRST ORDER AND SECOND ORDER

Both within and outside of the therapeutic encounter, the depth of change can vary. Although first-order and second-order change are defined a bit differently by different authors, the essential meaning is consistent (Sperry, 2022; Watzlawick et al., 1974). *First-order change* is linear, surface-level, uncomplicated, straightforward change that takes the form of an adaptation or adjustment. For example, one client may learn new communication skills to better get along with her daughter, while another client may learn to be assertive with his supervisor.

Second-order change, on the other hand, is more profound. It is a sweeping, deep structure or core change within an individual (Lyddon, 1990; Sperry, 2022). This kind of change fundamentally alters a person's core sense of self, mode of being, or essential worldview.

Second-order change radiates into and transfers across the wide array of a person's personality traits, activities, and interests. According to the CHANGES model, second-order change often involves intense initial turmoil or stress that is directly related to internal conflicts of considerable magnitude. These initial conditions are enough to threaten the person's equilibrium and psychological stability prior to the change itself. In other words, second-order change arises, often but not always, out of a crisis. It is also associated with advancement across stages of development (Gilligan, 1982; Hanna et al., 1995). Research has indicated that the precursors are intimately involved with the occurrence of both first-order and second-order change (Hanna & Ritchie, 1995).

An important goal for the fields of counseling and psychotherapy should be to develop new therapies that lead to greater magnitude and intensity of therapeutic change. When psychotherapy evolves to the point where almost any client who is free of organic brain damage can derive benefit relatively quickly, deeply, and with relative ease, the discipline will have taken a quantum leap. It is, arguably, our ethical duty to explore and develop new approaches that can lead to such results. The CHANGES model outlined in this book, applied to difficult clients, is not a quantum leap in itself but is based on the research of second-order, client-specific change experiences. It is offered to point the way forward to one possible, perhaps promising avenue of approach toward that goal.

MAJOR POINTS OF THE BOOK

Readers should consider the following central points as preparation for the chapters that follow:

1. The presence of precursors makes change possible.

2. The absence of even one precursor can inhibit therapeutic progress. When the missing precursor is activated, therapeutic progress can be made.

3. Client resistance, no matter how one defines it, indicates the absence of precursors.

4. Precursors regulate the rate, intensity, and magnitude of therapeutic change. The more they are present, the more likely change is to occur.

5. Therapy with difficult clients often involves a different set of skills than therapy with clients who are motivated or involved in the therapy process.

6. With many difficult clients, it is helpful to first establish precursors that are missing or deficient before proceeding to routine therapy approaches.

7. Difficult clients need a therapist with particularly effective relationship skills as well as a depth of empathy that surpasses what is necessary for willing and involved clients.

8. A therapist with inactive precursors can negatively affect therapeutic progress, inadvertently blocking client progress in a number of ways.

9. A remarkable number of techniques can be used to activate and enhance precursors.

10. Therapeutic change is a life skill that can be learned, practiced, and taught.

ORGANIZATION OF THE BOOK

This book is divided into five sections. It should be noted that all client names and other identifying information have been altered throughout the book to preserve confidentiality. Part I introduces the model. Chapter 1 introduces the technical, philosophical, and practical foundations of the CHANGES model.

Chapter 2 examines and reframes the basic idea of client resistance to treatment approaches, interventions, and strategies.

Part II is arguably the heart of this book, with eight chapters that describe clinical applications of the CHANGES model. Chapter 3 lists important guidelines and tips for relationship building with difficult clients. In Chapters 4 through 10, each precursor is defined and described according to how it brings about change. The clinical markers of each precursor are provided to help therapists detect their presence and absence in clients. Finally, each chapter includes techniques and practices for precursor activation, with case vignettes and transcriptions used to show techniques in action.

Part III describes the use of the CHANGES assessment form. Chapter 11 is devoted to the use of the form with difficult clients and provides several examples. Chapter 12 describes the use of the form to determine the level of precursors of a therapist working with a particular difficult client. In this chapter, examples are given of how a lack of activated precursors for the therapist in relation to a particular client can have a direct bearing on the climate, tone, and success of therapy.

Part IV is the specialized clinical applications section. Chapter 13 looks at therapist precursors in light of supervision practices, reframing the idea of countertransference as therapist interference. We endeavor to demonstrate how therapist reactions to clients can be leveraged for therapist insight and growth and how therapists can more effectively manage personal issues that inevitably arise in work with difficult clients. Chapter 14 discusses multicultural issues from the viewpoint of oppression. An oft-overlooked characterological outgrowth of oppression is discussed with the goal of supporting liberation among clients who identify with oppressed groups rather than facilitating mere adaptation or adjustment to oppressive conditions and environments. Chapter 15 reviews applications of the CHANGES model related to addiction and substance use, introducing the grand reframe of addictive behaviors and providing a litany of techniques and strategies for use with difficult clients in both individual and group substance use treatment.

Finally, Part V reviews the major advantages of the CHANGES model, proposes a metatheoretical framework based on the principles set forth in this book, identifies potential business applications using the proposed CHANGES Assessment for Businesses and Corporations, and examines some avenues for future research.

We are honored to present this material to you, dear reader, in hopes that the CHANGES model lends further insight into therapeutic change processes along with tools to facilitate said change.

ACTIVATING CHANGE
WITH DIFFICULT CLIENTS

1

Toward a Model of Change for Difficult Clients

Therapeutic change is the raison d'être of psychotherapy, serving as its most defining characteristic and its primary criterion for gauging success. Bereft of the concept of change, therapy practice loses its meaningfulness. Psychotherapists are first and foremost agents of therapeutic change, integrating relational skills with strategies and interventions to help clients attain beneficial ends. However, too much attention has been historically devoted to theories rather than what facilitates change itself (Gaines & Goldfried, 2021). If therapeutic change is such a crucial aspect of psychotherapy in practice, then it is extremely important to understand its basic nature.

This book examines what brings about beneficial change in human beings, regardless of whether one participates in therapy or not. Its promise lies in the fact that it concentrates on therapeutic change itself by centralizing client-focused factors that can be understood, identified, monitored, discussed, evaluated, and activated in the therapeutic encounter. As such, this book examines the capacity of individuals to activate therapeutic change, the many barriers to doing so, and the power of psychotherapists to catalyze this process using a wide variety of well-established techniques.

Lazarus (1990) opined years ago that psychotherapy was "still in the dark ages" (p. 356). In terms of what we know about the nature of change and how to help people achieve it as quickly as possible, this assessment remains more or less accurate today (Kramer et al., 2024; Silberschatz, 2017). Our collective difficulty in identifying mechanisms of therapeutic change has led some to quite appropriately label it the "black box of psychotherapy" (Zilcha-Mano, 2021, p. 516). Consequently, for psychotherapy to rise to a new level of effectiveness, it is

https://doi.org/10.1037/0000451-002

Therapeutic Change With Difficult Clients: Precursors and Techniques in the CHANGES Model, Second Edition, by B. D. Wilkinson and F. J. Hanna necessary to consider a range of potential paths that can lead to a more complete and dynamic view of how people change.

None of this is to suggest the field has not made significant advancements. In recent years, data-driven researchers seeking to advance psychotherapy have emphasized the value of randomized control trials to identify empirically supported treatments for specified symptoms and disorders (Philips & Falkenström, 2021). Neuroscientific developments have resulted in new psychotherapy intervention models (Cozolino, 2017; Smith et al., 2020), while integration-focused scholars have proposed a variety of unified psychotherapy frameworks based on the premise that metatheoretical modeling is needed to advance the field beyond its current, preparadigmatic state (Constantino et al., 2021; Marquis et al., 2021; Schiepek & Pincus, 2023).

Yet there is no solid evidence that psychotherapy outcomes are improving for clients in a consistent manner despite such advancements (Insel, 2022). The relative value of empirically supported treatments over myriad other approaches to psychotherapy remains questionable, as meta-analyses and metascientific reviews highlight concerns about replicability, effect size, and general efficacy (Machado & Beutler, 2016; Sakaluk et al., 2019). Significant questions remain as to the limits of neuroscience in the social sciences (De Vos & Pluth, 2016) and its applicability to psychotherapy practice (Insel, 2022; Paris, 2017; Wilkinson, 2019). In a tone quite reminiscent of Lazarus (1990), the psychotherapy integration movement has been described as "very much in its infancy" (O'Leary, 2021, p. 3).

There are, of course, many ways to approach and scrutinize these complex concerns, and there are no easy answers to the question of what makes psychotherapy work, or not work as the case may be. We do not claim to provide any definitive answers herein. However, we do wish to suggest that amid endless empirical, neurobiological, and integrative arguments about what precisely makes psychotherapy work, there seems to be considerably more emphasis on what therapists do than on what clients do. Scholarly interest in measuring therapist factors tends to outweigh emphasis on client factors (Fuertes & Nutt Williams, 2017). Wachtel (2018) argued that it is time to overcome our theoretical tribalism and "focus on principles and processes of change rather than branded packages" (p. 202). We agree; thus, we focus on change as a client-specific factor.

THERAPEUTIC CHANGE AND CLIENT-SPECIFIC FACTORS

Although therapeutic change is relatively easy to define at a superficial level, it is a remarkably complex, dynamic, and intricate phenomenon. As a working definition, *therapeutic change* is a beneficial, positive alteration in thoughts, behaviors, feelings, or interpersonal interaction that leads to improved or more effective coping or functioning and greater satisfaction with one's outer and inner life. In general, it is anything that constitutes an improvement to a person's life in terms of feeling, thinking, behaving, or relating. Therapeutic change is associated with simply learning to get along with one's supervisor, better managing one's time, or feeling better after talking about a problem. It can also be as profound as conquering major depression, recovering from addiction, overcoming the devastating effects of abuse, or finding meaning in a seemingly empty existence.

The motivation for therapeutic change can drive us to pursue love, travel the world, start a family, attend college, launch a career, pick up a hobby, or do myriad other things that human beings tend to believe will lead to greater satisfaction or fulfillment in life. It can also drive us to garner power, seek fame, acquire unnecessary possessions, and even use alcohol or drugs under the misguided premise that substance-fueled changes in feeling, perceiving, thinking, and behaving are a useful, if transient, form of therapeutic change. While the desire for therapeutic change is a fundamental aspect of human experience, not all paths to it are equal in effectiveness.

It is a mistake to discuss therapeutic change only in the context of psychotherapy and counseling. The fact is, people change all the time without therapy. We have known for nearly 75 years that a third of troubled individuals will improve on their own with no therapeutic intervention at all (Eysenck, 1952). We have known for nearly 40 years that about 15% of clients improve before engaging in their first session (Howard et al., 1986). If change occurs without an empathic therapist and without an identifiable theoretical approach, then change is largely in the domain of the person (Cuijpers et al., 2019; Hanna & Ritchie, 1995; Norcross & Prochaska, 1986a, 1986b). Therefore, a model of therapeutic change ought to account for and describe change outside of psychotherapy.

Common factors research has long demonstrated that extratherapeutic variables, or client-specific factors, account for 20%–40% of positive change outcomes in psychotherapy (Lambert, 1992; Peterson, 2019; Wampold, 2001). Client-specific factors include personal qualities, environmental influences, and what the client actually does in therapy and in life. There is considerable evidence that these are also the most important factors on which to focus a model of change (Bohart, 2000; Swift et al., 2023). After all, it is the client who does the work and who makes the changes. So, what kind of client is most likely to change? If we knew the answer to this pivotal question, we could likely predict who will respond to therapeutic interventions and who will not.

THE SEVEN PRECURSORS OF CHANGE

According to the CHANGES model, the client who is most likely to change is the client who has established the precursors of change in relation to a specified problem. A *precursor* is defined as a prerequisite or precondition that indicates an impending phenomenon. Therefore, a precursor of change is a specified precondition by which change may occur. The seven precursors of the CHANGES model seem to be present in clients who are actively engaged in the therapeutic change process. The seven precursors of change are as follows:

- *Confronting the problem* involves the steady and deliberate attending to and observing of anything intimidating, painful, or confusing, in spite of the inclination to avoid, shun, or act out. It is operative when a client looks at a problem squarely and directly and continues to observe, explore, or investigate it until the client grasps its essence.

- *Hope for change* is the client's realistic expectation that change can, and will probably, occur. It is not wishing, longing, desiring, or yearning. The hopeful client sees the possibility of change and the path to accomplish it. This recognition has the power to motivate even an apathetic client, especially if that client also has a sense of necessity.

- *Awareness of the problem* involves knowing that a problem exists and having a good sense of what that problem or issue is, as well as of the thoughts, feelings, and behaviors connected with it. Awareness is the opposite of denial or obliviousness. Without it, a person has no idea where to direct resources for change. With awareness, a client can pinpoint areas of dysfunction or need and identify relevant thoughts, feelings, and behaviors.

- *Necessity for change* is a felt sense of urgency or need that change takes place on the part of the client. In the person's assessment, current conditions are not at all satisfactory and must give way to a different set of circumstances.

- *Grit, or a willingness to experience anxiety or difficulty* indicates a readiness to feel the discomfort that accompanies change. Defensiveness, the diametric opposite to this precursor, is usually defined as an attempt to avoid anxiety. When grit is present, anxiety or difficulty is not resisted but directly experienced, with the knowledge that doing so is necessary for change to occur.

- *Effort or will toward change* indicates action actually taken toward solving the problem. It is the expending of energy and the movement made. It also involves will in the sense of making a commitment, coming to a decision, and initiating action. Effort manifests in two domains: the mind, in changing one's thoughts and attitudes, or the world, in coping with real-life situations.

- *Social support for change* consists of being engaged in confiding, supportive relationships dedicated to the client's well-being and improvement. Social support paves the path toward therapeutic change when those relationships function to enhance and inspire the presence of each of the other precursors.

The "CHANGES" acronym is designed to enhance therapist recall of the seven precursors. The model is rather like a display case, as the primary objects of attention are the precursors themselves alongside their interactions. As such, the CHANGES model does not sequentially arrange the seven precursors in their order of potency or in the order in which they occur. The precursors are present in clients in different configurations for different moments of change, and for the same person, different precursors may have varying degrees of influence from one instance to the next.

Since the precursors are a client variable, they are active in the change process both in and out of therapy. For instance, people who improve without therapy have often accurately identified a problem (awareness), become dedicated to overcoming that problem (sense of necessity), read a book (confronting), talked to a friend (social support) who made things seem not so bad (hope), and engaged in actions to facilitate change (effort) despite their discomfort (grit). As Prochaska et al. (1994) once put it, "It can be argued that all change is self-change, and that therapy is simply professionally coached self-change" (p. 17).

The CHANGES model maintains that every person has a complex configuration of waxing and waning precursors related to any given problem. It does not matter if the person is in therapy or not. If a client is in therapy, the counselor's theoretical orientation is inconsequential so long as the precursors are activated. Contrary to popular belief, talking about a problem does not always constitute "the talking cure"; talking is not always enough to produce change. Many clients talk about problems indefinitely, session after session, but nothing seems to change. This is not so much the fault of the client as a faulty understanding of therapeutic change itself.

If people possess, develop, or implement the precursors in the CHANGES model, then change will occur with or without a therapist. Logically, if change can occur without an empathic therapist who employs a psychological theory in practice, then (a) change is largely in the domain of the person and (b) it is the primary responsibility of therapists to identify and facilitate the activation of precursors. The CHANGES model thus represents a common factor approach to identifying the principles of therapeutic change itself rather than the more widely recognizable common factors of therapy. Armed with a well-founded grasp of therapeutic change itself, the role of the therapist is to help clients activate the seven precursors of the CHANGES model related to a given problem.

Notably, the precursors also precede, regulate, and influence the better-known change processes cataloged in psychotherapy. Most of these change processes are associated with classical theories; examples include insight, catharsis, changes in beliefs or thoughts, reinforcement, exposure, desensitization, problem solving, the act of acceptance, working through transference, and the corrective emotional experience. Without the precursors, these intervention-based change processes are unlikely to result in lasting therapeutic change. Client variables such as motivation and involvement are also widely regarded as important to the therapeutic change process, yet these too are dependent upon the precursors in many circumstances. The precursors can give definition, detail, and applicability to research findings on motivation, involvement, and other client variables.

VALUE OF THE MODEL FOR THERAPY WITH DIFFICULT CLIENTS

The test of any model of therapeutic change is whether or not it will apply to difficult clients. In the context of this book, a *difficult client* is a person for whom change is not forthcoming. The CHANGES model is presented precisely for the purpose of working with people who find change to be difficult, intolerable, or even a source of pain, inconvenience, or failure. When change is not forthcoming, the CHANGES model suggests this occurs because there are too few precursors present and operative in a client. As such, a difficult client displays what might be called *change deficits*, which indicates some lack of skill, ability, desire, and/or willingness to enact therapeutic change processes. A therapist using the CHANGES model can help difficult clients by providing education about the precursors of change and using techniques designed to activate the precursors.

Of course, there are many other ways to define "difficult," some of which do not fit with our approach in this book. Many difficult clients have been referred to as "resistant," a carry-over from psychoanalytic explanations of unconscious transference issues. When Freud (1910) said, "The patient who comes seeking desperately for help soon bends every effort to defeat help being given" (p. 54), he meant that resistance is an inner dynamic that leads people to repress and avoid painful or uncomfortable material in the unconscious. In such a context, virtually everyone displays some kind of resistance, and we maintain that this is a valuable way to understand some difficult clients.

However, a less specialized and more widespread use of the term insinuates that a lack of therapeutic change is due to client recalcitrance, active/passive aggressiveness, or ambivalence. A good working definition of *resistance* in this vein is "The patient's efforts to obstruct the aims and process of treatment" (Walrond-Skinner, 1986, p. 298). Although this is certainly accurate for some clients in some cases, therapists run the risk of impairing their empathy by framing difficult clients as having a characterological deficit in general. There is a long history of attributing poor client outcomes to self-sabotage rather than the complexities of sociocultural and relational factors. It is also far easier to blame clients than to recognize and acknowledge our culpability as therapists.

Change is difficult. Attempting to keep things the same is generally easier than making things different. While some people may view change as a worthy challenge to overcome, many others find the prospect of change threatening, upsetting, disturbing, overwhelming, painful, ill-advised, impossible, or even just plain silly. Some clients are uninformed about the benefits of change, feel undeserving of positive life changes, or vigorously engage in self-protective maneuvers to prevent change. Like communication or social skills, some people never learned how to change or to accept help to change. We have encountered some clients who never learned the fundamental lesson that therapeutic change is possible, much less valuable and helpful. Whatever the reason, if a person does not find the prospect of change appealing, then change is unlikely to be forthcoming.

Interaction and Interdependence of the Seven Precursors

The major psychotherapy theories identify the following as primary human motivations: reducing anxiety (Freud), attaining a life goal (Adler), self-actualization (Rogers), making sense of the world (Kelly), meeting needs (Murray), and reinforcement (Skinner). Even a casual study of these motivations reveals the importance of each and the liability of excluding any. Attempts to take something enormously complex and reduce it to one basic cause or principle, once referred to as "single principle imperialism" (Koch, 1981), is not a viable option in our search for understanding the dynamic nature of therapeutic change.

Human beings are too complicated to assign single principles to explain behaviors and motivations. In kind, therapeutic change should not be unduly oversimplified as if it operates in a linear, stepwise fashion. The precursors are not symmetrical, proportional, or equal in potency. They are also not sequential. Any given precursor can take the lead in one change experience, only to be far less prominent and consequential in another. The CHANGES model operates with a rotating form of circular causality. Instead of a static, two-dimensional patchwork quilt, the model is closer to a dynamic three-dimensional quilt where each patch changes in size, volume, area, and color in accord with the idiosyncrasies of a given client in a given situation (see Figure 1.1).

As common factors of change, the precursors are interdependent variables that overlap in both meaning and function. They can combine and recombine in

FIGURE 1.1. The Precursors and Their Interconnection, Interaction, and Interdependence on Each Other and Therapeutic Change

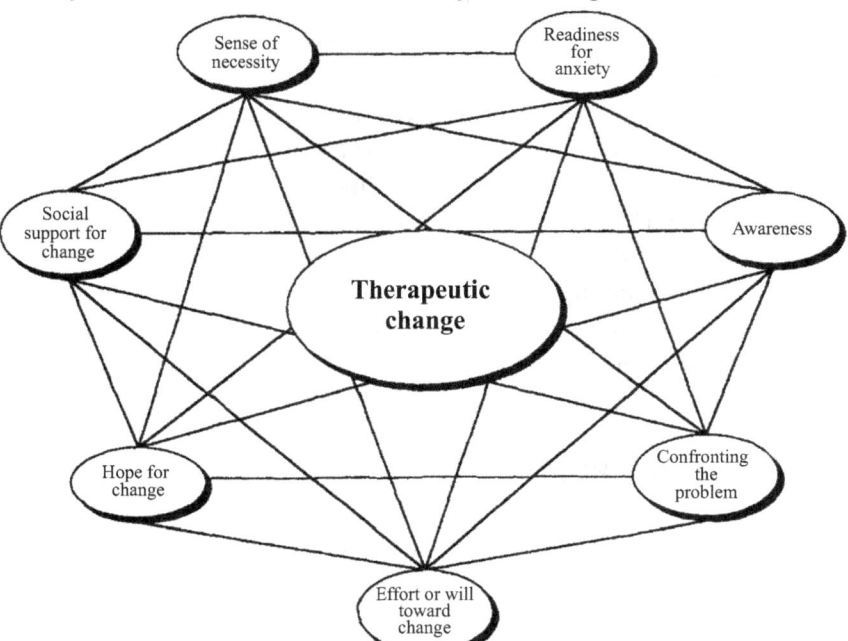

an extraordinary number of ways, and they vary in degree of presence from case to case or problem to problem. For example, a client who has reached a therapeutic impasse has an adequate presence of two precursors, awareness and a sense of necessity, but is largely lacking in all the others. Clients with this combination are quite common, and their lack of progress can be confusing without reference to the precursors. Yet when other change ingredients, such as confronting and being willing to experience anxiety, are addressed, change may occur. In a similar vein, deficits in awareness and necessity can be bolstered by social support and hope, while adding a sense of necessity can drive confronting the problem to greater depths and inspire grit, or a willingness to experience anxiety and difficulty.

Precursors are not static but can wax and wane throughout various stages of therapy. They can be powerfully present one day and nowhere to be found the next. They can vary in strength from minute to minute in the same session, which supports the need to study microprocesses in research. If a client does not trust their therapist, the precursors can almost literally be observed to diminish when that client enters the presence of the distrusted therapist. Many teenagers find it difficult to engage in therapy and act out or protest when they are told they must work with a counselor with whom they feel no rapport. Precursors vanish on the spot. Even with therapists whom they do trust, clients can bring a different level of precursors each day to therapy.

In addition, different precursors can vary in intensity and magnitude in different areas of a person's life. For instance, a person may be high in awareness but low in the sense of necessity when it comes to the need to quit drinking. On the other hand, when it comes to saving their marriage, that same person might have a high sense of necessity but very little awareness of the problems of the marriage. Each person can have a different configuration of precursors for each particular problem, which is one reason therapeutic change in general is so difficult to reliably map.

Finally, the precursors include, undercut, and incorporate the major theories of therapy. They are both transtheoretical and integrative without being dependent on the major theories, although our understanding of the precursors is certainly enhanced by theories and vice versa. These precursors are functions or conditions that can be found in a person's mindset (in the case of hope, grit, and sense of necessity), in one's environment (in the case of social support), or as metacognitive acts (in the case of awareness, effort or will toward change, and confronting the problem).

AT THE BASIS OF THEORY

Goldfried (1980) once wrote, "There exist certain timeless truths, consisting of common observations of how people change. These observations date back to early philosophers and are reflected in great works of literature" (p. 996). He further noted that these are "robust phenomena, as they have managed to survive the distortions imposed by the therapists' varying theoretical biases" (p. 996). The CHANGES model represents a compiled set of such change characteristics. The precursors are prior to and underlie all of the major theories of psychotherapy, making them applicable across theories in a manner that aligns with the psychotherapy integration movement. Researchers and clinicians long sought to improve psychotherapy along the lines of theory. In search of a new, global theoretical perspective, the field has accumulated over 500 schools of thought (Goldfried, 2019), of which 50 or so might be considered major approaches.

Eventually, the lofty ideal of the global theory of psychotherapy lost its luster, and a shift toward theoretical integration was underway (Stricker & Gold, 2013). The shift probably began with the classic study by Smith and Glass (1977), which found no evidence that any one of the major theories is more effective than any of the others. Soon after, the field entered a posttheoretical era more akin to "a maturing, scientifically based art rather than of an ideologically based sectarian mission" (Omer & London, 1988, p. 178). There has been little evidence to dissuade integrative researchers from the idea that all major schools of thought, from psychoanalysis to existential to cognitive behavioral, are equivalent in effectiveness under appropriate conditions (Wampold & Imel, 2015).

As a result, we now have a host of approaches that are characterized by categories and terms such as eclectic, integrative, transtheoretical, and containing the common factors of therapy. The early integrative movement revolutionized the landscape of psychotherapy. Wachtel's (1977) theoretical integration of behavioral and psychoanalytic therapies showed how two seemingly incompatible theories can work together in relative harmony. The development of technical eclecticism (Lazarus, 1976, 1996) streamlined psychotherapy by formalizing an emphasis on effective techniques with a minimum of theory. The common factors approach identified what each major theory has in common, seeking the middle path between advocating techniques and combining theories (see Frank & Frank, 1991; Grencavage & Norcross, 1990). Additionally, the transtheoretical model set forth by Prochaska et al. (1994) indicated how therapeutic change takes place in and across various stages of therapy.

Yet this is just the tip of the iceberg. The process of integrating or combining theories and treatments has added greater complexity to the theoretical picture and, in some ways, rendered the original problem worse than ever. To be clear, we maintain that original theories and integrative approaches continue to provide a treasure trove of insights concerning psychotherapy and human behavior. The CHANGES model is neither antitheoretical nor anti-intellectual. However, an emphasis on theories, whether in isolation or in combination, tends to inadvertently sustain the clinical fixation on the common factors of therapy rather than the common factors of change itself.

The CHANGES model encourages a therapist to incorporate any or all theories and techniques, as appropriate, into practice. Each theory presupposes the activation of the precursors in clients, although they seldom recognize or identify the role of precursors in the process of change. Across all psychotherapy theories, the precursors of change are always presupposed. Read the hundreds of successful case studies cited by therapists in books and articles, and the precursors are observably operative within and across all of those clients, regardless of the espoused theory.

Psychological theories play a critical role in the common factor process of providing an adaptive, psychologically derived, and culturally embedded explanation for distress, as well as a guide for implementing rituals and methods to enact something helpful (Frank & Frank, 1991). However, such explanations and methods are only of value when the client is invested in the change process. Confronted with a difficult client who has no precursors established, the finest therapists in the world will find their most advanced methods and explanations falling on deaf ears.

Realigning Psychotherapy Theories Around Change

It is well recognized that dogmatically insisting upon the "Truth" of any psychotherapy theory is a mistake born of philosophical naivete (Wampold & Imel, 2015; Yadlin-Gadot, 2016). Many theories take positions that were abandoned by the discipline of philosophy long ago. Traditional cognitive therapy, for example, subscribes to the view that reasoning is more important than behavior or affect in approaching various psychological problems. Such a view has its roots in the centuries-old philosophy of rationalism, the idea that the world is based on rational principles and amenable to rational speculations and explanations, as held by the likes of Descartes and Spinoza.

In terms of neurobiology, the assumption that affect and cognition engage independent brain regions or unique neural circuitry has long been framed by affective neuroscientists as one of "seven sins in the study of emotion" (Davidson, 2003, p. 129). The modern neuroscientific understanding that the brain is a large-scale, coordinated network means that we can no longer naively suggest that cognition, emotion, and perception are independent faculties (Pessoa, 2023). In cognitive therapy, dialogues on the role of emotion in the therapeutic process began to shift at the turn of the century (Samoilov & Goldfried, 2000), and the cognitive primacy hypothesis (i.e., the view that access to affective content is contingent upon cognitive categorization) is now widely acknowledged as an insufficient thesis at best (Reisenzein, 2019; Stevens, 2024).

The ostensible opposite of rationalism is empiricism, or the idea that we must rely on the senses to understand the world. Ultimately, empiricism led to a philosophy known as *logical positivism*, in which its original intent was to abandon any metaphysical and theoretical speculations that could not be verified by scientific inquiry. Popper (1963) once told Nobel Laureate Peter Medawar that logical positivism takes the naive position that "The world is all surface" (Medawar, 1984, p. 101), indicating that mental states need not be considered. For years, the use of the term *mind* was looked down upon in behaviorally oriented psychology circles as shortsighted and unenlightened

(Hackert & Weger, 2018). Contemporary research, however, has made it ever clearer that our perceptions and sense experiences affect, and are interdependently affected by, our thoughts and beliefs (Pessoa, 2022). Philosophy abandoned logical positivism decades ago (BonJour, 2009), but experimental psychology remains bound to positivist assumptions (Mayrhofer et al., 2021).

The problem herein is not with therapeutic practices per se but dogmatic adherence to particular theoretical vantage points as "right," "true," or "correct" assessments of the human condition. Current theories of psychotherapy neither capture nor contain truth any better than older ones. They contain too many elements of metaphysics. Both religion and psychotherapy theories are inextricable from metaphysics, one of the most perpetually perplexing domains of human knowledge (O'Donohue, 1989; van Inwagen, 2024).

Metaphysics is, simply stated, the seeking or study of knowledge that is beyond the capacity of science to verify. Most theories of psychotherapy contain metaphysical elements that cannot be verified by science, such as the id, the self-actualizing tendency, or the collective unconscious. The self is also a metaphysical construct that Adler (1956), as well as the philosopher Hume (1739/1978), poignantly questioned. Kant (1787/1929) showed in his classic *Critique of Pure Reason* that reason alone cannot solve metaphysical problems. James (1907) repeatedly showed in his treatises that reason could not solve metaphysical problems. James, whom Whitehead (1925, 1938) hailed as one of the four most important philosophers in history, developed pragmatism as a dialectical means of coping with and transcending metaphysically driven theoretical and conceptual conundrums.

Pragmatism, in a psychotherapy context, is a dialectical mode of thinking that fluidly moves between and among theories without any attachment beyond the immediate therapeutic situation. In the Jamesian tradition, what is true is so in terms of its pragmatic value. For instance, the highly praised idea of human free will is a metaphysical position that has pragmatic value in therapy. The problem is that our fascination with theoretical explanations—which are inextricably bound up in metaphysical presuppositions—delimits our focus on what produces change. It is in James's pragmatism and radical empiricism that the CHANGES model approach finds its truest inspiration.

James (1904/1977) wrote a brilliant series of articles in the first decade of the 20th century called *Essays in Radical Empiricism*. Both Russell (1972) and Whitehead (1925) believed that in those essays, James had discovered the long-awaited solution to the centuries-old Cartesian dualism of mind versus matter. Essentially, James showed how all of life, space, time, relationships, objects, and even awareness boil down to pure experience. James (1965) was clear that radical empiricism involves taking a phenomenological stance, such that "The only things that shall be debatable among philosophers shall be things definable in terms drawn from experience" (p. 105).

Rather than continuously engage in and elevate speculative metaphysics (see Henriques, 2019; Hibberd, 2014, for examples), an approach based on James' philosophy of radical empiricism might liberate psychotherapy from its longstanding conceptual entrenchment (Hanna, 1994). From a Jamesian perspective, if therapeutic change is at or near the essence of psychotherapy, perhaps there is good reason to focus the development of therapy models and speculation around therapeutic change itself, what produces it, and what enhances it (Goldfried, 2019). This is the heart of the precursors approach, and it is no surprise that some researchers have been advocating this for decades. However, the integrative question remains: What do we do with all of these theories?

Theories Are for Clients

The renowned family therapist Whitaker (1976) believed that theories were ultimately destructive to therapy, claiming that "My theory is that all theories are bad except for the beginner's game playing, until he gets the courage to give up theories and just live" (p. 154). Whitaker believed that adherence to a theory is a way of avoiding the basic anxiety of not knowing what the truth about human beings really is. Strean (1993) was even more direct:

> It is helpful for practitioners to study carefully their affinity to a particular theoretical perspective or therapeutic model as well as their abhorrence of other perspectives and models. When our clients idealize and/or denounce certain individuals, or certain "isms" with a great deal of affect, we try to help them resolve their infantile attachments and overdetermined hatred. (p. 14)

The CHANGES model aligns with common factors and regards classic theories of psychotherapy as better reserved for use by clients than by therapists. Clients, for example, have much to gain by understanding that thinking influences feeling and behavior. Of course, cognitive theory is not absolute truth, but many clients have used its germane ideas to effectively overcome difficulties.

As Frank and Frank (1991) observed, the healing process seems to require some kind of rationale or myth to serve as an explanation of a psychological problem, and the theory of each therapeutic approach provides a different rationale or myth. Thus, depressed clients can benefit, for example, from the 19th-century James–Lange theory of emotion, which states that if one acts confidently or happily, one eventually begins to think and feel that way. Similarly, clients can respond positively to existential and gestalt explanations, just as they do with those of Adlerian and family systems.

Theoretical explanations have healing value in themselves—as reframes— and should be readily available for clients who might be able to benefit from them when their situation warrants. Of course, students and practicing therapists should also study them, but not to the degree that they would actually believe in the ultimate truth of any one of them. Dialectical philosophers such as James, Heidegger, and Husserl have shown that theories possess no truth value in and of themselves. Theories are for clients, and the realization that the so-called truths of psychotherapy can be framed and jargonized from a variety of perspectives can liberate therapists from entrenchment in a given theory. That liberation allows for a fluid, dialectical movement between and among therapy approaches, with the needs of the client dictating the therapeutic approach chosen—a primary assumption in many psychotherapy integration circles.

The precursors underlie and run through the background of therapy theories, but they are seldom focused upon as goals in and of themselves. We are not suggesting that the CHANGES model should be the central focus of all approaches; that would be quite inaccurate. However, emphasis on the CHANGES model is particularly relevant when working with difficult clients who lack the precursors necessary to make standard therapy approaches successful, as is discussed in the next chapter. In ongoing efforts to improve therapeutic outcomes, therapists and researchers alike would do well to recognize the critical role played by the precursors as common factors of change.

AT THE BASIS OF TECHNIQUES

Techniques abound in psychotherapy. Role-playing, guided imagery, the empty chair, identifying and disputing dysfunctional cognitions, behavioral contracting, systematic desensitization, flooding, and self-monitoring are just a few. Just as the various theories assume the existence of the precursors, psychotherapy techniques are implemented with the assumption that the precursors are present in the clients who engage in techniques. However, this assumption is almost never stated as such. In the broad psychotherapy literature, the precursors are only seldom mentioned in the context of being necessary for techniques to work. Implementing techniques with a client who has no precursors in place is not much different from doing therapy with a sleeping client.

Just as theories might be oriented around change, it may also be advantageous to orient techniques around change itself in the form of functions such as the precursors. As in the case of theories, the precursors are also at the basis of techniques: constantly assumed but seldom acknowledged.

Techniques are thus dependent on precursors of change for their effectiveness. If a client has no sense of necessity, is not willing to experience any difficulty in therapy, thinks that there is no problem at all, and will not look at it or do anything about the problem or issue, it is naive to assume that a technique will lead to therapeutic change. The therapist must shift to helping the client activate precursors so that the technique in question can take hold. If precursors are present and the relationship is sound, then various techniques are likely to be effective.

One must also keep in mind that techniques used to activate precursors will work with some clients some of the time, but they will not work with all clients all of the time. They also will not work with the same client at all times. It is important that therapists not be bound by a manual or formula when working with difficult clients. Therapist creativity and spontaneity are crucial. One's therapeutic toolbox should be filled with options suitable for a wide variety of clients and situations. Knowing as many techniques as possible is optimum, as is being able to deliver them with timing, finesse, wisdom, and the proper amount of indifference or enthusiasm according to the needs and dictates of the moment. Of course, any reasonable techniques from the major theories may be called upon if and when they can be of therapeutic service to a client.

FRAMING TECHNIQUES AS EXPERIMENTS

Some difficult clients are hesitant to follow a therapist in a certain direction, particularly when the therapist frames it as a technique. The idea of being "therapized" is anathema to many. In gestalt therapy, techniques are typically framed as experiments (Polster & Polster, 1973) that allow therapists to be creative in the therapeutic process, launching techniques based upon the spontaneous identification of client needs, relational dynamics, and the climate of that particular moment. We have found that clients tend to be more willing to try something new when it has been framed as an experiment rather than a technique, although a client's level of commitment or engagement may remain low. Most techniques in this book can be framed as an experiment to encourage client involvement. To set up experiments, the therapist should always ask the client's permission to try something new and inform the client that they may end it at any time.

CHANGE AS A SKILL

The active agent conception of the human being views therapeutic change as something intentional and purposeful on the part of the client. Change is not necessarily something that occurs in a person according to a mathematical equation. It does not proceed in the same fashion as a physics experiment or the motion of billiard balls. Of course, mathematical equations and physics formulas do indeed describe much of the activity of the world, but they do not fully or adequately describe human beings. Specifically, they do not account for the fact that human beings are active agents who write the equations and the formulas, do the experiments, and set the billiard balls in motion. We understand only half of the process of change if we do not attend to the powers that set change into motion intentionally, purposefully, and with choices.

In psychotherapy, some clients are more than willing to talk about problems and describe their feelings but never seem to make a move toward change. In the midst of their dissatisfaction and unhappiness, one might ask why they are not willing to change. Yet sometimes, it is not a lack of willingness at all but rather a lack of knowledge or practice. We have found that people can learn how to change like they learn how to communicate or to have gratifying relationships. In other words, therapeutic change can be taught, developed, and honed as a skill.

Like nearly any other skill, some people have learned it and others have not, but everyone can learn how to cultivate it. Alternatively, some people have it but do not seem to know that they do, whereas others know they have it but are unsure how to intentionally engage it. Some people have learned the skill of change through hard-earned life lessons, accomplished in spite of low self-esteem and high adversity. Other people, unaware and unknowing, await change as something to magically arrive and are disappointed to discover that change is their own responsibility. These are all symptoms of a lack of precursors.

A primary message of the CHANGES model is that education is often necessary with difficult clients so they can know how therapeutic change works. Education about the change process itself provides a map and a rationale and is often effective (Bohart & Tallman, 1999; Eubanks & Goldfried, 2019). One of the fundamental mistakes made in psychotherapy and counseling is to assume that clients understand change processes. If they did, change might be accomplished much more quickly, easily, and on a routine basis. At first glance, it may seem silly to educate a difficult client about change when some may not care in the slightest. No doubt this is true in some instances. However, therapists using an active agent approach treat human beings as if they have choices and options. Change is one such choice, and if change looks to a client like it is in their best interest, that change will have a better chance of manifesting via psychotherapy.

METACOGNITIVE ASPECTS OF CHANGE

Many of the precursors of change are neither cognitive, affective, or behavioral. They are metacognitive. *Metacognition* can be defined as the psychological acts of recognizing, deciding, monitoring, and attending to self-regulation, self-instruction, and the processing of experience, memory, and attention (Flavell, 1979; Rhodes, 2019). It is knowing about knowing, thinking about thinking, or, in the case of memory, remembering that one once remembered. Most important for the investigation of therapeutic change, it can also be defined as the skill or ability "to be aware of being aware" (Singer, 2017, p. 608).

As a domain-general psychological skill tied to accelerated learning outcomes, metacognition includes processes like constructive and de-automated self-talk, intentional and self-directed goal formation, along with the vital areas of self-awareness and the de-automatization of habits and reactions (Eccles & Feltovich, 2008; Meichenbaum & Asarnow, 1979; Singer, 2017). Many metacognitive functions involve subtle acts of *willing*—intending the exertion of mental effort. The precursors most associated with metacognitive functions are awareness, confronting the problem, effort or will toward change, and grit, or the willingness to experience anxiety or difficulty. However, all precursors are arguably influenced by metacognitive beliefs.

Metacognition has been identified as a predictor of change across a wide variety of issues, from depression and anxiety to domestic violence to addiction to personality disorders (Carcione et al., 2019; Hamonniere & Varescon, 2018;

Seow et al., 2021). Insofar as metacognitive skills are not the same as cognitive skills, one person can be extremely intelligent but less capable of change than someone far less intellectually gifted but more metacognitively skilled. Perhaps this is why clients who intellectualize often find it difficult to change (Di Giuseppe et al., 2021). Metacognition is involved with other classic defense mechanisms, as well. Most therapists have seen instances in which deflection or repression is momentarily suspended, resulting in honest client engagement.

A metacognitive process is arguably occurring in such instances, as the cognitive beliefs connected with protecting the person's psychological system are metacognitively suspended or held in abeyance through an implicit decision process. Structural and functional explanations for such a process are plentiful in cognitive psychology (Jankowski & Holas, 2014; Kuhn, 2022; Leschziner & Brett, 2019), and alternative framings have been advanced in cognitive phenomenology (Arango-Muñoz, 2019; Norman & Furnes, 2016; Reggia et al., 2016; Wilkinson, 2023). Regardless of any such explanations, the CHANGES model supports the suspension or abeyance process so that therapeutic change can be launched through the activation of specific precursors.

The awareness precursor is among the most obvious of the metacognitive aspects of change. Sometimes a client decides to allow their perceptions to penetrate and enter the field of consciousness; this is essentially the decision to become aware of a problem, and it is highly metacognitive. For instance, a client may be surrounded by indications that their negative statements and behaviors are harming loved ones. That data does not register, however, until the person allows that data into awareness by selectively attending to that part of their life. That profound and fascinating process of allowing such data to register can sometimes be crucial to manifesting cognitive dissonance and the decision to stop destructive acts.

In terms of grit, the willingness to experience anxiety or difficulty is also a metacognitive process. Clients who are motivated to change must will themselves to experience the anxiety that accompanies the change process, as well as monitor their anxiety levels to avoid becoming overwhelmed. Willing and monitoring are inextricably linked in the process of enduring anxiety or difficulty, with research pointing to the interconnected nature of grit and metacognition in terms of achievement-oriented processes (Wang et al., 2023; Weintraub et al., 2023).

There is another highly relevant and important lesson that metacognition can provide to therapists. In many cases, clients are quite capable of actively influencing and changing their feelings and moods. Change of feelings can come about not only through the usual, well-documented cognitive and behavioral processes but also through direct and deliberate attention to feelings or emotions. Research on active–passive emotion regulation strategies consistently indicate that an active strategy leads to superior mental health outcomes (Birditt et al., 2020; Hipson et al., 2019; Silk et al., 2006) and that an active strategy enhances one's ability to directly modify emotions (Rholes et al., 1989).

The CHANGES model accounts for the possibility of such active and direct change. However, the term metacognition has its problems in this instance, and the phenomenon might be better described by terms such as dialectical thinking (see Slife, 1987; Wilken & Miyamoto, 2018) or wisdom (see Ardelt & Ferrari, 2014; Hanna & Ottens, 1995). No matter what we call it, this area has great potential for further research.

THE TRANSTHEORETICAL MODEL AND MOTIVATIONAL INTERVIEWING

The transtheoretical model of change (TTM; Prochaska et al., 1994) delineates five major stages of change: precontemplation, contemplation, preparation, action, and maintenance. Each stage requires the presence of the precursors to make progression to the next stage possible. This is part of how the CHANGES model actively complements the TTM's stages. The precursors are implicit and necessary not only in the beginning but during each stage of change. Prochaska et al. (1992) once noted that the stages are nonlinear and spirallike, involving regression back to earlier stages and launches forward to latter stages. When the precursors have waned, a client is likely to regress toward earlier stages. Overall, the precursors are critical in the process of moving clients from the stages of precontemplation and contemplation into the stages of preparation and action.

The TTM also identifies 10 change processes—five cognitive/affective and five behavioral—each of which is a categorical framing for relevant stage-based "strategies that may be composed of a seemingly endless number of techniques" (Gutierrez & Czerny, 2018, p. 203). In other words, each TTM process lets a therapist know what type of activity might best be used to facilitate movement from one stage to the next. For instance, consciousness-raising strategies like bibliotherapy might help move a client from precontemplation to contemplation or from contemplation to preparation.

While this is obviously a useful approach, TTM processes are fundamentally different from the precursors because processes only progress when certain preconditions are met. The precursors are preconditions of change itself. Processes are complex, iterative, and rarely linear. The process of reevaluating one's sense of identity in relation to a problematic behavior (e.g., learning to regard oneself as a "healthy nonsmoker") tends to occur in fits and starts, two steps forward and one step back, as they say. A single moment of insight rarely leads to lasting and transformational change.

When progress is being made, the precursors are in place. When progress is not being made, the precursors have waned. As clients move in and out of various processes, those shifts can be attributed to the flux and flow of the seven precursors from moment to moment or problem to problem. As such, the CHANGES model asks an important additional question: What client-specific factors must be activated for that client to consistently make therapeutic progress by steadfastly engaging in change-fostering therapeutic activities?

For example, imagine a therapist asking a client to read a self-help book. Upon finishing the book, the client moves from contemplation to preparation, stating to the therapist, "I'm fully aware of the problem now, and I'm ready to talk about what to do next." According to the TTM, we might say the consciousness-raising strategy of bibliotherapy successfully moved the client into the preparation stage of change. It is also fair to assume that the reading might have facilitated other processes, such as self-reevaluation, environmental reevaluation, and emotional arousal.

However, per the TTM, we can only say that reading the book either did or did not serve its purpose as a tool for facilitating those four processes of change. The CHANGES model pushes us to further distinguish between the client for whom that bibliotherapy strategy was effective and the client for whom it was not. To address that difference, we must examine the flux in specific client precursors during the period in which the therapeutic change process actually took place.

For the client who read the entire book voraciously over one weekend, perhaps there was already some basic sense of necessity that grew when she read its first few inspiring pages. The book then deepened her sense of necessity while also activating awareness and fostering hope. Fortunately, that client had deep reserves of grit that helped her keep reading through a tough chapter that "hit a bit too close to home," and so she continued to confront the problem by continuing to read despite her ongoing discomfort. Perhaps her effort was also being actively supported by a caring partner.

But what of the client who could not read a full chapter? Perhaps he did not really believe that the problem was so urgent that it required reading an entire book. Even though there was a sufficient sense of necessity for change that he sought therapy, there was not enough to make reading uncomfortable materials that "hit a bit too close to home" a worthwhile endeavor. As a result, there was no catalyst for hope to grow, as the client did not have the willingness to experience anxiety, confront the problem, and exert real effort. Without any social support, he continues to attend therapy but does not finish the book, telling his therapist he will get around to it next week.

Thus, the CHANGES model captures those client-specific factors that underlie strategy-specific processes within the TTM. Just as a change process has been defined in TTM as "any activity that you initiate to help modify your thinking, feeling, or behavior" (Prochaska et al. 1994, p. 25), the precursors in the CHANGES model can be defined as the client-specific preconditions that must be in place in order for any such activities to successfully modify thinking, feeling, or behavior such that therapeutic change occurs. Both the CHANGES model and the TTM identify the value of using techniques to facilitate change. However, the CHANGES model is unique in terms of identifying barriers to therapeutic change plus specific techniques to overcome those barriers.

While the TTM and the CHANGES model are models of change, motivational interviewing (MI) is not a model at all. It is a method used to engage clients in "a collaborative conversation style for strengthening . . . motivation and commitment to change" (W. R. Miller & Rollnick, 2012, p. 29). Leaning into the client-centered principle of unconditional positive regard and the use of reflecting skills, MI is an evidence-based approach to working with ambivalent clients (Rosengren, 2017). MI and the TTM both foster therapeutic change for difficult clients, with MI serving as an intervention style that can be applied within the TTM framework.

ASSESSMENT OF THE SEVEN PRECURSORS

As presented in Section III, the CHANGES assessment is an application of the CHANGES model and a therapy tool that helps clinicians determine which precursors need to be activated to bring about change. However, the assessment is secondary in importance to a deep understanding of the CHANGES model as a conceptual framework and the various techniques to activate missing precursors or to grow underactivated ones. The CHANGES assessment is a practical tool for gauging and monitoring degrees of precursor activation. For experienced therapists who grasp the fundamental nature and function of the CHANGES model, the assessment is easily internalized.

However, therapists who are becoming newly acquainted with the CHANGES model may find it helpful to use the assessment form in sessions. The assessment is rated by the therapist but may be completed with the help of the client when appropriate. It enables the therapist to see how the precursors overlap and interact and provides a relatively clear picture of what might be needed for a particular client to achieve change. Therapist and client can then work toward implementing and increasing missing precursors using the treatment strategy or technique suggestions provided throughout Section II. Again, the conceptual basis of the CHANGES model and its techniques take precedence, so we reserve a detailed discussion of the assessment for Section III.

CONCLUSION

As examined in this chapter, the CHANGES model is an example of how specific change processes can be identified in a context that owes allegiance to no particular theory. It is an example of how a therapy approach can focus on change itself and orient techniques, theories, procedures, and stages around specific change functions. The seven precursors are so fundamental that they lie at the core of theories, manuals, approaches, and procedures. This is not a global model of therapy, nor is it meant to be. But it may serve as an example of how techniques and manuals can be oriented around the therapeutic change process rather than treated as ends in and of themselves.

Consequently, one reason major schools of therapy are more or less equivalent is rather simple: They all have a fairly equivalent grasp on change itself. The same is generally true for techniques. Both theories and techniques require, draw from, and make use of the precursors. The absence of precursors means the absence of change. Any therapy, any procedure, or any approach that evokes, inspires, or brings to emergence the primary prerequisites of change will tend to be a valid therapy. And the therapist who encourages the presence of precursors will be an effective therapist regardless of training and theoretical background.

Insofar as up to 85% of what transpires in psychotherapy is common to all approaches (Cuijpers et al., 2019; Peterson, 2019; Strupp, 1996), researchers who compare therapies are not examining apples and oranges so much as tangerines and clementines. If psychotherapy is to advance as a discipline, it must be able to achieve therapeutic change more quickly, deeply, and efficiently. Advancements in theory and technique, while important, must be accompanied by a clearer and more complete understanding of what brings about change. To that end, therapists have a duty to understand why a client is not changing. Therapists must also be able to identify missing change factors in a client and then prescribe targeted strategies or techniques that can activate those change factors. Although it can be used with any client, the CHANGES model seems particularly valuable with difficult clients because a difficult client is one with few, if any, activated precursors.

2

What Makes a Client Difficult?

The primary duty of a therapeutic change model is to elucidate the process of how people change as well as how people remain the same. According to the CHANGES model, people change when the precursors of change are activated, and people stay the same when the precursors of change are inactive or underdeveloped. This means that when a client is responding well to therapy and undergoing change, there is little or no need to use the CHANGES model. Whatever approach the therapist is using is probably fine. We know from common factors research that all of the major approaches seem to work about equally well (Wampold & Ulvenes, 2019), with the exception of particularly effective applications for specified disorders, such as exposure therapy for phobias.

The secondary duty of a therapeutic change model is to show how change can be achieved where there are factors working against it. In other words, any model of change worth its therapeutic salt must highlight new ways to work with clients who have difficulty creating change. If precursors of change are absent or underdeveloped, the client may be regarded as "difficult." Our use of that term is not meant to pejoratively suggest a characterological deficit. Rather, it means there is a deficit in terms of the client's skill, ability, desire, or willingness to enact therapeutic change. A client is considered difficult when therapeutic change is not forthcoming. One difficult client may present as unmotivated and indifferent, another as aggressive and indignant, and still another as deferential and agreeable. However, all such clients may be considered difficult insofar as change is not occurring, and such change deficits are occurring because the precursors are not established.

Case examples have been disguised to protect client confidentiality.

https://doi.org/10.1037/0000451-003
Therapeutic Change With Difficult Clients: Precursors and Techniques in the CHANGES Model, Second Edition, by B. D. Wilkinson and F. J. Hanna

The irony is that if not for difficult clients, therapy could become quite automatized, and virtually any client would benefit from just about any competently applied theory. Indeed, chatbots trained using large language models to disclose humanlike emotions have proven successful with clients (Park et al., 2023). Such outcomes are not solely due to advancements in artificial intelligence, as people reported experiencing "therapist understanding" from mental health software prototypes long before the advent of large language models (Selmi et al., 1990). Similarly, bibliotherapy can be effective and helpful in a way that does not require a therapist (Christensen & Jacobson, 1994; Liu et al., 2022).

We demonstrated in the previous chapter that the reason for success when therapeutic change occurs is that the precursors are present and operational. Such change-activated clients can make substantial progress with people, chatbots, or even self-directed bibliotherapy. However, with difficult, self-undermining, manipulative, unwilling, or involuntary clients, the precursors are hardly present, if at all. Computer programs and bibliotherapy simply will not do the job. As such, the therapeutic mandate proposed in this book is to implement the CHANGES model with difficult clients so that more conventional therapeutic approaches can eventually be used once again.

DIFFICULTY AND RESISTANCE AS SELF-PROTECTION

The CHANGES model views resistance to change primarily as a mode of self-protection. Some people are so afraid of the world that they are hesitant to make any contact with it, let alone effect change within it. Perhaps this signals a kind of existential agoraphobia (Vahdani & Phillips, 2021). At some deep existential level, they believe making direct contact with the world is tantamount to experiencing pain and hold corresponding maladaptive beliefs that lead to further alienation from the world. Other people seem to believe that they do not have the capacity to alter either the world or their mind. Still others believe that they do not deserve the benefit of change, and through a lack of effort, they deliberately deprive themselves of change. Many passive clients are in this group.

Yet resistance can also be quite creative, such as when a client is perceived as difficult and disinterested in change in therapy but actively seeks therapeutic change through some misguided means. In other words, a client may honestly be trying to improve their conditions or fix a problem but is using flawed methods or inaccurate knowledge, as in the case of abusing drugs or joining a cult.

Thus, change is not always therapeutic. For some difficult clients, almost every experience of change they have ever undergone is associated with pain, suffering, loss, or oppression. Abuse causes change, as does violence and neglect. Even though psychotherapy holds no intention to produce these negative experiences, in a difficult client's mind, psychotherapy's tacit promise of change might be tantamount to the threat of pain by association. Therefore, in this private logic, all change (even positive change) can carry the implicit guarantee of being a painful, unbearable experience that should be avoided or deflected to protect oneself. Such a mindset is devoid of the precursors of change. Part of the process of establishing the precursors involves overriding such negative associations. Many techniques identified in this book are designed to do that precisely.

In the classic *Human Change Processes*, Mahoney (1991) noted that people who actively fight beneficial change do so because their beliefs and general outlook are so delicately in balance that change appears as a threat so great it could cause collapse and with it the loss of functioning and mental equilibrium. Interpreted in a different way, to the client for whom change is not appealing, the prospect of change, therapeutic or otherwise, represents the onset of a crisis. *Crisis* has been defined as an event or events that cause cognitive, emotional, and environmental turmoil so great that the person goes into a type of shock called "disequilibrium" (Janosik, 1986; Magnavita, 2006). Examples of such events are the death of a child, abuse, suicidal ideation, or tragedies caused by natural disasters. Crisis work consists not of enhancing the person's coping skills and range of functioning but of restoring that person to their precrisis level of coping and functioning.

Some clients experience a different kind of disequilibrium as a result of the perceived threat of change. They have feelings of instability and uncertainty, intense emotional swings, and a loss of perceived control (Pagnini et al., 2016). Clients of this bent understandably get angry, oppositional, and spiteful toward a therapist or anyone else who pushes them to change. Assuming that people are, to some degree, free agents, imposing change on a person, regardless of professional credentials, looks like punishment to a client who is not convinced that it will help. Such clients often fight hard to preserve whatever precious freedom and self-determination they have left. They dig in their heels and engage in a power struggle with the therapist, seeking to avoid any sort of surrender to a person they do not fundamentally trust. We have found that some of these clients are suffering from a previously unidentified trauma and are still trying to hold things together to get along in the world. From this perspective, it is wise to frame difficulty with change as a form of self-protection rather than implying that such clients are stubborn, defiant, or misguided.

Clients "Trained" to Be Difficult by Their Therapists

When a client is not changing, it is often for an excellent reason, and it could be that a therapist is indirectly bringing about the problem. The following case descriptions present a few examples of clients whose therapists played a key role in their difficulty. Two of these case examples will be reexamined in Chapter 12 in this volume, where the therapists are rated on the CHANGES assessment form.

Beth was a White, cisgender woman in her late 30s who was losing her home because of financial issues and losing her children to an ex-husband, who was falsely accusing her of abusing them. She was frantic. Her previous therapist had insisted that she explore issues of childhood, which were causing her current problems. The implicit promise was that if she resolved her childhood issues, her current problems would also resolve. Beth was an angry, suspicious, and bitter client who was still desperate for help.

Her new therapist found it perfectly reasonable that Beth was unwilling to explore her childhood and her emotions. What she needed from therapy was a problem-solving approach. Beth had been "resistant" to anything else and was very difficult to work with. But with the new therapist, she worked hard to resolve the real-time problems in which she was immersed. Beth's resistance was caused by her previous therapist's misguided insistence on the "proper" treatment.

A different example of therapist-initiated "resistance" is the case of Kurt, a 31-year-old male therapist, and his client Janey, a female university senior in her mid 20s. Janey was highly cooperative in answering questions in her early sessions with Kurt and initially seemed to value her therapy sessions. She freely and openly discussed her issues and problems. Her major complaint was that the men in her life verbally mistreated and did not respect her. She claimed to be worried about this issue and wondered if she would ever find someone who really loved her. She was articulate, easily identified her beliefs and feelings, and reported several seemingly important insights. On the other hand, there was a certain naivete about her that was reflected in her agreeableness as well as her tendency to smile while in pain and to laugh in a shrill, tinny tone.

After 20 therapy sessions, change was not apparent. Janey still allowed her current male partner to verbally mistreat her, and she complained of the same problems from session to session. Finally, she stopped attending sessions and did not return phone calls. In his final case note, Kurt identified that she had most likely terminated therapy due to her own "resistance to change."

In attempting to understand all this in supervision, Kurt discovered, reluctantly and with no small amount of embarrassment, that he harbored a hidden belief, formed in high school, that "attractive girls with fake laughter" who "smiled for no reason" were "stupid" and unlikely to achieve real significance in their lives. He realized that this implicit bias slipped out in various ways in his interactions with Janey, and although he never did or said anything overtly disrespectful, he never really empathized with her. Kurt had quietly minimized Janey's problems, delimited her capacity for change in his own mind, and failed to challenge her surface-level agreeableness. Janey had been an eager client in need of real support, but Kurt had created barriers to potential change.

A quite different example involves Jerry, a pleasant 30-year-old man who reported feeling "lost" and "wayward" about the lack of direction in his life. Although quite intelligent, he had no career plans, and nothing seemed to inspire him to want to do anything with his life. Nancy, his therapist, had 9 years of experience working in a university counseling center. In supervision, she reported that after 16 sessions, he was so "totally passive" and so "resistant" to help that she could not get him "to do anything" at all about his problem.

When asked to report her real feelings about the client in supervision, she was embarrassed to report that she found him "irritating" and "maddening" to work with, and she disliked the way he talked so slowly and deliberately, as though he were "picking each word, one by one." To her credit, she felt quite badly about her feelings toward him, but she also said that she was not able to help and suggested referring Jerry to another therapist.

The supervisor recommended that she write down all the people in her life of whom Jerry reminded her. The next week, she reported with a sense of both relief and astonishment that Jerry reminded her of her sexually abusive brother, from whom she had cut herself off 20 years earlier. After this supervision, she no longer considered Jerry to be resistant or difficult, and he began to make progress. In fact, she began to like him. At one point, Jerry told her that she seemed "nicer." This therapist learned a valuable lesson.

Such examples show how clients can be difficult because of the therapist's faulty perceptions or an inappropriate or ill-advised approach. The therapists were not immediately aware of their own contributions to their clients' perceived resistance. It is extremely important to emphasize this aspect of difficulty and resistance in therapy.

Clients Difficult All on Their Own

In many cases, the client is difficult despite the best efforts of the most competent therapists, as described in the following three case examples. Diagnoses from the *Diagnostic and Statistical Manual of Mental Disorders* are deliberately omitted in what follows so that a distinct picture of the client can emerge without clinical labels. We reexamine these cases in Chapter 12 in this volume.

The Story of Tommy
Tommy, age 29, was tall, handsome, charming, humorous, and thoroughly self-centered. He was married to Julie, whom he described as a loving and devoted wife and caring mother of their three children. He and his wife had been "fighting," and she insisted that he go to therapy.

Tommy hated himself for cheating on her at every opportunity, but he seemingly would not, or could not, stop. He would sometimes criticize her for being "oblivious" and "foolish," but when challenged, he would say, "My wife is a saint." He also said it was "only natural" for men to cheat on their wives. He reported that one of his friends had advised him to seek therapy because he was so unhappy and because he was "throwing away a good woman." A salesperson who regularly made house calls as part of his work, Tommy was so good at concealing his activities that Julie had no inkling of his promiscuity. Tommy, meanwhile, showed neither preference nor prejudice regarding the women he seduced. He was addicted to charming and exploiting women for sex.

Tommy boasted of his sexual prowess and said that such talents were wasted on a wife. Then, in almost the same breath and in an explosion of guilt, he ruthlessly criticized and condemned himself for being a liar and a phony.

He believed, as a Christian, that he was headed "straight to hell" for his many affairs. His fear of hell seemed to trouble him more than his infidelity, much more so, it appeared, than any potential harm done to his family or marriage. Tommy had been to three therapists trying to rid himself of his anxiety. He had apparently competed with and fought his therapists at every turn. In a tone of voice that combined both bravado and shame, he claimed that none of his therapists were of any help at all. His current therapist deduced that his apparent interest in therapy amounted to the improbable goal of reducing his anxiety without changing his behaviors. Beyond what he stated, his chief goal for therapy seemed to be reassurance that he would indeed make it to heaven, that his behavior was really okay, and that he was a good person. He had also confided in his minister but found no support for his promiscuity.

The Story of Joy

Joy identified herself as an "asexual former showgirl" from the Lake Tahoe region in Nevada. She was in her late 30s with dark hair and bright blue eyes. She was heavily into the occult and new age pursuits, believing that she was clairvoyant and psychically gifted. She had been involved with several new age cults. She was actively and avowedly celibate and freely admitted to a contempt for men. She also claimed that she was destined to find her "soul mate" sometime in the next year. She had been to many psychics and astrologers but had decided to seek therapy as a way of opening the psychological blocks that stood in the way of her realizing her "destiny" as an occult "adept."

In therapy, her insistence on staying "positive" was so strong that she avoided any disclosure that was associated with negative emotion or inferred weakness, as such things ran counter to the list of new age affirmations that she repeated to herself each day. She seemed interested only in discovering how she could undo the lingering negative "vibrations" of the destructive people of her past. These included her family, ex-husband, and many of what she called "false friends." She assumed that psychotherapy could teach her how to completely cut herself off from all negative emotions and influences, especially her parents. Joy was also highly demanding and wanted instant results. Quite rigid in her thinking, she often lectured her therapist on new age principles, which she said were superior to those of psychotherapy. Not surprisingly, Joy reached a rather dramatic impasse in her therapy after eight sessions, showing considerable impatience and correctly claiming to have derived no benefit.

The Story of Ricky

Ricky was 18 years old and a member of a street gang. He was tall, handsome, and muscular and had been placed in an outpatient adolescent drug and alcohol treatment program when he was 17. He was addicted to crack cocaine and was on probation for its possession and sale. He was a father to at least three children born of adolescent girls. He reported matter-of-factly that all women loved him, and he blatantly and proudly admitted, after some coaxing, that he liked to impregnate young girls. It was also clear that he had supplied many young people with drugs and had committed other crimes, although, according to his probation officer, he had not been brought up on charges.

He had an outwardly pleasant demeanor and smiled in a cocky, self-assured way. He had a coldness about him—a deeply disturbing lack of warmth or engagement that oftentimes evoked visceral reactions of intimidation among the therapists in the program. Ricky never exhibited any overt violence. However, with any kind of confrontation of his behaviors or attitudes came a subtle nonverbal threat of intimidation. He had a way of cocking his head and curling his lip in a silent, smiling snarl whenever questioned about his lifestyle or attitudes. These defiant behaviors seemed to open a window into a deep, smoldering hostility. Ricky was highly intelligent and manipulative. He displayed an extraordinary sense of entitlement that was, of course, part of his criminal mindset. In therapy, it soon became clear that he was immersed in a deep hatred of the world and people in general. Therapy to him was a form of control and punishment to be outwitted and thwarted at all costs. He often told his therapist, "You best not mess with my head."

Difficult Indeed

The examples in the previous section describe people who were extraordinarily difficult to engage in therapy. Standard therapeutic approaches were of no help, and each client was adept at strangling the therapeutic change process. Even those who recognized that change was necessary did not want the type of change that psychotherapy offered.

ROOTS OF DIFFICULTY: IMPLICIT LEARNING AND MALADAPTIVE BELIEFS

Difficulty or resistance to change is a consequence of beliefs that arise through implicit learning and are typically formed so early in life that the seeds of its formulation are sown before one learns to speak. *Implicit learning* involves the preconscious, nonintentional formation of knowledge, concepts, and beliefs about the environment as well as causal-relational structures between objects and events (Reber et al., 2019). Through implicit learning, people formulate assumptions upon which an entire meaning system can rest (Cleeremans, 2019). These assumptions are often highly emotionally charged and, if challenged, evoke vehement reactions ranging from protest and defiance to betrayal and hurt. If those primary, fundamental assumptions do not change, then neither will the person.

It is generally understood that the experiential, preverbal nature of implicit learning makes it "verbally inaccessible" (Hartmann, 2019, p. 264) and thus difficult to articulate via standard talk therapy. Trauma-focused somatic therapies have arisen to address how embodied, implicit learnings interfere with healthy functioning (van der Kolk, 2014). The fact that so much psychotherapy is narratively driven may explain why therapeutic change is so often difficult for clients with early life traumas. Fortunately, implicit learnings also tend to manifest cognitively as maladaptive, irrational, or pathogenic beliefs about the nature of reality and fundamental aspects of living (David et al., 2009; Gazzillo, 2023). They take the form of preverbally formed yet verbally identifiable judgments on subjects like awareness, love, people, self, problems, the world, or life.

Examples of some of these fundamental preverbal beliefs that directly affect the psychotherapy process are "interactions with people cause pain," "awareness of a problem only makes it worse," and "people only care about themselves." There is an old notion that one should never discuss religion or politics in casual conversation; such topics, like many discussed in therapy, evoke deep emotional responses or what is generally recognized in cognitive behavioral therapy as "hot" thoughts (McKay et al., 2021). In our experience, implicit knowledge can be changed but only with care and extreme courtesy, and usually, permission from the client must be deliberately and openly sought beforehand.

The Story of Kathy

Kathy had a doctoral degree in psychology and ran her own private psychotherapy practice. She was extremely self-aware and articulate. Somehow, she came to be convinced that no one would ever be there for her when she really needed them, not even her best friends. When asked, she said that even when her friends had been supportive and there for her, she always considered it surprising and unlikely. She had felt deep emotional anxiety over this issue and had consistently framed and described it as a problem in trusting others. Being familiar with her highly admirable qualities and knowing her to be a trusting person, the therapist eventually became highly suspicious of this view. When the therapist asked if trust might not be the real problem, she became upset and insisted that trust had been a problem all her life.

The therapist first asked Kathy if she noticed how upset she became when asked the question. Kathy nodded. The therapist then asked her if she would be willing to explore that but noted that if at any point she thought it was a waste of time to pursue, to make it known and they would move on. She agreed. The therapist asked her to hold on tightly to that feeling of upset and protest toward the question and to follow it into her mind. Being highly aware, Kathy was easily capable of such a directive, so the therapist encouraged her to allow any memory images to emerge that might be related to this feeling. She began to cry. She was soon relating memory images in which she was in her crib, crying and waiting for her mother to come to her. But her mother never came, and she remembered being horribly alone and deeply despondent, abandoned, and unloved. It was during this time, she said, that she formed a belief that no one is reliable and that people cannot be counted on to be there in times of need. She estimated that she was about a year to 18 months old.

Of course, it is not important whether the memory is accurate, if it actually occurred, or if that was her actual age at the time. Adler (1956) noted that early memories need not be verifiably true for a person to obtain therapeutic benefit from examining them. It is the maladaptive belief about people that was at the heart of the problem, regardless of the story content.

After this session, Kathy called her mother and told her about this early memory. Her mother, as Kathy later related the story, was quite surprised and expressed how bad she had felt listening to her baby cry for long periods. She said that she did not attend to her because the conventional wisdom at the time was to avoid spoiling the child by deliberately letting her cry, which allegedly would make the child more self-reliant. Seeing and dismissing the maladaptive belief was of value to Kathy but having her mother more or less verify the memory was of greater significance.

THERAPIST VARIABLES INFLUENCING THERAPEUTIC SUCCESS

Research into differential therapist effectiveness has consistently demonstrated that some therapists are more effective than others when it comes to creating positive therapeutic outcomes. Evidence first surfaced when Strupp and Hadley (1979) found that college professors untrained in psychotherapy were just as effective as experienced professional therapists. Many of the clients in this study had challenging disorders, yet there were no appreciable differences in effectiveness. Five years later, a meta-analysis comparing paraprofessionals to professionals (i.e., licensed psychologists, psychiatrists, social workers) found that "paraprofessionals must be considered as effective additions to the helping services, and in many cases they are more effective than professional counselors" (Hattie et al., 1984, p. 540). Level of education and years of professional experience were not significant in determining effectiveness.

Years later, Stein and Lambert (1995) found that professionals fared only slightly better than paraprofessionals and stated that "given the enormous, national investment of physical and human resources in graduate programs, it is quite remarkable that more compelling evidence is not available that demonstrates that graduate training directly relates to enhanced therapy outcomes" (p. 194). Such classic studies have withstood criticism over many years, and the results remain relevant: People who have only 20 or so hours of therapy training can be nearly as effective as professionals with advanced degrees, hundreds of hours of training, and years of experience.

Studies demonstrating a measurable impact of therapist experience on client outcomes have tended to have negligible effect sizes (Kraus et al., 2016; Walsh et al., 2019). Instead, research shows that the most effective psychotherapists facilitate change regardless of the presenting concern (Nissen-Lie et al., 2016), consistently over time (Kraus et al., 2016), regardless of years of experience in the field (Delgadillo et al., 2020), and that they might be identifiable from the earliest point of training (Edmondstone et al., 2023).

What do such studies really tell us? According to the CHANGES model, the dilemma boils down to two essential points. The first is that some people are somehow more fundamentally capable of helping clients change, regardless of education or training. In other words, professional training seems limited in its capacity to train some people to be more effective change agents. The second point is that if we more fully understand therapeutic change as a process in and of itself, perhaps we can better grasp what therapists must do to help make it happen.

Therapist effectiveness has little to do with GRE scores, high grade point averages, number of publications, research skills, or the ability to pass exams or write dissertations (Castonguay & Hill, 2017). Therapist effectiveness is not dependent on the university attended or the type of training program but rather on the personal characteristics of the therapist (Edmondstone et al., 2023; Firth et al., 2015; Goldfried et al., 1990; Peterson, 1995). Of course, this raises the question of what it takes to not only facilitate change but also to train and prepare professionals to be effective change facilitators.

Wisdom and the Wise Therapist

There is indeed a concept that accounts for the mostly unspoken and largely unspecified skills that differentiate the average therapist from the highly effective therapist. The concept is called wisdom (Grossman et al., 2013; Hanna & Ottens, 1995; Sternberg & Glück, 2021). This ancient concept is imported from research in developmental psychology and has great explanatory power. Researchers generally describe *wisdom* as a high degree of knowledge and expertise regarding the living of life itself. It is not the same as intelligence, although the two complement each other quite well. Characteristics of wisdom include empathy, compassion, metacognitive skills, perspicacity, self-awareness, and self-transcendence, among many others (see Table 2.1).

It may well be that lack of wisdom is at the core of the puzzle concerning why years of experience as a therapist does not seem to reliably predict effectiveness (Skovholt, 2017). One of the characteristics of wisdom is to resist habit in or automatization of thought and behavior routines (Sternberg & Glück, 2021). Take two therapists with 20 years of experience. One continuously self-reflected, learned, and improved therapy skills for a full, rich 20 years of experience, whereas the other had 1 year of therapy experience that was then automatized and repeated 20 times. In the latter case, the therapist more or less went through the motions of therapy on autopilot, with the net result of no longer improving their skills (Dawson, 2018; Dumont, 1991).

The effective therapist tends to be a wise therapist. Of course, intelligence is certainly handy and helpful, but when it comes to the skills necessary to be effective, the characteristics and thinking styles that make up wisdom seem more relevant than those of intelligence (Levitt & Piazza-Bonin, 2016). Yet we accept people into graduate training programs with criteria based on intelligence rather than wisdom. Could it be that graduate-level trainees end up with the same general level of wisdom as paraprofessionals because wisdom is not taught in graduate schools? After all, if wisdom is randomly distributed across the

TABLE 2.1. Characteristics of Wisdom

Wisdom characteristic	Definitional element
Empathy	• strong sense of the feelings and outlooks of others
	• understands others from their subjective point of view and from a perspective that is not self-centered
Concern	• compassion for others
	• cares for the welfare of living beings and the environment
Recognition of affect	• recognizes the interdependence of cognition and affect
	• aware of own emotions and feeling states
De-automatization	• resists habitual, automatic behavior and thinking patterns
	• emphasis on awareness of actions and responsible choice
Sagacity	• strong listening skills
	• deep insight and awareness into human beings and relationships
	• self-knowledge and capacity for self-transcendence
	• ability to learn from mistakes
Dialectical reasoning	• recognizes the power of context and the interplay of opposing views
	• fluid and intuitive reasoning
	• ability to consider all sides of an issue
	• orientation toward beneficial change
Efficient coping skills	• copes smoothly and efficiently across a range of people and situations
	• ability to find fulfillment and meaning in life
Tolerance of ambiguity	• recognizes ambiguity as intrinsic to the nature of being in the world
	• ability to perceive, appreciate, integrate, and use shades of gray
Perspicacity	• ability to "see through" situations
	• capacity to avoid being fooled or deceived
	• intuitive understanding and accurate interpretations of their environment
	• ability to look beyond appearances
Problem-solving skills	• identifies and frames a problem such that the solution is efficient
	• capacity to reframe problems and situations
	• expertise in the use of transferable metaphors
Metacognitive capacity	• ability to recognize presuppositions and assumptions
	• awareness of awareness; knowing of knowing; thinking about thinking
	• capacity to direct awareness, behavior, and emotion toward change

Note. From "The Role of Wisdom in Psychotherapy," by F. J. Hanna and A. J. Ottens, 1995, *Journal of Psychotherapy Integration*, 5(3), p.199 (https://doi.org/10.1037/h0101273). Copyright 1995 by the American Psychological Association.

population, then it should be rather evenly distributed among professional and paraprofessional therapist samples as well (see Hanna & Ottens, 1995).

Regardless, a wise therapist may well be the most capable of inspiring and implementing the CHANGES model. Pure intelligence is not oriented around skills such as listening, empathy, and interpersonal expertise (Skovholt, 2017). Thus, the crucial difference on which to place a research focus may not be the professional and paraprofessional, but the wise and not so wise. The difference may well lie in the ability to facilitate the precursors. With regard to research, it may be time to explore some research avenues implied or indicated by the CHANGES model.

Training the Wisdom Out of the Therapist

Lazarus (1989b) observed that formal education and training in psychotherapy and counseling can take a person's natural therapeutic warmth, wisdom, genuineness, and empathy and degrade them into a stylized professionalism that is detrimental to a would-be therapist's natural skills. He used the metaphor of "taking a can of spray paint to an artistic masterpiece" (Lazarus, 1990, p. 352) to describe how academic training can spoil a student's natural helping skills and suggested that much of what is taught to graduate students about doing therapy amounts to "deadwood, superstition, and plain rubbish" (p. 352) rather than useful knowledge about what is actually effective.

From the perspective of the CHANGES model, graduates of many training programs primarily learn a professional language; an array of theories, research findings, research methods, and ethical principles and behaviors; and a carefully cultivated professional demeanor, but they are not necessarily taught how to facilitate therapeutic change itself. There are therapists and trainees at all levels who, for example, do not use session time in ways conducive to arriving at solutions or strengthening therapeutic relationships with the goal of change. There are people working in community agencies without even a bachelor's degree who are natural therapists with a knack for helping clients change. Such natural therapists tend to have wonderful relationship skills, make perceptive decisions with a sense of precise timing, and tailor their interventions to client needs.

None of this is to suggest that graduate training is unimportant, as effective training programs can and do enhance psychological mindedness, refine presence, and provide a launch point for skilled interpersonal work with clients. However, it seems that what is most important is quite simple: The therapist must have the skills to help bring about change. According to the CHANGES model, the skillfulness of a therapist may be little more than the ability to inspire, engage, and enhance the presence of precursors in clients. Such therapists can orchestrate and implement change ingredients with a client through empathy, warmth, persuasiveness, techniques, reframes, metaphors, and general wisdom about human beings and life. The therapist could be the family doctor or the professional therapist in private practice. It could be the school counselor at the local high school or the recovering alcoholic who works for near minimum wage at the local community substance use treatment center. Whether a professional or paraprofessional, the presence of these characteristics in a person indicates a capacity to become an agent of change and a fine therapist.

Fundamentally, there are a certain number of well-off people who can be helped by almost any well-intended therapist using almost any sound approach (Wampold & Imel, 2015). Bartenders and hairdressers routinely perform this function. Some astrologers, psychics, and channelers act as therapists as well (Lester, 1982). If all that is needed, according to Frank and Frank (1991), is a myth to explain healing, astrology and channeling can certainly serve that function. People claim to gain benefit from these offbeat, at best, and at worst harmful therapies (Singer & Lalich, 1996). Why? That is the point of this book. If the precursors of change are present, that person is likely to change. If the precursors are not present, change is unlikely. As such, the most important skill of a therapist is the ability to activate the precursors within the CHANGES model.

CONCLUSION

Study the vast number of theories, procedures, and techniques used in psychotherapy, and one finds that most assume some degree of motivation and involvement on the part of the client. In the previous cases of Tommy, Joy, and Ricky, involvement was lacking in all three, and motivation was either absent, in the case of Ricky, or alloyed and misdirected despite a stated interest in change by Tommy and Joy. Techniques typically used with clients, such as role-playing, the empty chair, identifying and disputing irrational beliefs or dysfunctional cognitions, behavioral contracting, desensitization, and so on usually will not work with a client who is unmotivated and uninvolved. Without involvement and motivation, few techniques are likely to be effective, in spite of the therapist's level of skill. That is why positive outcomes seem to be related to these variables.

Clients who steadfastly refuse to engage in role-plays often judge such an exercise as useless. The empty chair is viewed with particular disdain by such clients, and the same can be said for many other techniques. The potency of powerful change-producing techniques such as these is irrelevant when a client is uninvolved or unmotivated. Many of these clients are tremendously difficult to engage. A few are almost inaccessible. The skills needed to work with such clients and engage them in therapy are seldom taught in graduate programs and are almost always learned on the job. Thus, the ability of psychotherapy to reach such clients more quickly and effectively represents one of the growth paths of the entire discipline.

There are a host of styles of being difficult. Many clients desperately want to change but find the process too painful and fight it at each juncture. Others are not forthrightly resistant or difficult at all; they would change, but they just do not see the point. For yet others, change seems a pleasant prospect but involves too many sacrifices to appear desirable. Another style is to see change as a hindrance to an established way of being. These people often see the therapist as an enemy intruder, there to confuse and confound. For many people with criminal histories, change is the same as an admission of weakness and guilt and is to be avoided at all costs. It can also be a threat to their "freedom" to do whatever they want, whenever they want, to any victim they choose. Another style of difficult client simply does not believe that change is possible—for anyone—and therefore devotes nothing to it, other than lip service, to a judge, employer, or spouse, as the case may be.

In view of all of these issues, the field is clearly in need of a broader and deeper understanding of why some people change and others do not. This a primary goal of the CHANGES model. The following section is dedicated to examining how therapists can accomplish this task, by examining each of the seven precursors in the CHANGES model along with myriad techniques to systematically grow client motivation and involvement in the therapeutic change process.

II

THE CHANGES MODEL, STRATEGIES, AND TECHNIQUES

3

Orienting the Relationship Around Change

I t would be a mistake to place one's trust solely in techniques when working with difficult clients because without a strong therapeutic relationship, techniques are likely to fall flat or not take hold (Cochran & Cochran, 2015). When client motivation is absent, the therapist's primary task is to get the client to participate or cooperate in therapy. Getting an unmotivated, disinterested client engaged in therapy requires a different set of skills than applying the steps of a particular theoretical approach, technique, or manual. In such cases, the ability to be persuasive and influential is often necessary to get a client on track. Empathy must be sufficiently advanced that the client feels understood by the therapist, even when the therapist does not at all agree with the client. The therapist may even experience nausea or visceral discomfort while empathizing with clients who display unsavory or destructive attitudes. Nevertheless, without the ability to reach and make that vital connection with a difficult client, little or no change is likely.

If a client does not respect a therapist, then premature termination is likely. That respect depends on various factors, but a major factor seems to be whether the therapist truly understands the client. Therapists have known for a long time that "feeling understood" is at or near the heart of how a person experiences empathy from another (Van Kaam, 1966). Adler (1927) gave perhaps the most descriptive definition of empathy when he portrayed it as seeing with the eyes of another, hearing with the ears of another, and feeling with the heart of another. Research indicates that empathy, warmth, and genuineness are related to a large percentage of the gains attained in therapy regardless of the therapist's

---

Case examples have been disguised to protect client confidentiality.

https://doi.org/10.1037/0000451-004
Therapeutic Change With Difficult Clients: Precursors and Techniques in the CHANGES Model, Second Edition, by B. D. Wilkinson and F. J. Hanna

theoretical orientation (Elliott et al., 2018; W. R. Miller & Moyers, 2021). When it happens, in therapy or out, the empathic person is valued by the other.

Thus, it is of central importance to respect and work from within the client's frame of reference, as Rogers (1951, 1957) repeatedly emphasized. Difficult clients who feel understood by a therapist no longer find it easy to summarily dismiss the approaches or observations of the therapist. Conversely, it is likely that many people can accomplish change faster on their own than with a therapist who is not empathic and does not engage a client in a viable working relationship. A therapist can know all the most innovative and brilliant techniques, but if they are not adept at empathy, they are likely to lose clients (W. R. Miller & Moyers, 2021) or have clients who do not change. We have talked with many therapy dropouts, and many of the complaints went like this:

- "My therapist never saw where I was coming from."
- "My therapist kept telling me what was wrong with me and never understood me."
- "My therapist's 'know-it-all' attitude bugged me."
- "My therapist made me feel stupid."
- "We just never connected."

The therapeutic relationship is filled with complexities and subtleties that research still seeks to understand. Many mysterious aspects remain. For starters, we do not know what empathy really is beyond a few surface definitions (see Maibom, 2017, 2020). Is it the process of experiencing another's inner world through a tangible and embodied connection (Manganaro, 2017)? Or is it a simulation-based, cognitive representation that we use to imagine what it would be like to have this person's experience (Decety & Jackson, 2004; Marsh, 2018)? One mode involves phenomenological contact, whereas the other is inferential. Is it both or neither? Each of these perspectives on empathy is based on a different set of metaphysical assumptions (Hanna & Shank, 1995; Maibom, 2017), and at this point, we really do not know. But empathy is so crucial to successful therapy that a more complete understanding could make therapy more effective.

INCREASING THE PRECURSORS THROUGH THE RELATIONSHIP

It would be simplistic to view the precursors as separate from the therapeutic relationship because they are interdependent. According to the CHANGES model, the therapeutic relationship is a necessary precondition for the activation of precursors, which in turn support therapeutic change. Therapeutic core conditions alone are insufficient to facilitate change until precursors are activated in the client. In this respect, the purpose of the therapeutic relationship is to provide a setting in which the precursors can be established and stabilized in a client, difficult or otherwise.

Of course, this is not as simple as it might initially seem. Weaving change through the relationship requires tremendous skill, particularly when a client is ambivalent about change. We have repeatedly found that techniques only occasionally work with a guarded and defensive client who still does not trust the therapist or the therapy process. The most enthusiastic and otherwise competent therapist can try a potent therapy technique on a difficult client, only to have it land with a "thud," to no effect at all. When this happens, it is often the relationship that is lacking.

Successful therapeutic relationships involve more than interpersonal trust. Again, inspiration and persuasion (see Afonseca et al., 2023; Frank & Frank, 1991) are also involved. Clients who do not feel supported and encouraged by a therapist are more likely to drop out of therapy (Friedlander, 2015), seek and accomplish change on their own, or find another therapist. Furthermore, a client can have a wildly different configuration of precursors with different therapists. It is the therapist's duty to tailor the relationship to provide an environment conducive to developing such functions as hope, effort, and confronting the problem.

As far as the CHANGES model is concerned, if the relationship is not established as a working alliance, the precursors may never develop or stabilize. The therapist must develop and refine the relationship so the precursors can incubate and grow to the point where the client can exit therapy in an improved state of coping, health, or functioning. What makes the therapeutic relationship therapeutic at all may well be that it activates the seven precursors, and a relationship that does not activate the precursors is not therapeutic.

Lazarus (1993) called on therapists to be an "authentic chameleon"—in other words, to provide a relationship that meets the client's needs without losing one's own genuineness or authenticity in the process. Some clients require a businesslike collaboration, whereas others need a lot of encouragement and nurturing. Either of these groups would probably find the other style unsatisfying. However, being an authentic chameleon goes beyond merely supplying the appropriate style. In the context of contemporary research on the therapeutic relationship, it also involves being able to match a client's worldview in an empathic and understanding way so there is as little "personality clash" as possible, in spite of interpersonal differences (Clark, 2023).

PURPOSE OF THE RELATIONSHIP: ACHIEVING CHANGE

Linehan (1993) often observed that successful relationships and interactions with difficult clients are brought about by teaching them what kinds of behaviors lead to therapeutic change. She referred to such behaviors as "therapy enhancing" and noted that they should not be expected of clients but should instead be taught. In this same vein, when a client learns that change comes about as a result of cultivating the precursors, the relationship becomes based on change principles. Therefore, a client's agreement can be procured to allow the therapist to gently or firmly point out when one or more of the precursors are being ignored or avoided. Timing is crucial, of course, but it does help to keep a client on task.

In addition, if the client knows and is reminded that the entire interaction is based on change, much less ambiguity is allowed into the relationship. There will be fewer opportunities to lead therapy astray by initiating casual conversation designed to avoid therapy involvement. The purpose of therapy is not often readily apparent to difficult clients. This is largely because the difficult client is not thinking about therapeutic change and therefore sees a relationship with a therapist in ways that often have little or nothing to do with psychotherapy being a means of facilitating change.

The easiest way around this is to clearly establish that the purpose of the relationship is to achieve change, even if change is framed as the goal of happiness for the client. Anything that strays from this purpose is seen as interfering with therapy and can be named as such. So, when clients suggest business dealings, casual meetings, romantic interludes, or conversation about sports, the purpose of therapy can be gently reiterated. In extreme cases, the therapist may even suggest that therapy be terminated on the grounds that the purpose of change is not being served and make a referral if appropriate.

ESTABLISHING THE THERAPEUTIC RELATIONSHIP WITH DIFFICULT CLIENTS

The following sections outline strategies for increasing empathy with a wide variety of difficult clients. Although some of these may be obvious to certain readers, the list forms a comprehensive overview of how to work with clients who care little for therapy, are not interested in seeking help, or are so fragile they are intimidated or threatened by the very prospect of change, no matter how much they might benefit from it.

There are many styles and patterns of difficult clients, so these strategies are not appropriate for all clients at all times. Therapists can refer to this list if needed when the appropriate moment arises and as appropriate for the client's needs at that time. We make no claim that any of these suggestions are original to this book; many therapists have adhered to and followed these suggestions for decades.

Being Courteous and Requesting Permission

Even though therapists and counselors are professionals, many difficult clients see routine actions by therapists as intrusive or even rude. From their perspectives, therapists regularly engage in meddling and prying behaviors. Courtesy can clear the way for probes that might otherwise be rebuffed. In many instances, it can be considered a basic courtesy to ask permission before posing a question or making a statement. Clients will usually agree, thus entitling and empowering the therapist to do so. One might also ask a client if there is a particular way to be challenging or confrontational that they would not perceive as rude or intrusive. In response, clients often give clear instructions that make the job much easier.

Asking permission is best done before asking deeply sensitive questions, and the therapist should add that the client does not have to answer. Clients nearly always agree. Asking permission has two advantages. One is that the person becomes prepared or ready for the question, which increases their willingness to experience the anxiety involved. The other advantage is that the client notes that the therapist respects the client's inner world. This is a form of communicating empathy in and of itself.

Part of asking permission is to be courteous about how one goes about it. This does not sound like much, but some difficult clients are going out of their way to answer such questions at all. For many, answering deeply personal questions involves a lot of effort in an area in which they have little practice or experience. Statements such as, "Do you mind if I ask a question you might find sensitive?" prepare the client for the question and show respect for their dignity and right to privacy.

Being Persuasive

Beyond core therapeutic conditions, persuasion in the service of therapeutic change is a uniquely crucial therapeutic skill in work with difficult clients (Anderson et al., 2020). Frank and Frank (1991) observed that persuasion is a common factor of all therapy approaches, operating in diverse ways but always present. Rhetoric plays a necessary role in facilitating change with difficult clients, as the stylistic use of language and its delivery influence how clients view problems, situations, and events (Frank, 1987). Compelling psychotherapy research in discourse and conversation analysis serves to highlight the legitimate value of persuasive rhetoric (Avdi & Georgaca, 2007; Peräkylä, 2019; Smoliak & Strong, 2018). As Jerome Frank told me (FH) in 1996, persuasion is inseparable from effective therapy, and methods of rhetorical influence should be taught in graduate school.

However, misperceptions of what constitutes persuasion may serve as a significant barrier to using the CHANGES model, which maintains that it is the role and responsibility of therapists to help clients activate precursors and facilitate change. If a therapist is dissuaded of the value of persuasion or otherwise regards persuasion as mere advice-giving or, worse yet, manipulation, then it will be difficult for them to make use of the model and techniques in this book with intentionality. Such negative reactions to a "call for persuasiveness" might be born out of recognizing that power in the therapeutic encounter is inherently imbalanced and that it is the therapist's responsibility to empower clients (Totton, 2018). Therapists must indeed avoid the needless power struggle that occurs when a client perceives the therapist as taking a "one-up" position that conveys an unspoken "I know better than you" message.

Yet persuasion is different from manipulation, just as rhetoric is different from grandstanding. The difference stems from intent, as guided by our ethical codes and professional norms. If therapists are trying to facilitate change, it is incumbent upon them to grow their skill as artful rhetoricians who can persuasively articulate the value of the change process itself (Anderson et al., 2020). Through the art of persuasion, therapists can encourage clients to do more of what is working, deemphasize what is not working, and promote the value of personal growth, mental health, and well-being (Anderson et al., 2016). Persuasion also plays a pivotal role in expectancy effects (Goodwin et al., 2018), hope (Griffith & Dsouza, 2012), and psychoeducation (Stice et al., 2008).

Most transcribed client–therapist dialogues in this book demonstrate persuasiveness, and many of the techniques herein require artful use of persuasion to be effective. Good timing, tact, and word choice all require a capacity to "read the room" in a manner that captures the context or prevailing mood of a particular moment. Facilitating client movement toward change without impinging on freedom of thought, identity, or autonomy is thus a fine art indeed. Being persuasive is not about getting your way or acting as though you know better than others. As such, therapists would do well to follow the proofs set forth by Aristotle on three modes of persuasion: personal character (ethos), stirring of emotions (pathos), and coherent or logical argumentation (logos; Bartlett, 2019). In alignment with our professional responsibility as ethical stewards of therapeutic change, the artful use of rhetoric in psychotherapy should proceed in a wise, caring, and truthful manner.

Validating Positive Qualities

A client does not have to have a high IQ to be smart. Clients who are perceptive, shrewd, or have street savvy should be validated for it. For example, when a therapist encourages a client to explain how a problem came into their life, they can say, "Come on, you are very smart. You know what's going on here." Any positive quality that the client displays can be used to facilitate therapeutic progress. Much of this approach to therapy involves discovering and revealing those positive qualities and genuinely admiring them in a client. Such positive qualities can form the platform upon which the precursors rest and find stability.

Additionally, positive qualities should be expounded upon at reasonable length whenever possible so the therapist does not come off as merely ingratiating. For example, if a client says, "I'm a bad person. I always hurt the people around me," then simply saying, "I think you're good" is not enough. The quality of goodness is more fully demonstrated when a therapist responds,

> Sounds to me like you're actually quite a good person. Bad people don't care about whether they hurt others. They just hurt them and don't bother to think about it. I would say that you're actually a good person trying to figure out how to be better. What do you think?

The therapist then waits for an answer so the client has a chance to vocalize agreement or otherwise engage in the process.

Such validation can have extraordinary effects in terms of stabilization, removing self-doubt, building the relationship, and helping a client feel more deserving of positive changes. This practice should be done constantly in therapy to create an ever-increasing list of positive qualities. Some clients initially object, but it can be helpful and quite humorous to all when they acquiesce.

Giving the Client the Option of Telling the Therapist to Back Off

After getting permission to intrude or confront a client, a therapist can say, "If I am bothering you, tell me to back off, okay?" This will often ease the tension of the question or the therapist's persistence by returning a sense of control to a threatened client. This can also be effective with clients who are intimidating, some of whom, when they hear the option of telling the therapist to back off, will consider it beneath them to admit that mere questions could ever bother them.

A client who is manipulative may indeed tell the therapist to back off. When this happens, the therapist readily agrees to do so but then asks if the client is getting uncomfortable. The therapist can also ask if this discomfort occurs often, and when it does, in what kinds of situations and with what kinds of people it occurs. This must be done casually, as these moments can be delicate, requiring good timing and proper phrasing based on client needs and the situation.

Attending to Metalogue, Then Bringing It Into Dialogue

Metalogue is a term we have adapted from its original use by Gregory Bateson (Bateson & Bateson, 1987) to refer to the unspoken conversation that the client may be having with a therapist. Because human beings have only one tongue but process their thoughts in parallel—that is, in many separate streams at a time (Metzinger, 2004; Ornstein, 2003)—many of these thought streams are never given voice. Clients are unlikely to express silent, self-statement thoughts, such as, "I wonder if I can trust this person," or "Why is she looking at me like that? She doesn't like me," or "I wonder if I can fool this guy." These thoughts may be occurring simultaneously, even as the client answers the therapist's questions.

With particularly difficult clients, there may be a different metalogue containing self-statements such as, "Therapy's a bunch of crap," "I wish I didn't have to be here," or "I hope she doesn't say anything about my drinking." These latter statements can be clear thought content to the client, even if they are simultaneously pledging to be cooperative with a reassuring smile.

Attending to metalogue statements has two advantages. The first is that it saves valuable session time by directly addressing not only the presenting complaints but deeper, unspoken issues. The second is that by doing so, a client will come to respect the therapist in a way that facilitates disclosure and cooperation.

The therapist attends to the metalogue through an inferential process. For example, a client may reassure the therapist that she wants to get better yet is not showing effort, confronting the problem presented, or being willing to experience anxiety. The therapist might ask the client, "Do you mind if I ask you a question?" The client will usually say something like, "Sure, go ahead." The therapist then says, "Please tell me if I am wrong, but I get the sense that you really don't want anything to do with this therapy thing. Is that right?" The therapist does not have to be right but may just be close enough that, for the first time, a real and genuine dialogue takes place. By bringing the metalogue into dialogue, therapy becomes more vital and interesting as well.

Reflecting Meanings Before Feelings

It is easy to plunge right into exploring a client's feelings, but this may not be appropriate with clients who are unwilling to experience anxiety or unpleasant affect. For such clients, feelings are not particularly accessible. It is often helpful to initially reflect meanings instead. Frank (1987) observed that "All psycho-therapeutic endeavors, whatever their form, transpire entirely in the realm of meanings" (p. 293). Getting a sense of the meaning system of that client can help in accessing feelings later. Casual expressions of opinions can be extrapolated and subjected to an inductive reasoning process that leads to a person's core cognitions. This is also a way of being able to match a client's worldview in a way that expedites the process of self-disclosure and the formation of a viable relationship.

For example, a male client once made a sexist statement about women, smiling a knowing, "brotherhood" type of smile to subtly suggest some form of comradery with the therapist in the moment. Rather than confront the client on his sexism, the therapist found it more effective to explore and discover his attitude toward people in general. The therapist's response was, "Do you mind if I try and sort out where you are coming from?" Following the client's hesitant nod, the therapist continued: "If you think that about women, then is it fair to say that you generally believe some people are meant to be taken advantage of by others?" This client said, "Well, yeah, I do, sort of." The therapist paused and said, "Well, I guess my question for you then is to which group you figure you belong: those who get used or those who do the using?"

This opened up a fruitful exploration of how this client had been used by others and how all his life he strove to become one of the users. This then led to a discussion of whether being a user was admirable and who the users were in his life that he strove to be like. Of course, it turned out that the people he was striving to imitate were people that he despised. This explained a lot of the self-hate that he disclosed later in the therapeutic process.

It is often true that even casual statements on mundane subjects can activate an inductive reasoning process, which in turn can support the isolation and identification of maladaptive beliefs about self, people, problems, or life in general. With a client who withholds information, it sometimes helps to evoke brief opinion statements on politics, sports, or even religion and from there, move deeper toward the underlying presuppositions of the statement itself. Whether one is a conservative, a Democrat, or a Dallas Cowboys fan, casual opinions can open windows into a client's deeper issues and problems. If a person says they are a conservative because their father was, the therapist can issue a challenge aimed at discovering whether the client ever made any independent decisions or whether it is a good idea to be one's own person.

This approach is sometimes highly valuable in easing a client toward detaching from sources of harmful or dysfunctional beliefs.

Increasing Therapist Capacity for Empathy

Increasing one's capacity for empathy seems to be more of a therapeutic duty than a mere suggestion. However, one particular angle on the topic of empathy is seldom discussed in the literature: How much is enough? Does a great therapist have a great amount of empathy? How much empathy does a client need for change to be accomplished?

Certain exercises can help a therapist increase empathy. One is to practice assuming the roles of other people, specifically those one knows or has known. It is also important to be able to assume the role of people with personality disorders such as narcissistic, borderline, or antisocial disorders. Personality disorders that have delusional aspects, such as schizotypal and paranoid, also make for excellent practice. Therapists can demonstrate their ability to think in a disordered way without agreeing with that way of thinking. Clients usually know this and can use the therapist as a model.

Carl Whitaker, the renowned family therapist, often advised being able to think like schizophrenic clients to be better able to work with them. North (1987), a psychiatrist who was once diagnosed with catatonic schizophrenia, stated that this experience made her better able to help such clients because of her ability to empathize with them. Of course, being able to assume the viewpoints of people with these disorders is not the same as having had them, but it certainly can help a client to feel understood. It is also important to clients to know that the therapist is at least attempting to see things from their perspective.

It is often helpful to a therapist to do an empathy check by simply asking the client if they feel understood. This can be done in general or specific ways on specific points. Statements like, "I am trying to see where you are coming from here," and adding, "Am I getting it?" serve this purpose. Simply asking, "Do you think I understand you?" is another empathy check. These serve a dual purpose: to help the therapist ensure that they understand the client and to communicate to the client that the therapist is attempting to truly understand.

Telling the client things like, "You are ultimately the expert on you" also serves this purpose by acknowledging that clients have access to information about themselves that is not available to anyone else. If the client informs the therapist that they do not feel understood, this can open the door to honest conversation and a potential disclosure of information that enhances the relationship.

Another exercise is to role-play a difficult client with a colleague or supervisor by fully assuming the client's meaning and value system and answering questions while playing that client's identity. A therapist should be able to role-play that client so thoroughly that they eventually begin to have a feel for what it is to be that person, in addition to the diagnosis or problem.

A final exercise involves the therapist role-playing the client during the session and checking with the client to determine whether the therapist is really grasping their perspective on life and living. As part of this role-play, it may help to have the client assume the role of therapist. This can help raise self-awareness in the client. Although some difficult clients will eschew this kind of approach, some will take to it, and it can be quite humorous if done lightheartedly. To the degree a therapist can empathically act as a client in role-play, it is important not to slip into caricature. Therapists should be thoughtful about how they convey the expressions, mannerisms, and vocalizations of a client. The same goes for trainees, who often need guidance on the subtleties of character development in role-play exercises.

Establishing the Client's Meaning System or Worldview

This strategy is an extension of the previous one and is related to a little-known school of cognitive therapy called *philosophical psychotherapy* (Mills, 2001; Sahakian, 1976). Based on what clients tell a therapist, even casually, an entire meaning structure can be deduced and proposed to the client (see McMullin, 1986). For example, a client casually declares, "You know you have to look out for number one in this world." A deductive response might be, "So if you are number one, does that mean that no one else in the entire world is as important as you?" A few clients will agree, and others may respond with a "not quite" answer. These are easy enough to handle with standard cognitive approaches. However, many difficult clients will boldly and shamelessly answer, "Of course I'm number one; who else could be?" In this case, an entire meaning system can be structured in a hierarchy.

Consider the example of William. He was 35, depressed, and said in the first session that looking out for himself was his primary task in life. His therapist drew a pyramid on paper, drew in various levels, and placed William's name at the apex or top level. Then the therapist asked who would be number two and so on down the levels. The therapist asked what sort of treatment people deserved at each level of the hierarchy. This helped to discern William's entire moral or ethical philosophy.

Like many clients of the narcissistic style, William calmly and directly said that people low in the hierarchy can be manipulated, cheated, and otherwise mistreated. The therapist asked if he himself was ever low on someone else's pyramid. He nodded hesitantly but seriously. This opened an inroad into his world. The therapist inquired whether he was ever manipulated, cheated, or otherwise mistreated by that person or persons. When he nodded affirmatively, the therapist asked if it hurt or caused him anxiety or difficulty. Once again, William nodded. From this point, the therapist was able to construct his meaning system, which included a view of the world based on contempt for and resentment toward others.

The therapist asked permission to reflect that viewpoint back to him for verification. With William's consent, the therapist stated,

> Please tell me if I'm wrong, but it seems that for you, life seems to be played in terms of who outsmarts and outmaneuvers the other and is based on each person causing

pain and hurt to others in the process. And whoever does it best wins. So, if no one else is looking out for you, then you have to make yourself number one in order to survive. Is that close?

William replied, "I guess so." Because William had already admitted that he was depressed, the therapist asked if this lifestyle worked to make him happy. When William said, "Not really," the therapist asked if they could use therapy to find a lifestyle that could. Although not productive of change on the spot, this empathic approach placed William on the path to awareness and a sense of necessity for change.

Operating Within the Client's Meaning System or Framework

Once the client's worldview is somewhat defined and outlined, it can become a pivot for various interventions. Techniques can be introduced and framed from within that perspective. It is not helpful to expect a difficult client, who is minimally involved in therapy anyway, to learn a new lexicon. From the perspective of many difficult clients, a therapist's use of jargon-filled explanations can look and feel suspiciously like an attempt to convert them to a new religion.

For example, the same "number one on the pyramid" technique was once used on a different male client who was highly self-centered and self-serving. The therapist got a good idea of the client's meaning system and began to work within it. Later in therapy, the therapist seriously and solemnly reframed the client's existence as the "Unknown King," noting that because he was the most important person in the world, he should be ruling the human race and should be given anything and everything he desired. The client looked at the therapist long and hard. After a pause of several seconds, the therapist said,

> And if that's true, then you must be a tremendously unhappy person who is never respected, meets frustration and disappointment at every turn in life, and believes other people are ignorant, foolish, and petty. After all, they don't recognize that you are the king.

From that point forward, the client began to make progress slowly toward change.

Redefining the Problem

There is always a fine balance between addressing a client's presenting concerns and resolving the almost inevitable deeper issues underlying them. Contrary to some views on this, it can be done briefly. When a client is low in precursors, their explanation of the problem is usually naive and inaccurate. A young woman being physically abused by her husband says it was her fault. A man with antisocial personality disorder says people do not like him because he is "too intense."

On the other hand, there is often a grain of truth in the explanation. A battered woman says that she cannot leave her husband because he needs her. Surely, he does, but that is not the problem. A man who stalks a woman says that he knows that if only the woman would get to know him, she would come to love him. Maybe in theory, but that part of him is so hidden by pathology that the real "him" may never emerge for the woman to see. A kernel of truth is the seed of delusion.

Difficult clients should indeed be acknowledged and understood from within their meaning system, but therapists must be aware of the fact that the meaning system is probably deeply flawed. Clients in general, and especially those who are difficult, fail to account for unconscious motives and beliefs.

Bringing Down Defense Systems From Within

When encountering a well-defended client, it sometimes helps to envision gently bypassing their walls of defense and peacefully entering the city. The goal is to be given an entrance point into the city itself. It will usually be given only to someone who is perceived as a friend. A therapist is the enemy of what Winnicott (1960/2018) called the "false self." In this context, the false self is what erects those defenses and guards the walls. The therapist's purpose is to restore or establish the greatness of the client's "real self," that which is open to experience and not entrenched, bunkered down, or ready for war. Once inside, the therapist usually perceives that the outwardly forbidding ramparts and walls nearly always look delicate and fragile from the inside.

To get past the walls, it sometimes helps to present oneself as a consultant to help improve the design and engineering of the walls. Validate defenses, even hostile ones, by pointing them out and asking if they are effective and what could make them more so. For example, one could say, "I have noticed that you do not like anyone being too inquisitive toward you and that you highly value your privacy. I respect that. Do you find that you like keeping people at a distance?"

People have excellent reasons for erecting defenses. Paradoxically, if the reasons are validated and encouraged, it sometimes reduces the need to erect them. One can also point out the energy drain that comes with keeping the defenses active so much of the time. If a person is tired, that could be reframed as due to their devoting a considerable amount of mental energy to defending instead of living.

Respecting and Encouraging the Client's Autonomy and Freedom

Respecting and encouraging autonomy and freedom is helpful with nearly all clients, but especially with criminal or antisocial clients. Regardless of any debate on determinism and free will, research has shown that appealing to the prospect of change as a free choice has considerable therapeutic value for clients (Kanfer & Grimm, 1978; Lavik et al., 2018). In fact, this has long been shown to be one of the few effective strategies with antisocial clients (see Kierulff, 1988; Samenow, 1998; Simourd et al., 2016). There is a catch, however. Criminals have learned they can violate a wide range of societal norms and dictates. They know they have the freedom to do so, and they live for it. This seems to be not so much a cognitive calculation as a palpable thrill or sensation that reinforces antisocial behaviors. It is as important to address the thrill or sensation of freedom, and the beliefs or attitudes connected with it, as it is to examine their irrational beliefs about criminality in general (see Benn, 2021; Samenow, 1998).

Perhaps the most important step toward working with the criminal mindset is to understand two things. First, the criminal seeks the admirable goal of absolute freedom of behavior—the ability to do whatever, whenever, and however. A criminal client will often combine the first goal with the contemptible goal of being able to have complete disregard for responsibility, accountability, and the well-being of others. This is often a core aspect of their flawed meaning system (Benn, 2021).

Encouraging Uncooperativeness as a Protection of Freedom

This is paradoxical, but it is also true. If a client with limited precursor activation steadfastly refuses to disclose anything of real substance, it might be of help to momentarily suspend the effort to get the client to self-disclose and instead talk about why the client likes to be uncooperative. It often turns out that some clients are so protective of their freedom and autonomy that being uncooperative is merely an attempt to retain the dignity and integrity that comes with being free. If this is the case, the therapist can offer to make an agreement with the client:

> I'll make a deal with you. The minute you feel that I am taking away your freedom in any way, please tell me. I have no interest in doing anything of the sort. If anything, therapy is meant to strengthen and increase your freedom. What do you think?

Once this is done, it is surprising how much a client will allow a therapist to probe and challenge.

Answering the "What's-in-It-for-Me?" Question

Difficult clients are often uninterested in therapy until they can answer the question, What's in it for me? Whenever possible, engage the client in the first session. There are many ways to do this, depending on the style and disorders of clients themselves. Maybe the best option is to offer a sense of hope, even if the client does not admit to lacking it. It is not necessary to promise any resolution of problems, of course, but it often helps to present the possibility of change or better conditions.

Many difficult clients view therapy with more than a little trepidation or suspicion. They are not likely to become involved in the process until they answer the What's-in-it-for-me? question. When it becomes apparent that they can gain some benefit from participating, their interest level will pick up to that degree. In the beginning, the answer to the question might be horribly mundane, such as "to satisfy my probation officer," but even that is a start.

Displaying Compassion and Caring

Compassion may be the most underrated element in all of psychotherapy (Gilbert, 2020; Lewin, 1936). Many clients have told me that the only thing that kept them going was knowing that someone cared about what was going to happen to them. If a client knows someone genuinely cares, this functions as a ticket or sanction to improve and get better. When someone else cares, it allows a person to feel deserving of improvement. So many people believe that if they are not loved, they are unworthy of happiness or joy. Thus, a demonstration of care by others can serve as an indication of a person's significance. This could be one explanation for why people with borderline and narcissistic disorders are obsessed with obtaining the love and admiration of others.

Alternatively, some difficult clients are extremely adept at getting people to hate them. It serves the inverse purpose of finding significance, as the false self further solidifies the core belief of unworthiness or insignificance (Masterson, 1988; Oberst & Stewart, 2014). A savvy therapist will be on the lookout for this unconscious tactic since it shuts down the change process immediately.

Moderating Compassion With Antisocial Clients

With clients diagnosed as antisocial, compassion and caring require a slightly different approach. These people are often accustomed to manipulating people who care about them. Many believe that showing love or caring is a sign of weakness. Thus, they tend to peg a warm, caring therapist as someone who is easily manipulated and unworthy of respect. For a therapist to openly display warmth and caring can be a mistake with some of these clients. With others, it is a wise and important approach. Clinical judgment needs to be exercised, but a fairly reliable indicator is showing some genuine warmth and watching to see how the client responds.

Addressing Problems in Chunks

If too much contradictory, destabilizing, or painful material is opened too soon in sessions, clients will tend to withdraw and feel disempowered and threatened by the depth and extent of the problems. It gives the "rug-out-from-under" feeling, and one's inner world appears to be poised at the brink of a void. The problem no longer seems manageable and is a cause of reduced hope.

The solution is to address things in chunks. The aim is to handle only what the client can confront without being overwhelmed. Sometimes, a client is difficult precisely because their tolerance of pain is so low. Additionally, clients can be "trained" to be difficult when they are asked to confront or change too much at once. Asking a client to confront too much material actually reduces the confronting precursor. Finally, a client can feel degraded or demeaned by a therapist who outlines a vast map of psychopathology. The relationship can be severely damaged, and a premature termination may be imminent.

Expecting Client Hesitancy After Great Effort

Nearly every therapist will recognize this phenomenon: A great session finally occurs with a difficult client, and you are pleased that a breakthrough has occurred, yet in the next session, the client is withdrawn, uncooperative, or perhaps even belligerent. In some cases, especially with people diagnosed as borderline, there may be extreme hostility and defiance toward the therapist for "tricking" them into disclosing or working. This can be upsetting to a therapist who does not know that such behaviors should be expected.

Thus, after a session in which a client does much confronting and exerts great effort, do not plunge further ahead but assess where the client stands with what was done. Enjoy the plateau. The client may not be ready for more just yet. Pacing in such situations is of the utmost importance.

Setting Boundaries

Each therapist has their own limits on what they will accept from clients in terms of middle-of-the-night telephone calls and the like. It is important to define limits that neither impede nor threaten therapeutic change. Therapists should instruct clients that they will not always have time to talk, that taking "no" for an answer will sometimes be necessary, and that keeping agreements and agreeing to cancel rather than skipping sessions is desirable behavior (Linehan, 1993; Pope & Keith-Spiegel, 2008).

Although extremely rare, threats of physical harm from a client—whether thinly or thickly veiled—should not be tolerated under any circumstances. If the client is already on probation or parole, therapists should inform the police of any threats (the therapist should be in contact with the probation or parole officer anyway). It should be made firmly clear to the client that despite compassion, empathy, caring, and the like, no boundary violations of this variety will be tolerated, especially those of security.

It is equally important for female therapists to make it clear that sexual comments or innuendoes will not be allowed. Some difficult male clients are adept at using graphic sexual language in a session to give themselves a cheap thrill and make the therapist uncomfortable. Any actions like this require immediate attention, and termination may be necessary if it continues. Grounds for termination should be made clear ahead of time with some difficult clients. With borderline clients especially, the range of acceptable and unacceptable behaviors needs to be set clearly and concisely so the client can be reminded, with as little ambiguity as possible, when they have gone too far (Linehan, 1993; McCloskey et al., 2021). At the same time, it is important to soothe a client's feelings about observing limits while not compromising the limits themselves.

Matching the Client's Emotional State

Match the client's emotional state but with one vital additive—interest. For example, if a client is sad or dejected, the therapist does not have to be melancholy and helpless along with the client. However, if empathic contact is present, the therapist will resonate with the client's emotions enough to reflect back that sadness. This empathic resonance helps the client accept the therapist and their input.

The danger is that the therapist can sink into sympathy and lose the empathic contact. After all, some difficult clients have backgrounds so devastating and tragic that a therapist's empathy can easily degrade into sympathy. One route of escape from this is through the element of interest. We have found that a strong and powerful sense of genuine interest on the part of a therapist, focused on a client and their condition, can be contagious. A therapist's interest can stimulate a client to also be interested without any verbal persuasion. In many cases, especially when coupled with humor, a therapist's contagious interest can help a client to be lifted, or at least dislodged, from entrenched emotions or mindsets.

Opening a Therapeutic Window

Much of working with difficult clients is probing here and there, trying this approach and that, searching for an entry point, an inroad, or a window to open that makes the client accessible. This is a difficult phenomenon to describe, as it is highly subjective. In any case, in working with difficult clients, one becomes familiar with canned responses, disingenuous behaviors, and flat, feigned, or exaggerated affect. Many clients have become hardened to any external inspection and have a response for just about any potential intrusion. But every now and then, a probe or a confrontation will bring a hesitance, a response that reveals a soft spot in the armor. A client may look at you with a sensitivity or genuineness that was not present and indeed may not have ever been there before.

When a therapeutic window is opened, a therapist must enter through it soon, for the client may close it with a new defense formed in a matter of moments. For example, some angry, defiant teenagers are proud of their anger. Although anger management strategies can get them to talk about their anger, many such clients will change little, if anything, about it. The teenager might even brag about their anger as though it is a prized possession. An example of opening a therapeutic window with this type of client is to ask, "Have you ever been hurt?" The answer is typically yes. This makes the client pause. The window can then be further opened by asking, "Is that hurt related to your anger?" and then, "If you didn't have the hurt, what would happen to the anger?" This approach will often open a window that allows entrance beyond anger into the client's inner world. It changes the relationship and initiates the change process (see Hanna & Hunt, 1999), as opening the window and entering smoothly are part of bringing down defenses from within.

Looking for and Connecting With the "I Behind the Eye"

In instances where a therapist has experienced a sense of connection with a client, it is quite revealing to ask oneself what got connected. Was it two brains? Two worldviews? Two selves? Two multigenerational family systems? Phenomenologically, the therapist may perceive something in a client that forms the basis for a relational exchange. It may appear as though one has made subtle yet deep contact with a client through a maze of turbulent thought patterns, raging emotions, and destructive behaviors.

Thinking too much in respect of clinical labels sometimes risks obscuring the actual person behind a series of professional templates and categories. When it comes to establishing relationships, it is probably better to suspend the labels and templates so one can get a sense of connection with the person. Gendlin (1992) described the person as the "I who looks at you from behind the eyes" (p. 453). That "I"—the real person—can be accepted unconditionally, even though negative behaviors and thoughts are seen as needing change. Unfortunately, sometimes it takes a year or so for that "I behind the eye" to show up in a therapy session, and sometimes it may not happen at all, especially with antisocial clients. But for the therapist who knows how to locate that "I," it may happen sooner.

Developing Perspicacity as a Wisdom Characteristic

Clients with antisocial or conduct disorders often respect therapists who are suspicious. "Bullshit" is a common term in casual conversation in this culture (Frankfurt, 2005). Its use is ubiquitous among antisocial clients, and most learn at an early age how to dole it out. Their peers ridicule them when they are susceptible to it, saying, "You idiot, you believed that bullshit?!" They will test therapists by tossing out falsehoods to gauge their sharpness or gullibility, and a degree of tacit respect is given to a person who can recognize it. One of the characteristics of an effective therapist, especially with this population, is what Sternberg (1990) called "perspicacity," or the capacity to see beyond appearances, to not be easily deceived or fooled.

Antisocial clients will be forced to respect a therapist who has a well-functioning, reasonably accurate "bullshit detector." This may not be sufficient by itself to get such a client to be compliant or to work in therapy, but it is essential to establishing a relationship and cannot be underestimated. The same is true in working with clients who use alcohol and drugs, another population notorious for dishonesty and deception concerning drug use and behaviors. It is difficult to teach, but I have observed that even initially naive therapists can cultivate it through experience.

Matching the Therapist With the Client

An intangible therapeutic factor largely unaccounted for by research is that some clients do better with particular therapists. Much of it seems to be related to shared worldviews (Davis et al., 2018; B. S. Kim et al., 2005; Lyddon, 1989), as clients and therapists who share general outlooks or beliefs seem to do better together in therapy. Of course, the therapist's personal responses and issues also play an important role, as will be explored in the next chapter. Yet there are simply times when one counselor will develop natural rapport with a client whereas another therapist will not. In such cases, switching therapists for the client's sake will likely help bring about change sooner.

Using the Concentric Circle Technique

When working with difficult clients, it is common for therapists to wonder how close they really are to a particular client as well as how deeply such clients are allowing the therapist into their confidence. In other words, it is helpful to know the level or degree of a client's self-disclosure. Lazarus (1989b) described a remarkably helpful and effective technique for finding out how far a client has "let one in." This adaptation is done by drawing five concentric circles with the core or innermost circle labeled as Circle 1, and the outermost perimeter labeled as Circle 5. The therapist then asks the client to conceive of the core self as being in the center, at Circle 1, where their most private and personal information is held. Circle 5, at the outer perimeter, is where the most superficial and insignificant information is—that which everyone knows. The therapist can ask the client directly, "Into which circle have you allowed me?" After finding out, the therapist can ask, "What would it take for me to get into the next circle?" or "Whom have you allowed into circle 1?" or "For a person to get into circle 1 with you, what do they have to do or be like?" Clients can be surprisingly honest in using this technique. It takes little effort but can be highly productive.

Using Different Therapy Modalities

The three major therapeutic modalities are individual, group, and family therapies. Each has its own particular and peculiar set of benefits not readily available from the others. Many difficult clients need all three, if and when appropriate. Individual therapy may not be the mode a particular difficult client needs most. For example, an alcohol abuser may be more in need of a group with similar issues and problems than an individual setting. Chances are they may need both—and family therapy as well. Children and adolescents can greatly benefit from family therapy, not to mention parents. Each modality provides a unique opportunity to build relationships with a therapist, with peers, and with family members. These skills can then be used in everyday life to build a social support network, possibly leading to a logarithmic effect on change.

A CLOSING NOTE ON THE THERAPEUTIC RELATIONSHIP

A strong therapeutic relationship is the foundation for positive changes to take place in psychotherapy. The CHANGES model requires the establishment of relational factors such as empathy, warmth, and genuineness in order to work with difficult clients. However, there are a number of interpersonal skills and communication techniques that therapists can utilize to foster engagement and enhance rapport, as seen in this chapter. Therapists should keep the importance of the relationship foremost in their minds in sessions, as it can be all too easy to forego empathic contact with a difficult client once the therapist initiates a challenging technical intervention. In moving from contact to intervention, therapists must not lose sight of the subjective personhood of the client.

4

C: Confronting the Problem

The term "confronting," as a precursor of change, has nothing to do with hostility, opposition, antagonism, or provocation. It also has nothing to do with challenging a client on an inconsistency, hesitancy, or incongruency. Like most therapy techniques, challenging a client is an attempt to implement this precursor, but the challenge is not the precursor itself.

In the CHANGES model, *confronting* is defined as the active, intentional, sustained, and deliberate directing of attention or awareness toward anything that is painful, intimidating, or stultifying. Confronting thus involves a continuous examination or investigation of something in spite of fear, confusion, or any tendency toward avoidance or acting out. Almost anything at all can be confronted: mental images, memories, emotional pain, behaviors of all varieties, thoughts, thought patterns, beliefs, persons, places, objects, and relationships.

Confronting extends well beyond mere acknowledgment of a problem, as in the case of the awareness precursor (see Chapter 6, this volume). Confronting the problem is a dramatic and radical extension of awareness, involving sustained attention on a problem with the intent to penetrate and understand it. When one actively sustains and deepens awareness, one might be said to "enter into" the problem, looking and observing in a manner undeterred by confusion and undaunted by pain or intimidation. One essentially uses their attention and powers of perception to look into, through, and perhaps even beyond a problem or issue rather than skirting or dancing around it.

Case examples have been disguised to protect client confidentiality.

https://doi.org/10.1037/0000451-005
Therapeutic Change With Difficult Clients: Precursors and Techniques in the CHANGES Model, Second Edition, by B. D. Wilkinson and F. J. Hanna

METACOGNITIVELY "HOLDING THE PROBLEM STEADY"

Confronting is a metacognitive process that involves directing and regulating awareness in the context of choice. We have known for a long time that attention is selective (James, 1890/1981; van Ede & Nobre, 2021), and that it does not randomly come to rest on various phenomena. It attaches to and apprehends certain objects and things for the purposes of survival, pleasure, interest, and other influences. This metacognitive aspect of confronting is not found among the other precursors.

Confronting is thus uniquely metacognitive in that it requires sustaining one's attention in spite of the impulse to avoid, give in to confusion, or act out. It involves holding the problem steady in the mind such that it does not waver, wander, or disperse. When a person confronts an intimidating, painful, or confusing phenomenon, there is a natural tendency to turn away or avoid (Scalabrini et al., 2020). Whether the phenomenon resides within one's mind or in the world, the person must hold it steady in conscious awareness and closely contemplate it. If the person is unable to sustain active attention, the degree and depth of confronting will be severely diminished or impaired.

Research on sustained attention in cognitive science and neuroscience distinguishes attentional arousal from attentional allocation, with the latter informing opportunity cost models and information processing stances (Esterman & Rothlein, 2019). Opportunity cost models suggest it is only difficult to sustain attention insofar as there is a subjective cost: It feels better to focus on good things rather than bad things. As such, confronting a negatively valenced stimulus (e.g., personal problems) is generally less rewarding and more subjectively difficult than engaging a positively valenced stimulus (e.g., fantasizing). Significant motivation is required to offset this cost. In neuro-scientific terms, enhanced communication between the default mode and attentional networks is observed during rewarding activities, indicating "that when motivated, participants' internal thoughts may in fact be more stimulus-related" (Esterman & Rothlein, 2019, p. 177).

HOW CONFRONTING THE PROBLEM LEADS TO THERAPEUTIC CHANGE

As far as therapeutic change is concerned, holding the problem or issue steady in one's mind begins a fundamental shift from being at the mercy of the problem to being in control of it. While the mechanism at work herein is subtle, it is pivotal to various effective interventions and practices. If a person can exert control over the problem enough to hold it steady in the mind, they are more likely to be able to influence or affect it in the world. Consequently, some remarkable change processes occur as a result of confronting a problem. These processes can be considered from a number of perspectives, as outlined in this section.

Confronting and Systematic Desensitization

One of the most powerful procedures in psychotherapy is systematic desensitization, a cornerstone of behavior therapies. It is based on the idea that if a client is exposed to repulsive or frightening stimuli gradually and with increasing intensity, anxiety responses to the stimuli will eventually reduce in intensity or extinguish altogether. This procedure is especially effective in treating phobias (Fear, 2018). Wolpe (1958) attributed the effectiveness of systematic desensitization to what he called *reciprocal inhibition*, or the idea that one cannot be relaxed and anxious at the same time. Thus, if a person can relax in the presence of noxious or repulsive objects or scenes, such as a snake or a great height, the phobic reaction will diminish and extinguish. Whether done via imagination (in vitro) or real life (in vivo), research has demonstrated that systematic desensitization produces therapeutic change for symptoms of anxiety, depression, posttraumatic stress, dissociation, and psychosis, to name a few (L. A. Brown et al., 2019).

While reciprocal inhibition and exposure involve confronting to good effect, these processes are not synonymous with confronting as an act. What helps a client conquer paralyzing fear is the continued, steady, and deliberate perception of the noxious object or situation. One must be willing to maintain engagement with the phobic stimulus, which has been referred to in other quarters as "resolute perception" (Hanna & Puhakka, 1991; Vickery et al., 2023). According to the CHANGES model, therapy procedures involving exposure and reciprocal inhibition require confronting as a necessary condition for change. The confronting precursor is an essential change mechanism underlying exposure, reciprocal inhibition, systematic desensitization, and flooding.

Cutting to the Essence of a Problem

Husserl's (1913/1982, 1936/1970) philosophy of phenomenology is particularly insightful when applied to the precursor of confronting and neatly explains several aspects of the process of confronting in therapy. In the early 1900s, Husserl developed a methodology of seeing and observing that was meant to free a person of their preconceptions. His method was probably the most fundamental, basic, rigorous discipline for observation and awareness ever developed in the Western world (Herrnstein & Boring, 1965; Zahavi, 2017).

The method was, at its core, quite simple. One puts aside as many of one's preconceptions and assumptions as possible and views the issue or object with sustained awareness. The item or issue can be any object (mental or physical) or relationship or any other worldly or mental experience or phenomenon. This is done until a person reaches or penetrates the core or essence of that phenomenon, with the consequence of thoroughly understanding it. Husserl said this is no mere intellectual process, nor is it a theory. It is an experiential process that Husserl called the *eidetic reduction*, meaning that one arrives at the essence of the phenomenon under investigation.

In the philosophy of Husserl and others, such as Sartre, Heidegger, and Merleau-Ponty, phenomenology is an extraordinarily complex subject with an intricate language for describing various aspects and modes of consciousness. It involves a method of seeing and observing that is as primary and unbiased as is possible for human beings to achieve (Herrnstein & Boring, 1965; Zahavi, 2017). In the phenomenological method, one observes any mental or physical phenomenon or experience openly and freely, with minimal expectations and preconceptions, with the intent of understanding it at its roots. In a therapy context, a remarkably similar method is often unwittingly applied to such problems as a cruel boss, childhood abuse, depression, anxiety, and rage. As one continues to look and purely observe, eventually the phenomenon becomes clearer until one begins to have insights into its nature and character. This is a fundamental aspect of the method of scientific observation, and as Nobel Prize laureate Sir Peter Medawar (1984) noted, it is a process that seems to be as intuitive as it is intellectual; certainly, Husserl would have agreed.

Husserl's method is near to the essence of what occurs in many forms of psychotherapy. Therapists and counselors routinely and regularly ask clients to delve into an area of pain or uncertainty with the intent of coming to a more complete understanding of it. This is the case even if the understanding arrived at is that the phenomenon itself is too vague to be understood, as in attempts to figure out another person's intentions. Continued, intense, sustained inquiry and observation has profound effects in terms of change. Carl Rogers and other experiential therapists have referred to the continuous process of examining feelings and views of a problem as "peeling the onion." This is a fitting metaphor that describes the method of cutting to the essence of an issue, and it describes the process made possible by confronting a problem.

Cutting to the essence of a problem or issue does not have to occur verbally. It can be accomplished without putting words to experience. Many clients do this routinely, even if they may be thought of as having "cognitive deficits." In such cases, behavior change comes with the confronting but may not be verbalized in the form of an insight. As Arkowitz (1989) once noted, insight often comes after behavior change. Once again, it is the confronting that seems to be the catalyst.

Ancient Approaches to Confronting

Confronting is at the basis of Indian psychology, being well expressed in the ancient text of yoga psychology, the *Yoga Sutras of Patanjali* (Aranya, 1983; Feuerstein, 1989; Nguyen, 2016). Patanjali's yoga is widely recognized as the chief application of the principles of various psychologies of India. *Samyama* is the name of a technique used in yoga that makes direct use of intense and highly concentrated confronting of various phenomena to arrive at deep insight and transcendence of self. Similarly, confronting has been a cornerstone of Buddhism for 2,500 years (Rahula, 1978). Buddhist monks have been practicing a wide variety of cognitive–behavioral techniques for the same length of time (de Silva, 1985; Tirch et al., 2015). Confronting is a crucial aspect of these practices (Pandita, 1991), although in Buddhism it is more commonly referred to as *mindfulness*. Mindfulness is fundamental to the Buddhist concept of therapeutic change and is a fascinating subject in and of itself. In many ways, this precursor can be understood as the Western equivalent.

Simplicity and Complexity

A fascinating phenomenological aspect of confronting is how the more one confronts a problem, the clearer and less mysterious it becomes. At first glance, the issue becomes simpler, but this is misleading. What is more likely is that the problem, as it becomes more thoroughly explored, examined, and investigated, becomes less and less obscure and vague, so that its intricacies stand out in greater detail.

For example, in the case of a relationship that has gone sour, a client explores and examines all aspects of it in therapy. The relationship is quite involved and has many dynamics, outside influences and pressures, and personal and inter-personal perspectives. In therapy, the person examines the relationship in terms of empathy, love, roles, social interactions, mutual friends, parental influences, sexual relations, met and unmet needs, spiritual beliefs, and children, if any. In the process, the relationship becomes more and more crystallized until the person achieves an overarching view of it accompanied by a more thorough understanding. The relationship is still quite complex, but now the complexities are mapped and stand out with more clarity.

Reality Testing

Another aspect of confronting as part of the change process involves differenti-ating reality from illusion or, in some cases, delusion. Confronting is intrinsic to *reality testing*, a continuous process of verifying the accuracy of our perceptions (Goldstein, 2013). Reality testing is related to but moves beyond simple clarifi-cation of the problem. It is the work done to test whether perceptions and beliefs hold up to the proving ground of the experiential world.

Setting aside metaphysical speculations as to the nature of reality, it is often important for clients to compare what is actually present in the world to what is in their minds. For instance, if a client is suspicious that their spouse is cheating on them, it is useful to determine whether this is true, that is, whether the spouse is cheating in fact. Otherwise, the client may construct a false reality forever, leading to further dysfunction, despite the fact their belief is not accurate.

From a pragmatic perspective, reality could be said to be what remains after all our theories, beliefs, constructions, and perceptual filters about it are stripped away. This was precisely Husserl's goal in phenomenology and is often what happens in psychotherapy. It is far more functional to cope with a situation that is accurately perceived.

A Smaller Problem Space

Another curious, highly subjective phenomenon associated with confronting the problem is consistent with Lewin's (1935, 1936) conception of what he called the life space. The *life space* is that part of the person's perceived world that is taken up by events, circumstances, or issues that are absorbing attention. According to Lewin, some of these issues can appear large in a spatial sense, whereas others can appear small. In everyday language, we speak of "big" problems and "little" problems.

The act of thoroughly confronting usually makes a problem or issue seem less significant. Where a problem once loomed large and foreboding, it can seem smaller and more manageable after thoroughly confronting it. The problem becomes less oppressive as it is progressively confronted. Some clients convey that they feel "bigger" after directly confronting a problem. A problem can seem smaller, or the "I" of a person can seem bigger. Either way, the implications for therapeutic change are obvious. For example, resolving a conflict with one's teenage son or daughter might initially seem quite daunting, but after confronting the problem, it feels more like a difficult but manageable task. When a person becomes competent at confronting, depression or anxiety can be viewed in this same fashion. This is part of developing the ability to confront as a skill of change.

Removing the Power of the Problem

When a problem or issue is ignored, resisted, or denied, it takes on what can appear to be a life of its own, influencing the person in a variety of ways. For instance, a 45-year-old client named Dominica believed that she had a lump in her breast, which she feared could be malignant. She did all she could to divert her attention from it, avoid talking about it, and pretend it was not an issue. Meanwhile, when she did think about it, she would cry, thinking that her life might be over. When she entered therapy for another reason, she had been ignoring this problem for well over a year and a half, fully aware that things could get worse if not treated early. Little by little over the course of therapy, she began to realize that ignoring the problem was actually lending it power over her. She saw how it intimidated her and exerted influence over her in various ways. It affected how she treated her children, how she viewed her job, and how she saw herself. When she finally looked at the problem directly and thoroughly, she was, by degrees, no longer intimidated and immersed in it and acquired some overview of her life again. The mere act of deciding to see a physician gave her a sense of control, although it did not remove her fear. The lump turned out to be benign.

This aspect of confronting is related to the popular notion of empowerment. When the problem occupies a smaller region in the life space and begins to lose its ominous or intimidating quality, one becomes empowered to move out from under the burden of worldly or psychological oppression. It also enables one to extend one's range of influence, scope, or outlook beyond a painfully limiting set of circumstances to more comfortably deal with the challenges at hand. There is little question that such conditions contribute to the well-being of a person.

The more intensively something is confronted, the more it diminishes in size and power. When a problem or issue is continually contemplated, a person seems better able to endure it without becoming overwhelmed. This is at the heart of the change principle of exposure. The key is to be able to look and observe even while caught up in painful emotions or profoundly confusing circumstances. Confronting is a skill that can be taught, trained, developed, and practiced.

The "Vaccine Effect" of Confronting

Confronting the problem, especially when combined with awareness and grit, appears to have a mental effect similar to the effect that a vaccine has on the body. With a vaccine, patients are exposed to a harmless form of a virus under conditions the body can control. In psychotherapy, clients are placed in conscious contact with an area of emotional pain or other difficulty under controlled conditions so that harm will not result. Confronting the phenomenon can have a healing or strengthening effect. It seems to reduce anxiety, allow for insight and personal growth, give more clarity to thought, release painful emotions, and improve interpersonal functioning. Confronting adverse conditions in a controlled setting also allows a person to better adapt to and, by degrees, master their environment.

SIGNIFICANT MOMENTS OF CHANGE INVOLVING CONFRONTING

John had been in therapy for 10 months, attempting to resolve the loss of a relationship with a partner he had loved very deeply. During therapy, feelings of depression would only slightly lift before returning. Cognitive approaches were used in an attempt to change John's thinking, but change was not forthcoming. Meanwhile, he was obsessed with his former partner, thinking about her continuously. He reported that he had been depressed for as long as he could remember, saying that his life had been "dominated by sadness and anxiety" and that he had been to many therapists. Therapy had "only helped slightly," he said. Then came a session in which the therapist was questioning him on what aspects of the loss of his relationship were the most difficult.

Suddenly, for no apparent reason, John was aware of a vivid memory from his childhood, around age 6. He "was lying in bed" and "heard an airplane flying overhead." He was "terrified" that the plane was going to drop a nuclear bomb. As he relayed this to his therapist, he realized that his lifelong sadness and depression somehow stemmed from this moment. He remembered how frightened he was of a nuclear holocaust as a child during the Cold War and how this had negatively affected his entire outlook on the world. He almost instantly realized that the strong anxiety he felt about the woman was of the exact quality as the anxiety he felt about nuclear war as a child. He saw that his fear of nuclear war was remarkably the same as his fear of losing his romantic partner.

On seeing how silly this was, he said that his "sadness and depression disappeared and never came back." Following this, he no longer obsessed about his lost love and stopped compulsively talking about it. He said, "She wasn't the problem; this incident was." He claimed it was this session that, as he put it, "freed up my emotions" so that he could "live a more real life." John's story is a classic example of peeling the onion until the actual problem emerges.

In another example, 13-year-old Bobby developed a phobia of dogs. His therapist asked him about a particular dog he found to be scary. He shared that the dog, named Sam, belonged to a neighbor and that this apparently ill-tempered animal was constantly trying to bite him. The therapist asked Bobby to hold a picture of Sam in his mind and "not let him get away or bite you; just look at him." Bobby was initially reluctant to try, but with some therapeutic encouragement, he eventually experimented with the visualization and did quite well. As Bobby did so, his fear began to diminish. He was amazed that the longer he imagined Sam, the less fearful he felt. Bobby's struggle was a genuinely heroic demonstration of courageous confronting in therapy.

CLINICAL MARKERS: HOW TO RECOGNIZE CONFRONTING THE PROBLEM

Clinical indicators of the presence of confronting are fairly straightforward and, in many cases, immediately evident. When a client is actively confronting, there is a sense of perseverance in facing up to and continuing to observe. The person displays an animated excitement or composure in meeting the challenges of life or therapy. There is a steadfastness, alternatively described as a "doggedness" or "digging in one's heels" in seeing and studying an issue to its resolution. Such a person will show a spark of determination in holding attention on a problem. The person is honest and direct, and defensiveness is overridden by the desire to overcome obstacles and barriers. They accept feedback and often ask questions of the therapist that take the therapy to a deeper level.

Metacognitively, what to look for in clients confronting the problem is the ability to hold the problem steady in their minds to be inspected and explored. Such clients seem to have attention sufficiently free so they can direct it to virtually any area of their lives or life histories. They engage in little or no deflection and do not turn away from or avoid an issue, emotion, or problem. The person is able to selectively view virtually any phenomenon.

Cognitively, there is a confidence in a confronting client that says, "I can look at anything at all in my mind" without fear of being harmed, consumed, destroyed, or disintegrated. The person believes that confronting is an important act and part of the healing process and that studying a problem or issue will enable them to understand and resolve it. This person is convinced that the way out of a problem or situation is by working one's way to the core or essence of problems, issues, emotions, beliefs, and so on. But the client does not necessarily have to articulate insights so much as be inclined toward behavioral change.

The confronting person or client is a confident person who is stable in the ability to maintain perspective. Confronting ability is a sign of high ego strength, whereby a person does not easily wallow or stew in their emotions but is consistently able to keep a sense of awareness and presence even in the face or threat of pain, discomfort, or deeply disturbing circumstances. This person is not intimidated by strong feelings or emotions and often displays a sense of calm, composure, or even poise in the face of adversity or hardship. From the therapist's perspective, it is common to find oneself deeply admiring such a client, appreciating and perhaps even being moved or touched by the client's courage, fortitude, and perseverance.

HOW TO DETECT THE ABSENCE OF CONFRONTING THE PROBLEM

Clients who do not confront will protect themselves from looking at or contemplating an issue or problem in the belief that harm will result. They will be adept at deflecting challenges from the therapist by changing the subject or implying or directly telling the therapist that looking at or knowing about a problem is neither necessary nor helpful. Some of these clients may be adept at "talking around the problem" or "skirting the issue."

Such clients may wallow in their problems, becoming overwhelmed and ensnared. They hesitate or waver in the act of viewing and find it difficult to maintain focus. They tend to offer or even prefer superficial or shallow solutions and minimize the importance of examining an issue or aspect of their lives. Such clients often need a great deal of coaxing or encouragement and may be easily intimidated by the magnitude of even small problems. Clients who seldom achieve closure on issues may be lacking in this precursor. Cognitively, a client who does not confront has not learned that confronting a problem leads to its resolution.

One of the most difficult of all difficult client styles is the intellectualizing client. This client is often highly intelligent and possibly highly educated and can simulate confronting and make it look like they are deeply examining issues. These clients often mistakenly believe that confronting is one of their greatest strengths and will offer a host of reasons for why the problem developed. Such clients will use sophisticated vocabulary and even therapy jargon. They may be successful at "snowing" the therapist into believing they are in control when in fact they are using their intellects to protect themselves from exposure to—or in gestalt language, contact with—the painful emotions, difficulties, or problems present.

In such cases, the client is not confronting at all. Instead, they are compulsively analyzing or thinking about an issue or problem. Indirectly, intellectualizing can anesthetize emotional pain to a small extent, providing the secondary gain or reinforcer that perpetuates the dysfunctional behavior.

One of Perls's (1973; Perls et al., 1951) best known and important contributions to experiential therapy is his therapeutic notion that we ought to "lose our minds and come to our senses." The intellectualizing client has a thinking mind so hyperactive that it has stepped beyond its boundaries and taken over the functions of being and observing. Such clients' high intelligence and compulsive thinking sabotage their ability to penetrate the essence of a problem and achieve a viable resolution. For such clients to achieve change, they may need to learn that there is a difference between thinking and looking and that analyzing and contemplating are not the same endeavor (see Heidegger, 1927/1962). Fortunately, many intellectualizers will readily respond to a range of techniques that enhance this precursor.

TECHNIQUES: ENHANCING CONFRONTING

Virtually all of the techniques used in psychotherapy, with the exception of medications and pure operant conditioning, use the confronting precursor. A vast array of procedures, such as identifying and disputing dysfunctional beliefs, role-playing, the empty chair, social skills and assertiveness training, working through transference, interpretation, paradox, reframing, the use of metaphor, and the talking cure itself, all require the problem to be confronted directly or indirectly. In essence, any approach that calls for sustained, continuous, and deliberate attention to a situation, whether to discuss or cope with it, uses confronting. The techniques provided in this chapter specifically support confrontation with difficult clients.

There are some important points to bear in mind regarding confronting. Forcing a person to confront too much, too soon, is traumatic by definition. Across myriad forms of exposure therapy, it is well understood that bringing a client into contact with painful phenomena must be done with care and attention to the person's level of tolerance (see Richard & Lauterbach, 2011). Overwhelming a client with mental, emotional, or environmental material that is too much to confront will not only bring about early termination; it will cause harm. Thus, exposure to sensitive memories, feelings, or beliefs should be done gradually so the client will be successful and not view therapy as a source of failure and pain. The techniques and strategies in this chapter are designed to encourage, implement, and strengthen the confronting precursor.

The Strengths Metaphor

Confronting is not only a psychological act; it is also an ability. Like muscles with weight lifting, it becomes stronger with practice and discipline. Yet some clients seem to find confronting their problems not only difficult but abhorrent and repulsive. For many, the act itself is painful. This is especially the case with clients with personality disorders. Although such clients are often almost vilified as being uncooperative, manipulative, malicious, and intrinsically flawed, the truth may be that, at the core, they lack the skill and ability to confront such things as unpleasant thoughts, feelings, behaviors, and events. These clients are often in need of education concerning this and other precursors. Many have never learned that confronting, rather than being harmful, is the beginning of healing and a source of exhilaration.

Thus, the metaphor of strength can be used to show clients that the more one confronts issues, the better at it one gets. Although some people can confront a vast range of psychopathology in one grand sweep of consciousness, others can take in only small bits and portions at a time (and even then, with great difficulty). The difference, as in lifting weights or exercising, lies in understanding that the more confronting one does, the more capable one is of doing more of it and the more stamina and strength one develops.

Confronting the Hesitancy to Confront

Often, clients are aware of a problem area, such as alcoholism, depression, anxiety, or some compulsive behavior, but are unwilling to confront anything about it. In such cases, the therapist can offer an approach framed as an experiment. The therapist can openly inform the client that confronting the problem is not necessary. Next, they can ask the client to think about the problem and report all the thoughts and feelings that arise. The therapist again asks the client not to talk about the problem itself but rather whatever springs to mind when thinking about it. The client will often report disliking the subject and simply not wanting to think about it or any other problems. These statements can then be fully acknowledged and reflected.

This technique aims to identify the automatic thoughts, beliefs, and feelings that stand in the way of confronting. The therapist can divert the client and ask them to talk about not wanting to talk about or explore anything, fully understanding and reflecting back everything the client says. Eventually, the client may be more likely to confront the problem or issues and may do so spontaneously.

Confronting the Idea of Change Itself

The technique described previously can also be applied to difficult clients who find the idea of change itself uncomfortable or objectionable. The client can be asked, "Consider the idea of making changes [or one particular change] in your life." Next, the therapist can ask the client about what kinds of thoughts and feelings rise to awareness, including thought streams and unspoken verbal responses such as, "Go to hell," "That's a load of bull," or similar statements. It will often turn out that the idea of therapeutic change insults the person's character or dignity and that the mere suggestion of its need is a kind of criticism. Furthermore, the contemplation of change by a difficult client can bring up a variety of beliefs about change, such as "To change is to fail," "To change is an admission of being wrong," or "To change is to give up." When disputed, some fascinating clinical material that accompanies these beliefs is often encountered.

In Vivo Confronting

Talking in therapy does not always lead to the talking cure. Talk can be used to circumvent and even avoid problems and issues, resulting in the illusion of progress but never any real resolution. In many cases, the emotions, passions, and desires involved with dysfunctional behaviors must be aroused so they can be addressed in the present moment. Talk therapy does not always accomplish this. In vivo confronting is a variation of the well-tested and venerable techniques derived from the behavioral principles of exposure and reciprocal inhibition, which also recognize the limits of the talking cure. This technique is equally well explained by the concept of the resolute perception of particular issues and problems. The problem can be recreated in the therapy room in real time with therapeutic benefit, invoking the vaccine effect.

In vivo confronting is an adaptation of the classical behavioral techniques of flooding and systematic desensitization, as well as resolute perception. Of course, the classical application of these techniques is with phobias, and it is so well documented there is no need for elaboration here. However, these principles, all based on the confronting precursor, can be applied to compulsive behaviors, such as stealing, substance use, and compulsive sexual behaviors. In applying this approach, it is wise to inform the client of the procedure and frame it as an experiment that can be backed out of at any time.

The Story of Marvin

Marvin was a difficult, conduct-disordered teenager convicted of theft and placed in an outpatient program for adolescent criminal offenders. Because stealing was the problem that landed Marvin in the outpatient treatment program, the consulting therapist decided to use a technique designed to get Marvin to confront his compulsive stealing behaviors, which he had willingly discussed in group.

The therapist asked Marvin if he was willing to try an experiment regarding his urge to take things that belonged to others. Marvin agreed. At that point, the therapist pulled out a $20 bill and placed it in front of the client, turned his back on him (he was sitting between the client and the door, of course), and asked him to report his thoughts and feelings as he looked at the money. Marvin immediately said, "I want to take it, man." The therapist asked him, "What are you feeling in your body right now, Marvin?" He replied that he was feeling excited and pointed to his stomach. When asked, he added that this was associated with the challenge of getting away with something and doing something at which he felt competent (stealing).

The therapist asked him, "Marvin, is this the same feeling you get when you are in the street or in a store and you think about stealing something?" He replied somewhat contemplatively, "Yeah, it's the same feeling." The therapist asked, "When you have this feeling, are you feeling pretty good about yourself?" Marvin looked at the therapist and said, "Yeah, it's like I feel really cool, and I can take anything." A discussion then ensued concerning the relationship between stealing and his sense of self-esteem and self-worth and how his parents and uncle had tied these together. Marvin recognized this and was by now capable of elaborating on it. The therapist asked if this was how he gained respect from his peers. Marvin replied affirmatively to this, saying that among his friends, he was acknowledged as "the best."

The term "stealing" was now being used directly. Importantly, it soon became clear that, to Marvin, the most appealing aspect of stealing was the feeling, the excitement, and the challenge of taking something not his own. He reported that the biggest obstacle to quitting stealing was not the value of the item stolen but the appeal of the thrill and excitement that came with the mere prospect of stealing it. The therapist asked him, "Do you feel more alive when you are thinking about stealing something?" He quietly said, "Yeah." As a result of this experiment, the therapist asked if it would be okay to get a little more serious about producing that feeling, to which Marvin agreed.

The therapist placed a credit card in front of him (turned upside down and face down) and once again turned to the door. With his back to the client, the therapist asked if the feeling of excitement was there again. Marvin replied that it was indeed, and even stronger this time. He was asked to describe the feeling in detail, outlining where in his stomach he felt the feeling. Marvin did so. The therapist asked Marvin, "When you have the feeling, do you feel like you *have* to take something?" He thought a minute and said, "Yeah, it's like it's there, and I gotta do it." The therapist asked if he could feel good by not giving in and being ruled by the feeling. Marvin had never considered this.

The therapist took Marvin to a local store, walked around with him, and asked if he felt the excitement in his stomach. Marvin reported that, like always, he did. There was a pocketknife that appealed to him. Marvin was asked to describe the feeling and what it was like to watch the feeling and not be taken in by it or drawn into it. "Weird" was the word he first used to describe this new feeling. "Good weird or bad weird?" asked the therapist. "Kinda good," he said, "Like I don't have to give in to it just because I feel it." The therapist asked if part of this new feeling was a sense of strength. Marvin responded positively, and the therapist pointed out that perhaps the real strength was not in the guts to steal but in the strength to resist. He had already proved that he had the former but not the latter.

This was the beginning of Marvin's rehabilitation. In his case, it was not only his thinking but his need for sensation that needed attention. The success of this technique in Marvin's case was through establishing the confronting precursor by getting him accustomed to looking at and examining issues. After this, he responded more positively to both group and individual therapy. When dealing with people who engage in criminal behaviors, therapy is probably incomplete without addressing the sensations and feelings that accompany the acts (Samenow, 1998).

The Story of Rusty

Rusty, age 17, was addicted to crystal meth. He had been arrested several times for possession and had just spent 6 months in a youth detention center for dealing meth and other drugs. He had been expelled from three schools for behavior problems. His father was an angry man who weighed nearly 500 pounds. He was habitually abusive, both physically and verbally, toward Rusty; was on disability; and rarely left the house in their poor neighborhood.

In treatment, Rusty often said that he loved meth, could do nothing about quitting, and did not want to quit. The director of the program described Rusty to the consulting therapist as a noncompliant borderline client for whom the treatment program had been so far ineffective. He had already been in treatment in this outpatient substance use program for about 4 months, and his urine screens had consistently come back dirty. Rusty sometimes acquired money by breaking into cars or mugging people for their purses and wallets.

In the first session, the consulting therapist asked Rusty if he was willing to try an experiment. Rusty agreed, probably because of the novelty of having a new therapist and because of the chance to get out of group. After establishing an initial rapport, the therapist offered a small piece of chalk and asked Rusty to pretend that it was "crystal." Rusty was surprised at this but also excited to get the chance to talk about meth. "When you look at this crystal, Rusty, what are you thinking?" Rusty unhesitatingly answered, "I want some right now, man. You have no idea how bad." The therapist acknowledged this and said, "So you're craving the high at this very moment?" Once again, the immediate answer was, "Yeah, bad."

"Is there a place in your body where you feel the craving, Rusty?" Rusty considered this for a moment, looked up, and said, "Yeah, here," and pointed to the area in the upper part of his stomach. "When you look at that part of your body, what feeling is in there?" Rusty again considered the question for a moment and said, "I don't know ... emptiness." The therapist was encouraged by this answer, which indicated an unexpected degree of awareness. He asked, "Is that emptiness a good feeling?" to which Rusty replied, "No. I don't like it." The therapist went on, "And when you're high, what does the crystal do to that emptiness feeling?" Rusty said, "It's like it fills it up." The therapist asked, "So is it fair to say that you use crystal to fill up that feeling of emptiness you don't like?" Rusty thought about it momentarily, looked up thoughtfully, and said, "Yeah, I guess I do."

Continuing, the therapist asked, "How much does smoking meth actually fill up the emptiness feeling? All of it, or only part?" "Only part of it," was Rusty's honest reply. "So, you always have some emptiness inside you, and it bothers you. Is that fair to say?" Rusty agreed. "You know, Rusty," the therapist said,

> Counseling can show you how to fill up the emptiness in ways that won't land you in jail or in programs like this one, and there are no cravings like the ones you have right now. All you have to do is keep looking at and talking about your problems just like you did here. What do you think?

Rusty, deep in thought, said, "Yeah, why not."

This was the beginning of Rusty's road to recovery from his use of crystal meth. His urine screens were clean from that session onward. His continued abstinence was documented for 2 years after his graduation from the program, which occurred 90 days after that session. Of course, there is far more to this story.

This conversation was just the beginning, and many other precursors needed to be established in Rusty before his recovery strengthened and stabilized. However, the establishment of the confronting precursor in this session was what placed him on the road to recovery and was the key to all of his successful treatment. This case example shows how it is possible for confronting to be used to an advantage even with clients known for being difficult.

The Onion Peeler

The onion peeler, a powerful technique that uses direct confronting, is derived from Husserl's (1913/1982) phenomenological method and from various applications of existential and gestalt therapies (Perls et al., 1951). It can be quite intense and should be used only with a client who has a rating of at least 2 for awareness on the assessment form, and the grit precursor also contributes to its success. Additionally, it is powerful in enhancing the change process among clients who are not difficult at all. It is called the onion peeler because it strips away automatic thoughts, self-talk, beliefs, defenses, and feelings and helps a client arrive at the heart of the problem or issue. It evokes deep emotions and can produce insights that are central to the nature of the problem.

The onion peeler is a cyclical question that is repeated over and over again after getting an answer to each cycle. The central question is, "How does [fill in the blank with whatever the problem is] appear to you now?" Variations such as "How does it look to you at this point?" or "What seems most obvious about it now?" can also be used occasionally. Another variation is, "How are you experiencing [the problem] now?" These questions require the client to observe in order to answer the question. Remarkably, the problem will appear to change after several cycles, and possibly it will change again and again until the core of the onion is reached.

Before beginning the technique, it is important to identify or name the problem or issue with the client's agreement that this indeed characterizes the problem itself. This is where awareness is established. Once the problem has been identified, the characterization can be inserted into the body of the cyclical question. The client should be fully informed of the nature of the procedure, its purpose, and what to expect in terms of how it is done.

The problem itself can be almost anything. For example, the problem could be a person, such as an ex-spouse, current spouse, son, daughter, employer, probation officer, teacher, betraying friend, or abusive parent or relative. It can be a condition or feeling, such as depression, anxiety, loneliness, or helplessness, or it can be a situation, such as a lack of romance, homelessness, or an unpleasant marital or work situation. One can fill in the blank with alcohol, cocaine, or other drug of choice. "How does your body appear to you now?" can be used with some people with eating disorders. For clients who are on probation or parole, "How does [the particular crime] appear to you now?" can be used. Of course, therapeutic judgment should be exercised about the proper timing of these techniques.

As the onion peels, the question can be further refined as the problem appears to change or become reshaped, allowing for more focus. For instance, after asking, "How does your depression appear to you now?" 15 times or so, the problem reshapes itself, and the question becomes, "How does being alone appear to you now?" or "How does being a failure appear to you now?" With the client's approval, the refined version is then used. The technique itself can be used at many levels. At much higher developmental levels, well beyond the focus of this book, the sentence can be filled in with such items as the ego, life, meaning, god, or the world in general.

Every now and then, in between the cycling questions, the therapist is advised to add a processing question, such as "What's happening?" or "What are you experiencing?" or "How are you feeling about the problem?" This helps maintain the communication link between therapist and client and is often where the client will report insights, progress, or how the problem seems different.

Initial responses to the onion peeler question are often defensive, with answers ranging from "Who cares?" to "It sucks." The therapist acknowledges these responses, saying "okay" or "alright" and perhaps reflecting on the meaning or feeling involved. However, to be effective, the question should be returned to as soon as possible to continue peeling the onion. Later answers tend to be characterized by more intense feelings, such as deep concern or helplessness.

In the case of a highly defensive male alcohol abuser, for example, his initial answers to "How does drinking appear to you now?" were along the lines of not having a problem or not needing to drink. After about 20 repetitions, answers revolved around his loving to drink, and after about 60 or 70 questions, he was worried that he could not quit. Obviously, the technique can last several sessions, and if done smoothly, it should not be a grinding or abrasive process. It is always important to check with the client to make sure their interest in continuing the procedure is still present or if the client feels like progress is being made. If the client is not interested, the therapist should not continue.

How Could the Problem Be Worse?

We have focused on clients who deny their problem behaviors or attitudes and who avoid awareness or confronting by minimizing their dysfunctionality and presenting it as normal or even advantageous. However, there are clients at the other end of the scale who will not confront an issue or problem simply because it is deemed so terrible that it is unconfrontable and beyond their capacity to view, explore, or otherwise tolerate. With such clients, a technique can be used that develops the confronting precursor indirectly by imagining something even worse. By talking about how things could have been worse, the client is more or less forced to contextualize the event or situation. In seeing how things could have turned out worse than they did, the client may begin to build tolerance for the current condition as it is.

This is delicate work and appropriate only in particular situations where the client will not think their problem is being invalidated or rendered insignificant.

Thus, while fully and rightfully respecting the severity of the problem, the therapist can ask the client, "As terrible as this is, it seems you were fortunate that [a worse circumstance] did not occur." This can sometimes be appropriate for clients who have suffered a disability or family tragedy.

However, this technique is contraindicated for victims of physical abuse and sexual assault. For instance, rape has been minimized throughout history and across cultures (Daly, 1978; Feinstein, 2018). To lessen or dismiss the profound tragedy of rape by finding something worse would be destructive and harmful, only serving to perpetuate the ill-founded, ignorant, patriarchal tradition that contributes to ongoing violence against women. Thus, it is better to avoid this technique than to inadvertently do harm with it.

Mirroring

The mirroring technique involves presenting a physical mirror and asking the client to dialogue with it or to comment on what they perceive in it (Mahoney, 1991). Although its potential might not be immediately accessible with difficult clients, it can be used as a means to get a client to begin to confront the self and how they regard it. It has the advantage of showing a client how little actual confronting of their life has taken place. If done correctly, it can get a client to begin to confront dysfunctional traits or aspects of the self that are a source of shame, self-blame, guilt, or regret. It helps a person take stock of their life and goals and can be used to assess degrees of self-loathing.

Representational or Concretized Confronting

Some difficult clients find the prospect of confronting thoughts or problems to be too abstract. There are times when it is easier to treat problems and emotions as concretely as possible using objects or props to represent thoughts and images to enhance a client's understanding of confronting. This is often helpful with children but can be highly effective with adults as well. It is especially helpful for clients who are not adept at holding a problem steady in their minds so that it can be more readily and fully studied or examined. For example, if a particular client tends to deflect or avoid issues and problems, the therapist can point this out to them and represent the thought, idea, or image as a physical object to be used as a prop.

For instance, Elizabeth, age 45, was wealthy and unhappy and blamed a wide range of people for her "unhappiness," including her children and her parents. In her descriptions of the people in her life, she perceived them as wanting her to be unhappy and treating her in a way that was disrespectful and insensitive to her needs. Her depression was "their fault," and attempts to isolate beliefs related to her unhappiness had failed. Unfortunately, she repeatedly avoided her therapist's attempts to get her to confront her own actions as part of her situation. Other approaches to blaming had also been ineffective. Rather than pursuing this line further, the therapist pointed out her avoidance and attempted to concretize the problem to help her hold the issue steady.

THERAPIST: I've noticed that as soon as I bring up the possibility of how your attitude might play some small part in your unhappiness, you immediately change the subject or blame someone, like your husband or your children. Please tell me if I am wrong.

CLIENT: You don't understand—they are all mean and cruel to me. They hurt me over and over again.

THERAPIST: Yes, you feel that all they cared about was making you hurt and that you did nothing to bring this on. It just wasn't your fault at all.

CLIENT: Yes, that's it. I don't deserve this!

THERAPIST: I don't blame you for feeling that way. Isn't it interesting, though, that every time I mention the possibility that your own attitude might have some part in your unhappiness, you immediately change the subject?

CLIENT: But they were the ones ...

THERAPIST: Please pardon me for interrupting you, but do you see, you are doing it again. You don't have to agree with me. Just tell me if I am wrong.

CLIENT: About what?

THERAPIST: Do you change the subject every time I ask if your own attitude might play a part in your unhappiness?

CLIENT: Because it's not true.

THERAPIST: Fair enough. Can I have your permission to go on with this just a bit more?

CLIENT: I suppose.

THERAPIST: Please tell me if I am wrong. Is it fair to say you don't like the idea that at least part of your unhappiness has to do with how you might be thinking and acting at times?

CLIENT: I don't like that idea at all.

THERAPIST: I understand. Would you mind trying an experiment?

CLIENT: I guess so.

THERAPIST: (offering the client a pen) Let's pretend for just a moment, Elizabeth, that this pen is the thought that your attitude might have some role in your own unhappiness, okay?

CLIENT: Okay ...

THERAPIST:	I am going to hand the pen to you as though I were saying that thought to you again. As I do, please show me, with the pen, what you do with that thought.
CLIENT:	(throws that pen to the side of the room and looks at the therapist)
THERAPIST:	Is it like you don't want anything to do with that thought at all?
CLIENT:	Nothing.
THERAPIST:	(retrieving the pen and handing it back to her) Would you mind just holding it in your hand and telling me what feelings and thoughts you have?
CLIENT:	(looking at the pen and beginning to cry) Sure, I have made mistakes, but they are mean to me, and then I do things that I know aren't right, but I just can't help it.

In this fashion, the technique broke through some of Elizabeth's strong deflections to the point of opening a productive dialogue about mistakes she had made and her regrets and guilt about them. She slowly progressed toward examining and changing her beliefs and behaviors.

Concentration-Based Techniques

As with representational confronting, concentration-based techniques help clients hold the problem steady in their mind. One technique adapted from gestalt therapy (Perls et al., 1951) is a form of in vitro exposure that involves asking the client to hold a thought, image, feeling, emotion, problem, or situation in the mind. As with concretized confronting, the therapist asks the client to continue to look at the object in the mind, holding it steady and reporting on what occurs as they do so. The image of a boss, parent, or coworker are fairly standard examples. Third-wave mindfulness-based cognitive therapies regularly use similar techniques to reduce experiential avoidance and encourage varying iterations of acceptance (see Hayes & Linehan, 2018).

Such moments call for effective psychoeducation as well as conveying empathy and understanding to clients because holding a problem steady in the mind can seem contrary to common sense. As a defense, some clients believe that unconsciously jettisoning a thought or image from the mind is exactly what will relieve them of anxiety. They believe that if it does not stay in the mind, it won't hurt. In a similar vein, Gendlin's (1981) focusing technique is a form of confronting that helps clients direct sustained attention toward implicit and often murky, indistinct bodily sensations. In all such cases, confronting as sustained attention on the problem is the central precursor at work.

The Miracle Question

The miracle question technique originated with solution-focused brief therapy (de Shazer, 1985) but was actually used by Adler (1956) many decades earlier. Assuming that the person has a small degree of awareness of a problem, this technique can be a bridge to greater confronting. The miracle question goes like this: "Suppose one night, while you were asleep, there was a miracle and this problem was solved. How would you know? What would be different?" To be answered, this well-crafted question requires the act of confronting and clarifies the problem even further by requiring the client to look at the problem itself, then look through it and beyond it. It can also build the hope precursor.

A CLOSING NOTE ON CONFRONTING

At the very heart and soul of what brings about positive change as well as mental and emotional healing, confronting may be the most powerful therapeutic change mechanism. Virtually every therapy technique makes use of confronting the problem as a precursor of change. What we have presented here are strategies and techniques to stimulate the confronting of problems with difficult clients. However, the effective implementation of such techniques to activate confronting also enables standard treatment approaches to work more effectively. When clients confront a problem, dedication to the therapeutic process tends to increase and success is far more likely in the end.

5

H: Hope for Change

It is no surprise that Dante described hell as a realm bereft of hope. Without hope, life holds little in the way of inspiration or motivation. *Hope for change* is the realistic expectation that the future will be positive and experienceable (Snyder, 1994). Hope may be said to be a precursor not only of change but possibility. It inspires action and courage and paves the way for the realization of dreams, whether simple or sublime. Unfortunately, hope is widely mischaracterized as something akin to longing, desiring, and especially wishing. In our professional context, wishing carries the overtones of a collapsed sense of hope, in which one has, to some degree, bid farewell to the real world and has become resigned to an inert fantasy that derives its power from yearning.

Hope is about what can occur in reality, what can truly be accomplished, even if the odds are long or daunting. Competitive athletes, for example, live on a diet of hope that involves envisioning a realistic form of success, not some idle fantasy. The only thing that hope shares with qualities such as longing, wishing, or yearning is a concern for a better future. At its peak, hope involves not only seeing the future as experienceable but inviting or welcoming the future as preferable to the present (Aubuchon-Endsley et al., 2015).

Thus, hope is different from blind optimism, which is often unrealistic and can take the form of fantasy (Schmid, 2019). Hope is based on realistic vision and probability, replete with options and a plan to meet the future. Hope is intimately related to the ability to solve and frame problems in ways that lend themselves to solutions (Oettingen & Chromik, 2017). What Seligman (2006) called *learned optimism* is closely related to hope, which can be practiced as a skill. What may look like a fantasy future to one person may be a calculated, realistic possibility to another who has learned that no matter how bleak the outlook, there may be a

---

Case examples have been disguised to protect client confidentiality.

https://doi.org/10.1037/0000451-006
Therapeutic Change With Difficult Clients: Precursors and Techniques in the CHANGES Model, Second Edition, by B. D. Wilkinson and F. J. Hanna

hidden solution. Without a realistic element of calculation and discernment, however, dysfunctional fantasy is always a pitfall.

Hope seems to have profound effects on the human psyche. It can inspire a person to not only survive but to live more fully. It has been described as the activator of the motivational system in human beings (Seligman, 2006) that grows investment in the outcome of one's actions. Hope has been associated with enhancing a person's coping ability from a wide variety of perspectives (Schmid, 2019). Just as this book conceives of it as a precursor of change, hope has been described as a prerequisite for effective coping (Al-Yagon & Margalit, 2017; Ong et al., 2017). Jerome Frank (Frank & Frank, 1991) identified hope as the operative factor in the placebo effect: Symptom alleviation by placebo is common in studies of depression, and hope may be the active ingredient.

Conversely, a lack of hope can delay recovery and even hasten death (Frank, 1961). Cannon's (1942) classic anthropological study of "voodoo death" in such places as Haiti and Australia found that voodoo deaths occurred due to the expectancy effect, when fearful beliefs about "black magic" resulted in a complete loss of hope (Hahn & Kleinman, 1983). In the Nazi concentration camps of World War II, Frankl (1992) and Bettelheim (1960) identified the disastrous effects of giving up, or the absence of hope, on survival rates among the prisoners under extreme conditions. Nardini's (1952) research on American soldiers in Japanese prison camps during World War II showed that those who managed to survive demonstrated certain dispositional tendencies, including the hopeful expectation that conditions could be tolerated and that, eventually, they would be set free.

HOW HOPE LEADS TO THERAPEUTIC CHANGE

Hope's role in change is subtle, without the drama of some of the other precursors, such as confronting or effort. While hope and self-efficacy are often grouped together under the heading of client expectancy factors (Constantino et al., 2023), it has alternatively been framed in terms of perceived possibility rather than expected probability (Nelissen, 2017). In this respect, hope has an indirect or subtle influence on therapeutic change outcomes: It is responsible for alighting the path to change rather than for precipitating the walking of it.

In the CHANGES model, hope's real power is in its widespread effects on other precursors. Hope can enhance the intensity of other precursors and, in some cases, can be a catalyst that activates other precursors. The opposite is also true, of course, since the precursors are profoundly interdependent. Hope makes experiencing anxiety or difficulty more tolerable by indicating the positive payoff for the discomfort. It makes confronting easier through the knowledge that one will not become lost in a tangle of confusion and darkness. Hope jump-starts effort by making a positive outcome appear viable so that the end seems imminent and the effort expended seems well spent. Hope can be the wellspring that arises from, and even further inspires, genuine and avid social supports.

Hope can enhance a sense of necessity by bringing a person out of a state of apathy to the point of recognizing the urgency of the current predicament. A situation that once looked overwhelming and discouraging, with no solution or egress in sight, is radically altered with the introduction of hope. With hope, it still appears as a problem, but not a problem that is "tightly packed" and impenetrable. It is now "porous" with the possibility of options and alternatives and, most important, the potential for resolution. Yet a sense of necessity can also inspire hope when the necessity is so urgent that it forces a person to confront the problem and envision hopeful solutions.

Any problem or issue can be perceived as a threat or as a challenge (Oettingen & Chromik, 2017). When a problem is seen as a threat, one is more likely to withdraw, avoid, or otherwise defend against it. When a problem is seen as a challenge, one is more likely to approach it with interest or excitement. Challenges can be framed as opportunities. As a precursor, hope can transform a threat into a challenge. For example, the loss of a job might look like a threat through the lens of hopelessness and an opportunity through the lens of hope. A hopeful future is perceived as fluid rather than static, and problems are considered a source of potential gain rather than probable loss. Many have pointed out the remarkable way in which the word "crisis" is written in Chinese, where it is represented by two characters: one denoting danger and the other, opportunity.

SIGNIFICANT MOMENTS OF CHANGE INVOLVING HOPE

Anthony, age 17, was well over 6 feet tall, handsome, and charming. Unfortunately, he was also a member of a gang heavily involved with drugs and violence. His fellow gang members respected him for his fearlessness, ability to fight, and loyalty. Like so many adolescents in his situation, he said that he wanted to improve his life and help his little brother, who idolized him, as well as the aunt who had loved him and raised him after his mother was killed. He said he was tired of the fighting and "all the hard-ass bullshit." But he reported that it really didn't matter: "I'll be dead before I turn 21," he told his therapist softly and with great conviction. Then he added, "Besides, if I ever try to leave the gang, they will f—up my world."

The therapist told him three stories of other gang members who were able to leave their gangs and make something of their lives, and he became visibly more animated. The therapist also promised to "hook him up" with one of those men who had made great strides in improving his life. Anthony jumped at the chance to speak with this man. The possibility that he could help himself and his family escape a desperate situation inspired him. What was once a threat had become a challenge.

Tina, age 36, was held in psychological bondage by her husband. She was mentally immobilized by his dominance and verbal abuse. Her extreme dependence appeared to be induced by a brainwashing campaign carried out from the time they were "high school sweethearts." Having given up on her own chances for happiness and fulfillment, her chief concern was for her three children, who ranged from ages 8 to 14. During their 13 years of marriage, Tina's husband had convinced her that she was incompetent, powerless, insignificant, and incapable of surviving without him. She had been in therapy for six sessions, originally for her oldest child, a highly intelligent boy who was flunking out of his freshman year in high school. She had been extremely careful to avoid any mention of her relationship with her husband.

In the seventh session, which she attended alone, she tearfully spoke of her sense of being trapped by her husband and how she needed to "get away" from him but just did not know how. She was convinced, however, that this was not easily done. "I don't think I can survive on my own," she said fearfully but also with a strange sense of calm. She also stated with grim satisfaction, "He needs me."

In time, Tina eventually achieved therapeutic change when she saw that she did not have to be dependent on her husband. Hope dawned when she learned of other women who had moved out of similar oppressive circumstances and spoke with a couple of divorced friends who had been through similar situations. As she began to see solutions to her problem, she eventually gained the confidence to move out on her own. Her husband did not allow this without a lot of anger and fuss, but she eventually reported, "It's okay. I can handle him now."

Both Anthony and Tina developed a sense of hope when they recognized that other people in similar situations to their own had successfully created change. They subsequently explored their problems with a greater focus on solutions, and the possibility of change became increasingly realistic. They each began to imagine a future in which they were no longer helplessly trapped, and that future appeared experienceable, valuable, and worthy of pursuit.

CLINICAL MARKERS: HOW TO RECOGNIZE HOPE FOR CHANGE

The most important clinical indicator of the presence of hope is a sense of confidence that conditions will improve (Larsen & Stege, 2010). Change, in the form of therapeutic goals, is seen as genuinely attainable. The outlook will be realistically positive and, even in the face of adversity, the client will not become discouraged or apathetic. A hopeful client perceives a problem in terms of solutions rather than becoming entrenched in "awfulizing" the problem. That perception is accompanied by enthusiasm or even excitement about life (Schmid, 2019; Snyder, 1994). Perhaps the ultimate sense of hope occurs when a client grows thankful for lessons learned from a problem, and demoralization or distress is seen as merely temporary.

The following statements are clues to the presence of hope:

- "I know things will eventually be okay, but things are really difficult right now."
- "I know I will get through this, but it is so hard and I feel so terrible."
- "I have been through tough times before, and I can get through this, too."

A therapist can also test for hope by gently probing with alternative views. For example, if a client remarks, "I have absolutely no idea how to deal with this situation," a therapist can reply, "Do you have a sense that you will eventually figure it out?" A client inclined toward hope will indeed have that sense, knowing intuitively that a way exists but has not yet been discovered.

Hope and Humor

Hope also gives rise to *therapeutic humor* (Gladding & Drake Wallace, 2016; Sultanoff, 2013; Snyder, 1994), or humor that is insightful and uplifting and that transports a person out of a burdened mindset and into alternative perspectives that cause some degree of amusement. For instance, a male client with a verbally abusive wife once said with a sense of trepidation, "My wife said she's going to leave. I don't know what I'll do without her." The therapist smiled and replied with a somewhat satirical tone, "That's quite a problem. What will you do with all of that freedom and well-being?" The client suddenly laughed, and the seriousness of the moment eased a bit. He was surprised that he did so, and this fostered further discussion. The client's response also hinted that he was hopeful enough to eventually be able to see a future without her.

Humor, in this sense, can function as a therapeutic reframe of an otherwise oppressive problem. Ideally, therapeutic humor is directed at the ambiguity or quirks of life or the foibles of human nature. The kind of humor to avoid is that which is at the expense of another person, such as gloating over the misfortunes of others. Other types of destructive humor involve ridiculing another about looks, mannerisms, or lack of intelligence or skills. Humor based on stereotyping is, of course, another nontherapeutic variety. In any case, hope can give rise to humor and using humor properly can give rise to hope, reframing the problem just enough to lift the seriousness and rigidity of a problem to allow a healthy escape from an otherwise discouraging situation.

A therapist who is genuinely lighthearted and can tactfully integrate humor has a real talent. Clients generally look forward to sessions where the work is hard but fun and done in a setting that combines lightheartedness with learning. Timing and appropriateness are key, as it is important to fit humor into an acceptable framework for the client. While humor cannot be taught to therapists in any consistent way, modeling it in supervision may be a good approach (Gladding & Drake Wallace, 2016). In some cases, therapeutic humor can be conducive to an increase in awareness.

HOW TO DETECT THE ABSENCE OF HOPE FOR CHANGE

A client lacking hope will display an almost palpable sense of despondency or despair and probably a sense of apathy as well. They may believe that life is pointless and there is no significance in anything. Other common emotions are resentment and deep self-pity. Sometimes, a hopeless person displays a pessimistic humor that conveys bitterness or biting sarcasm. Such a client will question the worthiness of life and living. A fatalism, as though life is out of human control, may manifest and pervade statements and beliefs. The person may say in one way or another, "Things never turn out well for me," or "It doesn't matter what I do; it's always a disaster."

Such a person displays little confidence in their ability to solve problems. Discouragement and disappointment are always just around the corner for these unfortunate people, and their inclination toward resilience in difficult experiences is low. A client low in hope may display some degree of suicidal ideation without necessarily ever intending suicide. On the other hand, suicide may be imminent, and resolving this crisis will become the first duty of therapy. Clients low in hope may also harass themselves with self-doubt and express a general sense of protest against the seeming unfairness of life and the impossibility of ever being happy. To the truly hopeless person, life is a painful process and staying alive means the pain will continue. When hopelessness reaches its greatest depths, each passing moment is a kind of torment.

Farber (1968) suggested that suicide is an inverse function of hope. He described it as a disease of hope that proceeds from a "no exit" belief, wherein a person believes that death is the only escape from an intolerable situation or set of conditions. Ensuing research determined that suicide is more closely associated with hopelessness than depression (A. T. Beck et al., 1974, 1979), and the Beck Hopelessness Scale (A. T. Beck et al., 1985) developed to measure the likelihood of suicide remains in widespread use today (Kocalevent et al., 2017; Marchetti, 2019). Difficulties in social problem solving have also been linked to suicide risk, with perceived burdensomeness serving as a primary mediating factor (Chu et al., 2018).

TECHNIQUES: BUILDING HOPE

When the precursor of hope is activated, the vision of a bright, promising future brings with it the love of life and the joy of simply being. When coupled with other precursors, such as awareness, effort, and social support, the scenario begins to look like a poet's portrait of the undaunted human spirit. It does seem to be true that where there is hope, there is life. It is simply a matter of degree.

If a client leaves the first session with a sense of hope, the odds of their attending another session are much higher. Building hope involves directly empowering a person, helping them to become more capable and confident as part of perceiving a favorable, realistic future. The enterprise is largely dedicated to helping a client become more stable in the face of adversity and better able to focus on positive outcomes with the realistic expectation that problems and situations will turn out well. The client who is hopeful has sufficient coping skills to deal with problems and issues, as well as that fascinating quality that psychodynamic therapists refer to as ego strength. The hopeful person also has the capacity to see beyond problems toward a bright future.

The techniques and strategies in this section are designed to instill hope as a precursor to change by strengthening and empowering the person. When a client has hope, the other precursors can be positively affected by its pervasive influence throughout the range of that person's life. The gift of hope is the gift of a desirable future. Thus, hope building is done through any approach that can make the future more tolerable. The following techniques can help the therapist build the hope precursor in clients.

Overcoming the Influence of Negative Role Models

This technique addresses the impact of negative role models on client behavior, particularly among adolescents and young adults who are abusing drugs or alcohol. According to Bandura (1977), people tend to imitate or take on the roles and behaviors of the people whom they admire. This technique seeks to reduce the internal power that the influential person exerts on the client's mindset and provide a sense of hope for living more congruently. The strategy is simple since such role models tend to hold significant weight in the client's mind and lead the client to imitate particular roles, mannerisms, or behaviors.

Begin by asking the client about the most influential people in their life, with an emphasis on those people the client "most wants to be like" in terms of certain behaviors. For instance, if a teen client is getting into fistfights at school, ask about their role models for being tough and winning fights. If a client is using drugs, ask about their role models for drug use. Have the client list these people and, one at a time, provide a detailed description of each. Be sure to have the client include musicians, actors, and other media, popular, or subcultural figures of relevance.

Monitor what the client identifies as admirable about their role models, empathize with the client about those points of commonality, and ask the client if there have been negative outcomes or life struggles for any of those role models. In many cases, the client will hope for the accolades or perks that seem to accompany the behavior of their role model, such as power, status, money, or influence. Peer recognition is a powerful influence on behavior among adolescents and young adults. However, in other cases, the client will identify with the "crash-and-burn" aspect of a role model's life simply because this is how they seem to feel themselves. A 19-year-old budding alcoholic once told his therapist, "Kurt Cobain's my hero. He died, like, forever ago, but I understand him. No one got him, you know? But I do. I'll probably be dead before 30, too."

Whether related to drug and alcohol use or not, it is important to validate the perceived connection between the client and their role model before examining potential negative outcomes. Trying to undermine the influence of the role model can be difficult. It takes a certain finesse. Work with the client to examine the similarities and differences between themselves and the selected role model. Look for any differences that the client perceives as a personal deficit. It can be helpful to then note areas in which the client has a strength that the role model does not or to highlight behaviors of, and outcomes for, a role model that the client might find uncomfortable or distasteful.

At each step in the process, ask the client if they still choose to have the person be influential. Note any dysfunctional cognitions or beliefs that are connected to this person. Use a cognitive approach, including the cognitive therapy of oppression if appropriate, to refute and reformulate any harmful beliefs. For situations in which the role model has died or has been incarcerated, it can be beneficial to ask the client what they know that the role model did not know. Additionally, it can be helpful to put the admired person in the empty chair and conduct a therapeutic dialogue. Regardless, this technique has the potential to free the client from negative influences and move the client toward empowerment through an enhanced sense of agency and authenticity. Most importantly, the technique can have a profound impact on hope, as the client comes to recognize that their own fate does not have to align with the deleterious outcomes experienced by certain negative role models.

The Jamesian Device

James (1907) developed a theory of truth that is suited to personal knowing that does not rely only on objective criteria. This has an application in therapy that can greatly help some clients. Many difficult clients are remarkably hesitant to believe that anything positive about them may be true. James' definition of truth can provide clients with an internal measuring device that can indicate whether or not a particular belief or statement has any truth value. The therapist explains to the client that when a statement or belief is true for a person, it produces positive feelings and a sense of well-being and resonates and harmonizes within oneself. Even if the statement is negative, that resonance will take place, producing a feeling of peaceful acceptance "deep down inside." On hearing this idea, many clients immediately discount it as wishful thinking. However, when told it was originated by America's greatest psychologist (Korn et al., 1991), it is easier to accept, or at least less easy to dismiss.

For example, Michelle, a woman in her early 20s, was depressed and lacking in self-efficacy. She found it exceedingly difficult to accept any positive statements about herself from her therapist and would not engage in disputing negative beliefs. She told her therapist several times that it was nice to suggest such positive things, but she knew they simply were not true, and for that reason, she would not believe any of them. "I know," she said, "that there is nothing positive about me and that all the people who have hurt me were right."

At that point, the therapist introduced James's theory of truth and explained it in language that was meaningful to Michelle. The therapist then asked her if she would like to try an experiment. With a sigh, Michelle agreed. The therapist said,

> I am going to give you a statement to repeat to yourself out loud. When you repeat it, rather than think about whether it is true or false, I would like you just to watch and see how the statement makes you feel inside.

The therapist gave Michelle the self-statement, "I am a good person," a declaration she would not even consider previously. Michelle repeated it to herself a couple of times, looked up at the therapist hesitantly, and said, "It makes me feel kind of good to say that, but I am just kidding myself." The therapist asked, "Did it feel good deep down and give you a sense of inner peace?" Michelle, now on new territory, only nodded. "Well, Michelle," said the therapist matter-of-factly, "according to William James, you may very well be a good person."

Michelle was forced to consider this and, in the following sessions, tried out many other self-statements using her new internal measuring device. The therapist also told her she could use this tool in everyday life when someone criticized her or forced a belief on her. Such affirmations and positive self-statements had not worked previously. This experiential technique bypassed the difficulty she was having in terms of disputing her cognitive distortions. Of course, this internal measuring device can only gauge the validity of self-evaluative statements and not of environmental conditions or other people. Otherwise, it would convince paranoid or narcissistic clients, for example, that their ideas of reference are correct, making such clients even more difficult to treat. Examples of statements that should not be used in this technique are, "They are out to destroy my life," "I'm going to win the lottery," or "[fill in the blank] is in love with me."

Empowerment Strategies

In the enterprise of hope building, it is wise to take every opportunity to help a client feel capable and empowered to make changes. Many therapists have told me they sometimes do not know how to empower dysfunctional clients who seem to have little going for them. As part of empowerment, it helps to recall that even the most dysfunctional people occasionally do something functional and to concentrate on reinforcing that fact, rather than implying that they lack skills and have to learn new skills. In many cases, new skills do need to be learned, but it is easier to do so when these are built on a foundation of established skills. Two modes of empowerment are especially helpful in this regard: reframing negative behaviors as skills and converting a threat into a challenge.

Reflecting the Hopelessness

It is often a mistake for a therapist to refuse to accept the client's conviction of the hopelessness of a situation or condition. To work with a client who is bereft of hope, it is often vital for the therapist to reflect that hopelessness, conveying that it is fully understood and why. A client may be more inclined to listen to messages of hope when it appears that the therapist truly understands the grimness of the situation. Many hopeless clients seem to demand that their therapists see the hopelessness and feel it as well. To meet this demand, it is helpful to empathically paraphrase and summarize exactly why things cannot and will not improve. The therapist then invites the client to comment on the degree of the therapist's understanding.

For example, a therapist might say to such a client,

> Please tell me if I am tracking with you here. You figure that no matter what you do, things are going to be a disaster, and you will end up being a failure. There is no point in trying, and the only way out is by ending your life. Am I close to understanding how you see all this?

When clients are convinced that a therapist truly understands the depth and degree of their hopelessness and the internal logic of that hopelessness, then they may be more inclined to explore or consider alternative ideas or options.

Reframing Negative Behaviors as Skills

One of the most helpful ways of empowering clients is to demonstrate to them that their dysfunctional, negative behaviors can be reframed into positive skills that are available to them at their own choosing. All too often, the message received by people who behave in maladaptive ways is that the behaviors are "bad," or something that no good or worthy person would ever do. The key is to reframe negative behaviors as skills. For example, rather than inform a manipulative client that their behavior is destructive, the therapist can reframe it as a kind of skill that involves accurate perception and persuasiveness in getting people to do what they want.

Clients are far more willing to talk about their manipulative behavior when it is framed as a skill. The therapist can admire it as a hard earned and well-practiced skill that has served a useful purpose. The therapist can then suggest that the skill is actually underused and can be used in other, more positive ways. If one is a selfish manipulator, one can redirect or reverse that very same skill and become a helper. The same perception that is used to exploit a person can also be used to help. The same is true of the skill of counseling: If that skill were reversed or redirected, an effective therapist could become an extraordinarily effective verbal abuser.

Thus, the therapist can inform the client that up until now, that skill at manipulation has been used for selfish purposes, but if the client so wished, they could use the same skill in a positive way to become a corporate manager, salesperson, or counselor. When a client realizes that they already have the blueprint of positive skills, it builds hope by making the refinement of those skills seem like a realistic possibility. This technique can also be used with other "skills." Lying, for example, presupposes a creative ability to reshape and reformulate information. The negative behavior of verbal abuse, when reversed, can be validating, encouraging, and even inspiring. The blueprint is obviously therein. The challenge is in identifying how to constructively adjust its use.

Converting Threats Into Challenges

When a person is threatened by circumstances, problems, or conditions, hope can be adversely and sometimes seriously affected. The greater the perceived threat, the lower the degree of hope for a positive outcome. One strategy is to reframe a perceived threat into what looks like a challenge, thus rendering it more likely to be handled successfully (Oettingen & Chromik, 2017). If a threatening problem is perceived as a challenge, hope can be sustained or even enhanced.

The procedure involves two steps. The first is to find and identify the client's skills, of which they may not even be aware. If the client was a victim of oppression, for example, they may be highly perceptive of others, even if easily exploited. Similarly, being a survivor of abuse can be reframed as an ability to endure hardship as part of solving a problem. Ingratiating or people-pleasing behaviors require the skill of perception as part of knowing what people want. A host of skills can be recognized in clients, ranging from patience and strength to assertiveness and intelligence. A skill is a skill, no matter how developed it is. If a client recognizes it as a skill, hope may be enhanced.

After skills are identified, the problem itself can be addressed. The therapist suggests that the client's skills are especially suited to the problem at hand and are what is needed to solve it. When clients see their skills in other domains can be transferred to the current problem, hope can be increased, and the effort precursor may be enhanced as well.

The Story of Gwen

Gwen, age 38, was a salesperson for a major pharmaceutical company. She presented with what appeared to be a career issue of being bored with her work, and she was no longer willing to continue her career. She referred to her job as a "drug pusher" and said that it was not in harmony with her true nature. In spite of her depression, she had an inauthentic way of smiling through it and saying that everything was as it should be. In the second session, she hesitantly though enthusiastically revealed that she was studying with a group whose guru had magical powers over her well-being and spiritual development. She also revealed that the real reason she was in therapy was that her husband, Bill, had insisted on it. Bill believed that the guru was crazy and was convinced Gwen had fallen prey to his manipulations and that it was ruining their marriage. The guru himself, she said, was opposed to her receiving therapy and was not happy with it.

Gwen maintained a schizotypal belief system based on and reinforced by her guru, who had convinced her that even her dreams and moods were a result of his control over her mind. Part of this belief system was that the guru was putting her through uncertainty and depression for the purpose of spiritual "testing" and "cleansing" for her eventual enlightenment. Gwen had little self-efficacy and almost no faith in her own ability to achieve happiness and fulfillment. Her faith in the magical powers of the guru was a way of bypassing her helplessness so he could achieve happiness for her. Only he could do it. She vigorously defended against any perceived criticism of the guru.

In the third session, Gwen admitted that even though she had great faith in her guru, he was not making her as happy as she would have liked. However, she anxiously added that this was a "test" of her loyalty and resolve and that, in due time, she would be rewarded with a mystical experience of supreme peace and tranquility.

In the next session, the therapist recognized and reframed her resolve and her faith as skills. Taking great care not to threaten or attack her delusional system, the therapist reframed Gwen's belief in the guru and her presenting problem of wanting to quit her job as related to the deeper, more pervasive, and admirable goal of attaining self-knowledge and self-mastery. Gwen agreed that this was indeed her ultimate goal. The guru's test that had caused her so much distress was reframed as part of the challenge for her to come to know herself.

Gwen accepted the reframe, as it fit rather easily and comfortably into her delusional system. The therapist further informed Gwen that therapy was another path to self-knowledge and self-mastery that did not have to conflict with her spiritual beliefs and that therapy had the capacity to help her be happy and find fulfillment. The therapist did not challenge her spiritual beliefs; instead, they reflected to Gwen that her beliefs were from ancient sources and were not dependent on the guru for their validity. The therapist took great care not to invalidate the guru himself because it was clear that Gwen would likely terminate therapy if this were to happen.

This approach was consistent with her beliefs and delusions about her guru and allowed egress from her attachment to the guru and the cult in which she was entrenched. The basis of hope provided to Gwen early in the therapeutic relationship was the prospect that therapy could lead to self-knowledge and self-mastery. Crucial to her liberation from the guru was the recognition that the vast power she had attributed to him was evidence of her own power of belief and that she could begin to use some of it now instead of waiting. This was another great source of hope for her.

In time, she began to see that her intense dislike of her job was a source of self-knowledge in itself, and she no longer linked it with her guru's ridicule of such "lowly" occupations. She also took heart in her absolute faith in the guru, having reframed it as an insight into her admirable qualities of faithfulness, loyalty, and friendship. Most important, she began to see the guru's narcissistic need for admiration and control. Her faith in him progressively weakened as she regarded him in this realistic fashion. After about 15 months, she left her job and entered law school full-time, and she gradually ended her involvement with the guru and his circle of admirers. Gwen attributed her change to the promise of hope, the various reframes, and the relationship that kept her engaged in therapy in spite of her guru's admonitions to terminate.

Hope as Contagion

We know that a therapist's positive expectations of a client can impact the client's success in therapy (Sperry, 2022). The therapist's confidence can be contagious. When working with a client to build hope through empowerment, just believing a client can indeed get through an issue or successfully solve a problem will indirectly affect the client. This belief is communicated through the therapist's metalogue and dialogue; of course, it also helps if the therapist directly and often voices their belief in a client's skills or ability to deal with an issue.

Many clients have told their therapists that they successfully handled a problem because of the faith or confidence the therapist had in them. In this way, hope is contagious.

Hope Requires a Sense of Worthiness

It is important to ask clients whether or not they feel worthy of having good things in life, as unworthiness can act as a powerful obstacle to therapeutic change. Many difficult clients, when asked, report that they do not deserve to be happy and do not feel good about themselves or their lives because of mistakes they have made in the past. Ironically, such a stance serves as evidence of goodness or worthiness, while for many clients, it is perceived as the path to eventual redemption.

Regardless, if a client deems themselves unworthy of positive life experiences, change will not occur because the client has lost hope in the possibility of redemption. Clients in recovery and in treatment often say this is why they did not previously respond to therapy after years of treatment across multiple treatment programs. Again, the main reason clients feel unworthy is because they have harmed others in the past and punish themselves accordingly. Although this is sometimes an unconscious phenomenon, many clients are distinctly aware of the issue when pressed to discuss it:

THERAPIST:	Do you feel like you deserve to be happy?
CLIENT:	(shaking head) No, not really.
THERAPIST:	Would you like to feel deserving and worthy of a happy life?
CLIENT:	Yeah, sure. But I don't know what that even means.
THERAPIST:	If you did feel worthy, how do you think your life might be different?
CLIENT:	I don't know. I probably wouldn't be so depressed all the time.
THERAPIST:	That sounds pretty great, not being depressed. So, when therapists suggest things to do to reduce your depression, there's a big part of you inside that says, "Nope, not going to do it because I deserve to be sad." Is that right?
CLIENT:	Exactly. I don't deserve to be happy. I've done too many bad things.
THERAPIST:	So, you're not allowing yourself to feel happy?
CLIENT:	Man, you don't know me as well as you think. I've done *really* bad things.
THERAPIST:	Do you feel bad about the bad things you've done?
CLIENT:	Yeah, I do. I think about it a lot.

THERAPIST:	You know, the fact that you feel bad is just proof that you're a good person.
CLIENT:	(rolling eyes) Whatever.
THERAPIST:	Do you think a truly bad person would feel bad about hurting others?
CLIENT:	Probably not.
THERAPIST:	Bad people don't feel remorse or guilt. Good people do. You feel guilty, which means you're a good person. You've made big mistakes, but you're obviously still a good person because you clearly feel remorseful.
CLIENT:	I guess. It still doesn't change what I did, though.
THERAPIST:	No, but maybe you still deserve some good things in life. Maybe your path to redemption can include positive changes. Besides, it's hard to overcome our mistakes and do better by others when we're depressed, don't you think?
CLIENT:	Yeah, maybe.
THERAPIST:	So, I'll ask again: if you did feel worthy, how would your life be different?
CLIENT:	Maybe I'd do more good things for the world if I was just a bit happier.
THERAPIST:	Okay. What do you think about exploring the good things you could do?
CLIENT:	Alright, yeah. Let's give it a shot.

Hope is the wellspring from which all self-transformation occurs. If a client believes they do not deserve to transform, therapists need to resuscitate hope. Doing self-forgiveness work can help get a client to let go of the past and start to forgive themselves for the harmful acts committed toward others. Simply acknowledging that one is a good person can be transformative. In terms of addiction, therapists can ask a client whether their drug or alcohol use was a response to feeling worthless or undeserving of a good life. Self-forgiveness can be a powerful catalyst for sobriety. Other operative precursors in this technique are grit, confronting, awareness, and effort.

Creative Narratives: Relating and Rewriting

In some cases, therapists can begin work on the hope precursor by asking a client to tell the story of their life. There is no need to focus on tragedy or trauma, but only to get a view of life as the client perceives it. If the story is told tragically, the therapist can help the client reconstruct the story to retell it with a sense of hope, empathy, and understanding—as a story still in the making. If the story is told in a narcissistic fashion, complete with fantasies of brilliance or superiority, the story can be retold to show how difficult it must have been for others to appreciate such a great person. The retelling could include how important the development of empathy and compassion for others might have been so that the other people in the client's life would have been more communicative and appreciative. The purpose, again, is to open a therapeutic window.

The retelling of a life story can be powerful for some clients. It allows a client to become liberated from a stuck or fixed pattern of conceiving the self and surrounding contexts. When creatively and therapeutically retold, the story can allow therapeutic change to become part of the story itself, supporting the emergence of precursors such as willingness, awareness, and necessity.

Telling Stories of Recovery

Like Anthony, who struggled to imagine a future for himself, and Tina, who could not envision leaving her husband, many difficult clients have great difficulty conceiving the possibility of change. Telling stories of clients and people with similar problems who made positive changes in their lives can be helpful. Clients will often inquire about the person or client mentioned by the therapist, sometimes bringing them up months or weeks after the story was told. Stories can be introduced by saying, "You know, I once knew someone who was similar to you," or "You remind me of someone who was in a predicament similar to yours." Clients have sometimes told me later that a particular story about a person with a similar dilemma kept them going during difficult times.

Exposure to Others Who Solved the Same Problem

Group therapy can be remarkably powerful in building hope, with unique benefits not found in individual or family therapy. Yalom (1995) noted that hope is often instilled when clients observe their peers making therapeutic changes. Group therapy can communicate a client's potential for change in a way that goes far beyond encouraging messages from a therapist. In addition to groups, hearing speakers, watching films, or reading books that contain stories of change can also be a powerful source of hope. In treatment programs for adults or adolescents, bringing in people who have worked on similar issues to tell their stories of change is another effective strategy. I have observed several instances in which a sense of necessity arose in a client when a person inspired hope by relating a personal story. This is especially helpful, for example, with adolescent gang members who believe they have no future and no escape from their circumstances. It is also helpful for substance users.

Examining Maladaptive Beliefs About the Future

Because hope intertwines with positive expectations for the future (Wampold & Flückiger, 2023), hope building can take the form of examining maladaptive beliefs about the future itself and the context of those beliefs. If a client is habitually inclined to regard the future with suspicion, fear, apprehension, and anxiety, that client's capacity for hope will diminish. In many cases, if maladaptive beliefs are not addressed and disputed, the techniques in this chapter may not bear fruit. Distorted views and beliefs about the future can affect the smooth implementation of any program of therapeutic change, regardless of the theoretical approach. It is the therapist's job to help identify and properly phrase these beliefs with the client's assurance of accuracy before disputing them. The following are examples of maladaptive beliefs about the future:

- "The future holds nothing for me."
- "Only bad things are waiting for me."
- "The world is a cruel place to live."
- "No matter what you do, things will never really get better."
- "Life is a process of failing to realize one's dreams."
- "The future holds only what others want."
- "Other people dictate my future."
- "The passing of time is painful."
- "The future provides nothing but anxiety."
- "The future is filled with continuous disappointment."
- "The future is filled with unforeseen catastrophes."
- "I am unable to affect the future."
- "The future is a continuous threat to my well-being."
- "Hope is for fools."
- "Nobody has any idea of the future."
- "My life has been disappointing, and the future will be more of the same."

A CLOSING NOTE ON HOPE

As we have stated previously, all of the precursors are interdependent and interactive, and thus, the increase of one precursor can increase the presence of others depending on the circumstances. Of all the precursors, hope demonstrates this interactive quality as much or more than the others. For example, a client may lack a sense of necessity, but that lack may be due to apathy, specifically, in the belief that things cannot and will not ever get better anyway. Thus, for such a person, there is no point in entertaining any sense of necessity because hopelessness has rendered such action a waste of time. Hope can also stimulate the precursors of grit and confronting the problem where these qualities did not exist previously. It can be surprising and encouraging to client and therapist alike when motivation to change emerges alongside the rediscovery of hope. If there is anything at all magical about the therapeutic encounter, it is to be found in the moment of hope's resuscitation.

6

A: Awareness of the Problem

Many philosophers have framed awareness as the most fundamental aspect of life, its qualities extolled in wonder and awe since the time of the ancients. Generally speaking, *awareness* is the cognizance, recognition, or knowledge of any mental or physical object, relation, or event. As a precursor of change, awareness involves a client's recognition of, or clarity of perception about, a problem. Put another way, awareness is the identification or pinpointing of issues or relationships that need to be addressed as part of the therapy process and its tasks. It is the function that moves issues from the edge or ground of consciousness into figural focus. Plucking a problem out of the realm of the obscure and dropping it into the light, awareness illuminates and enables genuine recognition of the potential for change. It gives substance to shadow and form to oblivion.

People lacking in the awareness precursor have, for the most part, shut off the process of knowing and growing. When there is no awareness of the existence of a problem, therapeutic change occurs only by accident or through a process that does not require consciousness raising, such as pharmacotherapy or pure operant conditioning. It is therefore a vital element of the psychotherapy process. Without awareness, self-determined change would probably never directly take place. When awareness is present, only denial itself can be denied. Unsurprisingly, awareness has been identified as a common factor tied to the change process across the established psychotherapies (Drozd & Goldfried, 1996; Høglend & Hagtvet, 2019).

Case examples have been disguised to protect client confidentiality.

https://doi.org/10.1037/0000451-007
Therapeutic Change With Difficult Clients: Precursors and Techniques in the CHANGES Model, Second Edition, by B. D. Wilkinson and F. J. Hanna

DEGREES OF CONSCIOUS AWARENESS

Awareness is not an all-or-nothing phenomenon. It can be active to varying degrees, reflecting the extent to which an individual is consciously aware of a problem. The first degree involves uncertainty as to whether there is a problem at all. Whether framed in terms of defense mechanisms such as denial and repression or simply in terms of obliviousness, many clients are unaware and unsuspecting that a problem exists, even when the problem is severe. Few people who lack any awareness of a problem or issue seek therapy on their own, and most such clients have been referred by a spouse, judge, employer, or friend. For those clients, the first order of business is usually to identify a problem that needs attention.

The second degree of awareness denotes ambiguity as to the nature of the problem. The person may be aware that something is wrong but has no idea what that something is. Such awareness is often accompanied by a cognitive dissonance that initiates the change process. In such cases, a person may have a high sense of necessity and grit. However, without awareness to pinpoint the area on which to focus, the client will demonstrate a certain amount of vagueness about what to address. Such a person may come to therapy to try to determine if there is indeed anything to address at all. Often, this kind of client secretly wants the therapist to say, "You're fine. There is really nothing wrong and you can go home."

The third degree of awareness denotes a genuine clarity about the nature of a problem, including the ability to identify specific behaviors, emotions, beliefs, cognitions, and interpersonal issues in need of remedy. The more details a client recognizes in a problem, the easier it is to manage it and maneuver around potential pitfalls. Such awareness can include recognizing the origins of a problem and properly attributing responsibility for a problem without blaming.

HOW AWARENESS OF THE PROBLEM LEADS TO THERAPEUTIC CHANGE

Awareness is fundamental and integral to all the other precursors. To the degree that a client can learn to detect such things as emotional difficulties, unresolved issues, problematic behaviors, harmful relationships, dysfunctional thoughts, anxieties, and negative environmental stressors, the potential for change gains entrance into the realm of the imminently real via awareness. The capacity for awareness can be enhanced through therapy to great effect, even if it is seldom sufficient by itself for change to occur. To better understand how awareness leads to change, we look to various processes to better understand and support the advancement of awareness.

Metacognitive Aspects of Awareness and Change

Metacognition involves two primary functions: monitoring and control (Norman et al., 2019). Awareness is obviously fundamental to the monitoring function, which includes detecting, seeing, and observing, in one's "inner eye," cognitions, beliefs, and thoughts. Perhaps the most important metacognitive aspects of awareness are what needs to be observed and where to direct attention. Whether a client is avoiding or dealing with an issue hinges on awareness. In this regard, the awareness precursor is tremendously powerful.

Another metacognitive process related to awareness, known as *decentering*, involves shifting from being within subjective experience to reflecting upon that experience (Bernstein et al., 2015). Many clients are so enmeshed and immersed in a situation, behavior, thought, feeling, or sensation that they can contemplate or think of little else. One of the most valuable aspects of awareness involves the action of taking a step back and viewing a problem, emotion, or obsessive or compulsive pattern dispassionately (Bernstein et al., 2015; Goldfried, 1995). This essential action of stepping back is a prime ingredient of change, creativity, and mental health (Coffey et al., 2010).

A. T. Beck (1976) referred to such stepping back as "distancing," not in the negative sense of avoidance but in the sense of getting an overview. This has also been described as taking a broad or overarching viewpoint. By removing oneself from confusions and mental entanglements, one can get perspective. For cognitive therapists, it is the act of stepping back in one's mind and viewing thoughts or beliefs connected with an event or emotion from a self-distanced stance (Travers-Hill et al., 2017). Self-distancing is experientially synonymous with concepts such as cognitive defusion within third-wave cognitive behavioral therapy approaches (Hayes & Linehan, 2018).

In many instances, increased awareness is the metacognitive equivalent of learning how to negotiate one's way through a cognitive and interpersonal minefield. Each successive increase in awareness reveals the position and placement of other mines, which can then be avoided on the way toward freedom. Just as the shunning of awareness is the essence of defensiveness, the strengthening of awareness opens the door to exquisite feelings of vitality. The key to that vitality seems to be the belief that even the awareness of pain is better than no awareness at all.

Consciousness Raising

Increasing awareness is often referred to in therapy and counseling literature as *consciousness raising*, which has been cited as a common factor across therapy approaches (Prochaska & Norcross, 2018). Freud attributed awareness to the functioning of the ego. Of course, the concept of the ego and awareness was around long before Freud, and he himself studied it under Franz Brentano (Hergenhahn, 1996), who also taught the founder of phenomenology, Edmund Husserl. The philosophical discipline of phenomenology made consciousness its central focus of study.

Awareness was praised and celebrated in the *Upanishads* (Easwaran, 2007), one of the world's oldest known religio-philosophical works. It was also empha-sized by other ancient Asian philosopher–psychologists such as Buddha, Shankara, and Patanjali (Gupta, 1998; Hanna, 1993, 1995; Theise & Kafatos,

2016), who regarded conscious awareness as the passive witnessing of all phenomena of mind and the world. Western philosophers have long written about awareness in the form of consciousness; it is a theme in the writings of Plotinus, Kant, Husserl, and Sartre.

Consciousness raising is present in virtually every form of psychotherapy and counseling other than pure operant conditioning. It involves attaining clarity of perception of thought processes, mental images, feelings, emotions, interpersonal interactions, and environmental conditions. It also involves recognizing the effects of one's actions upon any of these aspects of living. It plays a critical role in existential and humanistic therapies, both of which claim a long tradition of emphasizing this phenomenon. Awareness as consciousness raising is an indispensable part of behavior therapy as well, which utilizes such techniques as self-monitoring and self-observation for the purpose of bringing a person to discern more fully and precisely the nature of behaviors or reactions, ranging from problem drinking and smoking to irrational fears or phobias.

Behavioral techniques that make use of exposure would hardly be workable if not for awareness, and it is here that much of therapeutic change originates. However, while it is true that behaviorists can manipulate change in a person through conditioned responses to stimuli, that change is entirely dependent on a largely unchanging environment to maintain new behaviors. For example, many clients change in inpatient drug and alcohol treatment programs, only to relapse when exposed to old environmental cues due to impaired meta-awareness (Ruimi et al., 2018) or lack of cognitive integration (Vafaie & Kober, 2022). In awareness, change only becomes stable and lasting when new cognitive structures are successfully integrated with older knowledge and experience.

Awareness Remains Consistent

One of the most remarkable things phenomenologists have discovered about awareness is its amazing consistency. When present, awareness itself seems not to change in its essential character, regardless of what is being contemplated (Merleau-Ponty, 1962), even during drug-induced psychedelic experiences (Yaden et al., 2021). In other words, the content of awareness changes and can be altered by various mental states and drug influence. However, as a function, awareness itself remains consistent. In the Tibetan Buddhist tradition of Dzogchen, this stream of consciousness is referred to as *Rigpa*, "which continues with no beginning and no end, without any break ... and constitutes the mental continuum of each Being" (Klein & Wangyal, 2006, p. 73). In the field of experimental psychology, Powers (1973) made a similar discovery about the consistency of awareness and expressed it well:

> Awareness seems to have the same character whether one is being aware of his finger or of his faults, his present automobile or the one he wishes Detroit would build, the automobile's hubcap or its environmental impact. Perception changes like a kaleidoscope, while that sense of being aware remains quite unchanged. (p. 200)

As we know, awareness can be directed toward the contemplation of a tremendous range of physical and psychological phenomena. Psychological phenomena include mental images, thoughts, desires, intentions, and even hallucinations and delusions. They include emotions as well, from sadness and grief to enthusiasm, joy, and happiness. Awareness of physical phenomena requires the senses to contemplate the sights, sounds, smells, tastes, and touch of, for example, music, mountains, oceans, city traffic, living beings, and inanimate objects. Physical sensations, for instance, headaches, dizziness, nausea, motion, goosebumps, and sexuality are other examples. Thus, awareness is tremendously consistent yet versatile, capable of attending to and beholding a fantastic array of phenomena without itself being altered in its essential character.

Empathy as a Form of Awareness

From the perspective of psychotherapy, empathy is intimately related to awareness. *Empathy*, or the inferential knowledge or perception of how or what another person is perceiving, thinking, or feeling, is a form of awareness. In the CHANGES model, empathy falls under the awareness category. People who have a reasonable amount of it are more likely to engage others in harmonious social interactions than those who lack the awareness necessary to recognize the cues and indicators of the thoughts, feelings, and responses of others. This has important implications for people with antisocial, narcissistic, borderline, and histrionic personality disorders, where lack of empathy serves as a fundamental aspect of psychopathology (Kajonius & Dåderman, 2017).

In some people, transformational change arises from sudden empathic awareness. When a client becomes aware that their temper scares and alienates their young children, that may be enough to enable them to start managing their outbursts. In such cases, awareness catalyzes all of the other precursors and launches the change process. But for most clients who find change particularly difficult, awareness is a helpful but insufficient catalyst for activating the other precursors.

SIGNIFICANT MOMENTS OF CHANGE INVOLVING AWARENESS

The following example of Claire's significant moment of change illustrates the mechanism of coming to awareness and the accompanying action of stepping back from the problem. As she put it, her awareness came "in a flash." After 9 years of marriage, Claire began to notice that she was becoming increasingly depressed. As time went by, she told her therapist, "It just became so obvious that I was in a state of depression." This depression was accompanied by a series of illnesses in the form of infections that were perplexing to several doctors. Although these illnesses were "more annoying than life-threatening," one particular infection did become rather serious. The combination of medicine she was taking as well as her depression had made her lethargic. Her husband was noncommunicative, and she had been consistently "rebuffed" whenever she tried to talk to him. He had also consistently refused her requests to attend marital therapy.

Her change began right after her most serious bout with an infection. "I was standing in the kitchen next to my kitchen stove—I remember staring at one of the burners," Claire reported. The "realization hit me that because my life was in such a disarray that I was dying ... not so much physically dying; mentally and emotionally I was dying." She went on: "I realized I had to take any step necessary to change my situation. I felt certain that divorce was the answer." Soon after that realization, she initiated divorce proceedings, and "all my physical problems dissipated ... the medication started to work." She reported that she "healed and felt great within 1 to 2 months." She had not had a similar illness since that time.

In summarizing her change, Claire explained, "I was denying myself an opportunity for true happiness. I couldn't say that I didn't matter anymore—life and being happy was very important to me." She also reported that she realized, "I'm the only one who can create my happiness." She arranged her life to maintain some control over it from that moment on. She recognized that the change was sparked by the initial awareness of her circumstances, which in turn stimulated the presence of other precursors, for instance, a sense of necessity for change. All of this culminated in her determined, focused, and intensely inspiring movement toward change.

CLINICAL MARKERS: HOW TO RECOGNIZE AWARENESS

Awareness of the problem is relatively easy to detect among clients. When awareness is amply present, the client is able to identify thoughts and feelings with ease. Such a client is alert and catches on to where a therapist may be going with a particular technique or series of questions. There will be certainty about the person, a poise that manifests as an air of assurance and confidence. The person may show that assurance even when depressed, discouraged, or stressed. The person will generally respond quickly to queries regarding behaviors, feelings, or thoughts and will often offer helpful details above and beyond what was requested.

However, they do not always change, so change itself should not be looked for as a clinical marker.

In this regard, the aware client can sometimes be among the trickiest of all difficult clients. When working with a client high in awareness, therapists are likely to believe that change is imminent. However, many articulate, self-disclosing, and insightful clients do not take any steps toward change. Such clients may be remarkably skilled at pointing out their issues and explaining their maladies, which can seem like a gift to the inexperienced therapist until it becomes apparent that change is nowhere in sight and may never occur. Some of these clients have been validated by previous therapists for their awareness but not for making changes in their lives. As has been noted, awareness, like the other precursors, is a necessary yet insufficient condition for change by itself.

Alternatively, a person with high awareness may not be particularly verbal or articulate but may demonstrate considerable awareness nonetheless. In such cases, the therapist should help articulate certain details that the client may recognize but need assistance in describing. With an empathic understanding of what the client is experiencing, the therapist may articulate that understanding while simultaneously asking the client to modify or verify, as the case may require.

The certainty accompanying this precursor manifests in the cognitive context as well. When awareness is high, the person can be certain of being uncertain. The person can easily identify thoughts, beliefs, conclusions, schemas, memories, perceptions, and most other cognitive phenomena. They will find it easy to see how cognition affects behavior and feelings and vice versa. In cases of high awareness, thoughts are generally clear, attention is focused, and the person can step back from a problem or complex of emotions relatively easily. This client will also be likely to identify not only the problem but also the circumstances surrounding the problem and, perhaps, the source of the problem. They will likely be adept at assigning or assessing responsibility for a given situation or set of circumstances and be able to identify contributing factors in interpersonal dynamics as well. It is often helpful to observe the degree of detail, coherence, or clarity in the stories the person tells related to the presenting problem. The way a person tells such stories can give clues as to the degree of their awareness.

People with high awareness are not likely to get lost in feelings or emotions. With little prompting or encouragement, they can extract themselves from entanglement in strong emotions and return to viewing the problem or issue. Clients with a high degree of awareness may report a variety of mixed emotions, such as simultaneous love and hate or concurrent sadness, helplessness, and anger. A person with a high degree of awareness will also be likely to accurately and poignantly describe inner conflicts about decisions as well as opposing intentions and purposes.

While aware clients who are not verbally inclined are unlikely to spontaneously articulate experiences, they will readily relate to reframes or reflections made by the therapist. Overall, a client with awareness is every therapist's desire. Even when change is not occurring, session time passes in a deceptively smooth way—a note of caution to not sing the praises of awareness in therapy too loudly.

HOW TO DETECT THE ABSENCE OF AWARENESS

The absence of awareness is one of the most frustrating conditions a therapist encounters outside of deliberate recalcitrance or deception. It is a form of psychological obliviousness, the hallmark of a difficult client. Vagueness and obscurity define the client's relation to their inner and outer worlds. Such clients will be consistently unclear, unsure, and, at worst, oblivious to all that surrounds them. They typically answer the therapist's questions with brief, noncommittal statements like "I don't know" or "I guess." Blaming is common among people lacking in awareness, not so much because of an inclination toward avoidance as because of an inability to properly designate influences and causes.

A client can be burdened by an array of issues and yet be largely unaware of how profoundly those issues negatively affect their life. To such clients, the mind and the world are shrouded in haze and obscurity. An example is the obsessive–compulsive client who repeats and checks behaviors, knowing only that "it has to be done." Another example is the criminal who has spent a lifetime learning to victimize others. His behaviors have been validated and reinforced repeatedly by peers and the environment, to the point where he believes the only improvement needed in his life is in his skills at deception and intimidation. Clients lack awareness in different ways, but in each, the pattern is similar: confusion, ignorance, or dogmatic beliefs dominate. Another indicator of low awareness is when a clearly problematic belief or behavior is regarded by the client as an asset. This is evident when the client takes an "ignorance is bliss" kind of stance.

Additionally, it is common for a client to have acute awareness of problems in some aspects of their life while being oblivious to others. This is sometimes referred to as *splitting* or *compartmentalizing*. For instance, a client may be quite aware of her feelings about a romantic relationship but only dimly aware of the gravitas of her behavior outbursts when arguing with her partner in public. Another client may be sensitive to his partner's emotions and reactions to various situations yet have little awareness of how his own behaviors and beliefs affect his relationship. Another common example of lack of awareness is the employer who is convinced that she is loved by all but is, in reality, poorly regarded by nearly every staff member. Such people are excellent candidates for group therapy since receiving interpersonal feedback on how one is perceived by others is among its greatest therapeutic benefits (Yalom, 1995).

Another important manifestation of the lack of awareness is a general pattern of minimizing, which involves behaving as though a genuinely important event or experience is inconsequential. Minimizing typically occurs when the client claims that a problem behavior such as lying or drinking is of little or no consequence, resulting in accusations that their spouse or employer, for example, are "overreacting," "blowing things out of proportion," or "barking up the wrong tree." Both minimizing and exaggerating a problem can indicate that awareness is limited.

Without the precursor of awareness, a presenting problem will seem vague, overly generalized, or indistinct, and therapy progress will likely be slow, tedious, and difficult. More importantly, therapy techniques are likely to be ineffective to the degree that clarity of the problem is not attained. Without a focal point for techniques, the entire exercise may appear pointless to difficult clients. Thus, it is often wise, in the initial stages, to devote some time to defining and clarifying the presenting complaint, problem, or symptom.

TECHNIQUES: CULTIVATING AWARENESS

If awareness is not present and operative to some degree, the other precursors will lack focus and power in producing change. Therefore, when working with clients low in this precursor, the therapeutic task is to build or cultivate awareness so that confronting and effort resources can be brought to bear on a known problem or concern. Bringing about awareness in clients who receive low ratings in this precursor can be challenging and demands considerable creativity on the part of the therapist. This section contains several approaches to cultivating awareness in the form of metaphors, reframes, and techniques.

Metaphors That Illustrate Lack of Awareness

As with the willingness precursor, metaphors can help a client recognize that a problem or an area of life needs attention, even when the client does not initially perceive the problem. Some of the metaphors that follow are rather graphic, even off-color. However, metaphors that are used effectively will illustrate how a client has overlooked or ignored important issues. Metaphors are also meant to normalize a lack of awareness so the client does not feel criticized. A difficult client will often perceive a direct statement about lack of awareness as an insult delivered by an arrogant therapist. Metaphors help avoid this pitfall when used with tact and timing in the proper context.

Successfully using metaphors in this context is limited only by a therapist's wisdom and imagination. We have seen many memorable cases in which therapeutic change emerged through the use of a simple but powerful metaphor. To produce metaphors with great change potential, understanding the client's frame of reference is essential. Clients often provide the best metaphors themselves, whether knowingly or unknowingly, and therapists should draw upon such insights in abundance.

Blind Spots in the Rearview Mirror

This metaphor is helpful for any client who has a driver's license. The therapist tells the client that people do not see everything on the road, and that is why we have rearview mirrors: so we can be more aware of what traffic surrounds us. Unfortunately, rearview mirrors have blind spots. Relying only on the mirrors will not reveal a nearby vehicle at certain angles. Sometimes, we have to turn around and look at the road directly.

Awareness also has blind spots, and to compensate for those blind spots, we sometimes have to turn around and look; that is, inspect our minds— for thoughts, intentions, and feelings—and our environment for what is happening around and within us. This metaphor is effective in getting a client to see that there may be things they are doing or thinking that have negative consequences and to indicate that it is the right time to check things out.

Bad Breath

For some clients, this graphic, albeit crude, metaphor can be highly effective in communicating how a person can have issues or problems they are unaware of. The therapist can ask if the client has ever known someone with bad breath who had no idea of it and needed to be told. The therapist can make the point that all people have blind spots. They can then seek permission to point out a possible blind spot for the client's consideration. If the relationship is reasonably secure, the client will often give permission, even though they may not agree that they have the issue. But by that point, the door has been opened for discussion through further use of the metaphor. Another point the therapist can make is that all of us rely on someone else for feedback at certain times in our lives. In the context of therapy, a therapist's function is to provide that feedback in a trusting, confidential climate.

Body Odor

This metaphor serves the same purpose as the bad breath metaphor and can be used if and when appropriate with clients for whom it is suitable. It can be effective in conveying the idea of how a person can have a problem but lack awareness of it, especially if it affects relationships with others. Body odor can be used as a metaphor for a "behavior odor," that is, a behavior such as being obnoxious or arrogant that can get a person into difficulty, but the person is so used to it that they can no longer "smell it" or be aware of it. It is a primitive but often useful metaphor.

The Mountain Overlook

Part of attaining awareness is to step back to gain a more global view of the situation or problem. A. T. Beck (1976) referred to this psychological act as self-distancing, while proponents of acceptance and commitment therapy discuss it in the context of cognitive defusion (Hayes et al., 2011). It is often needed when a client is so deeply committed to a particular viewpoint that they will not reconsider it. Stepping back can be suggested in therapy with the help of the mountain overlook metaphor. It is easier to understand a city by looking down at it from the top of a mountain than by walking a single street or alley. The therapist can ask the client to step back and provide what might be called "the big picture" of a situation. This process can be enhanced by outlining, mapping, or diagramming the problem to get a more complete perspective. The therapist can sometimes add new aspects to the map or diagram for client consideration as part of attaining an overarching view of the problem or issue.

Finding an Example of an Unaware Person

Nearly everyone knows someone with quirks, odd habits, or idiosyncrasies, of which, it seems, the person is completely unaware. It is sometimes helpful to use this observation to create an opening through which clients low in awareness can take a fresh look at themselves. The first step is to get the client to recall someone who had strange, harmful, or otherwise eccentric habits. Once recalled, it can be pointed out that virtually all of us have quirks we are not aware of. At that point, the therapist can respectfully ask if it is possible that the client might have some habits or actions they are not aware of. The therapist then asks permission to point one out for the client's consideration. This will often help initiate the process of enhancing the awareness precursor.

Reframes That Raise Awareness

Reframes are invaluable when trying to build client awareness of a problem. As a technique, reframes have been praised as a foundational element of all psychotherapies (Barker, 2013). The most effective reframes arise from empathic attunement and can be particularly powerful when formulated in accordance with the client's language, experience, and understanding.

Reframing Negative Behaviors in a Positive Light

Marvin, age 17, was court-ordered into an outpatient treatment program for adolescent criminal offenders after a theft conviction. After only a month in the program, he had acquired the reputation of being difficult and incorrigible. He was described to the consulting therapist as a "compulsive thief and liar." Marvin had little regard for boundaries and felt entitled to own any object he perceived. This client's father, apparently a career criminal, was currently serving time in prison, and his mother's whereabouts were unknown. He was being raised by his favorite uncle, who also appeared to be a habitual criminal offender. Marvin had little or no awareness of the consequences of his actions and would not tolerate any form of discussion about theft or stealing.

It eventually became clear that, as a child, Marvin's father, mother, and uncle consistently validated and encouraged him when he came home with something stolen. Stealing made his parents proud of him. It was a source of pride and esteem for Marvin. Once aware of the historical reinforcement of stealing behaviors, the therapist began to reframe his stealing as "being a good boy." Marvin found this amusing and often laughed out loud when the therapist said it. The therapist asked Marvin if he could use that phrase in place of the word "stealing." Marvin agreed. From his perspective, the reframe was much closer to reality and greatly contributed to the fast formation of a therapeutic relationship.

Eventually, awareness of his problem emerged as he explored the contradictory messages he had received from his parents, schools, courts, and society and the consequences of those contradictions. He also developed awareness of the problem as a multigenerational family issue. Marvin's story is further explored in relation to the confronting precursor.

Awareness as Savoir Faire

For many adolescents and even some adults, awareness can be a foreign term. A solid goal in educating clients on the benefits of awareness is to help them see it as a desirable and worthy pursuit. It can help to point out that many of the people the client admires already possess awareness in some form or another, even if it is in terms of knowing what people want or "what's cool." Reframing awareness as knowing "what's happening" or "what's going down" places it in a more desirable light for many clients. Eventually, the client learns that awareness is related to therapeutic change and leads to better coping strategies and success in life. When awareness is aligned with the client's personal goals, a greater level of hope develops as the future is perceived with increased clarity. The trick is to help the client see that greater awareness is what has really been desired all along anyway.

A Situation Rather Than a Problem

Some difficult clients respond negatively at even the hint that their issue is a problem. Some boldly proclaim, "This is not a problem!" It can be a mistake to assert that a client has a problem, as a common response is for clients to stiffen or become defiant or indignant. Although many clients with a lack of awareness will not admit to a problem, they may be amenable to reframing it as "a situation that needs attention." Thus, terms like "situation," "challenge," or "puzzle" can substitute for "problem" quite nicely. One can introduce the idea by questioning and probing the consequences of the situation if it were to continue unchecked. Of course, the initial response would be a superficial denial, but this will usually diminish to the degree the situation is defined.

Getting Lost in the Thought Stream

People who are subject to compulsive behaviors such as excessive shopping, sexual acting out, checking, and substance use often find themselves caught up in escalating desires and thoughts that lead to repetition of the unwanted behavior. Therapists can help clients enhance their awareness of the phenomenon by reframing these automatic thoughts as being "lost in the thought stream." This can be combined with a metaphor of being caught up in the river rapids of the mind, which carry one away helplessly. The metaphor can then be extended by introducing the idea that it is possible to swim to the shore as well as to remain on the shore of the river, observing the rapids from a safe, calm vantage point.

The client can be guided to identify the pattern of cascading thoughts, desires, and emotions that consume them, sweeping them away in the stream. It also helps for the client to observe and identify the environmental triggers that lead to an onslaught of desires, emotions, and thoughts. The therapist may even, in a controlled fashion, recreate the cascade in the session and help the client "swim to the shore," so to speak. The metaphor of "keeping one's head above water" can further symbolize how the client avoids becoming submerged in the rapids of desires and thoughts and reaches the stability of the shore, which is, of course, sustained awareness.

Confrontation

Confrontation is perhaps as old as therapy itself and requires no explanation other than to say that it is completely different from the confronting precursor. Virtually every school of psychotherapy has a version of it, except perhaps "pure" client-centered therapy in the vein of Brodley (2002), although even therein, it has been argued that confrontation takes place in its own form and fashion (see Kensit, 2000). Regardless, confrontations remain a classically effective way to bring a client to awareness. The key to confrontation is that it be done with compassion and empathy. Otherwise, unnecessary power struggles may occur.

One example of using confrontation to catalyze the awareness precursor involved Jeff, a 24-year-old man who had just completed a year-long prison stint for assault. He was emotionally volatile, with a history of escalating minor conflicts into dangerous situations. During his recent stay at a halfway house, Jeff admitted to planning how to harm an individual who allegedly stole his sandwich out of the refrigerator. He was subsequently referred to an inpatient facility by his parole officer for observation and assessment.

Jeff presented as arrogant and defiant in group work, but he also displayed a keen self-awareness when discussing resentment over perceived injustices during individual sessions. As seen in the following transcription, the individual therapist sought to validate the perceived injustice while tapping into Jeff's self-awareness to encourage a confrontation with how anger controls him:

THERAPIST: It seems like there are times when your anger gets out of control, like the incident with the sandwich. Can you tell me more about what happened there?

CLIENT: (shrugs) Look, I know it sounds stupid, but that sandwich was mine. And when I saw it was gone and found out who took it, something just snapped. I couldn't stop thinking about it.

THERAPIST: Your anger overtook you in that moment. Do you ever feel like your anger controls you, maybe more than you realize?

CLIENT: (pauses) Yeah ... I mean, I don't know how to stop it. It's like, once something sets me off, I can't stop it. People just need to stop messin' with me.

THERAPIST: Your support team at the halfway house said they found you pacing back and forth in the alleyway with a knife in your hand, cussing and talking to yourself.

CLIENT: It wasn't a knife; it was a scrap of metal. But yeah. I blacked out, man.

THERAPIST: If only people would stop messing with you, then you could control yourself.

CLIENT: Nah, I mean, yeah. You know, I *can* control myself. But people do stupid shit like steal my sandwich, and then they need to learn a lesson.

THERAPIST:	Ah, so you can control yourself *and* you wanted to teach that sandwich thief a lesson.
CLIENT:	Yeah, something like that. I mean, people can't steal your shit and get away with it. Then they'll always just steal your shit.
THERAPIST:	Makes sense. I do have a question for you, though, Jeff. Do you really think planning to shiv someone over a stolen sandwich makes sense? Like, is that really the best way for you to let people know not to steal from you?
CLIENT:	(laughing) Uh, no, that's j-cat [crazy]. I'd go back to the clink.
THERAPIST:	And you already said that you don't want to go back to prison. You mind if I share a thought with you?
CLIENT:	Yeah, what is it?
THERAPIST:	You're a smart guy who wants to be respected. You also don't want to go to prison for stabbing a guy over a sandwich. But the fact is, you were pacing around with a shiv and planning to do some j-cat shit because some dude stole your sandwich. Anger overpowers you sometimes, and you're going to land back in prison—over a sandwich—if you don't do something about it. I'd like to help you do something different so your anger isn't running the show ... so you can run the show. What do you think?
CLIENT:	(nodding) Yeah, I get it. I've gotta stop raging out. You got ideas?

Isolating Automatic Thoughts

Automatic thoughts are often habitually repeated in a thought stream, with no conscious decision to actively form them (A. T. Beck, 1976; Vago et al., 2022). The phenomenon carried a slightly different connotation for Meichenbaum (1977), who emphasized its dialogical aspect and referred to it as negative self-talk, another commonly used term in therapy. For all practical purposes, automatic thoughts and self-talk are the same phenomenon and can be treated in the same fashion.

With regard to the awareness precursor, therapists should be alert to automatic thoughts that relate to denial of the severity or even the existence of a problem or issue. There are two primary methods of accessing and attending to automatic thoughts. The first is to have a client repeat a dysfunctional statement to the therapist, doing so out loud and with conviction. The second is for the therapist to repeat the statement directly to the client with the same level of conviction. In either case, the client then reports what thoughts arose when the statement was made, and the therapist writes the thoughts down so they may be examined and disputed later.

In the case of a client with a drinking problem, a therapist might choose the second method. The therapist can say to the client,

> I am going to make a statement to you. Please understand that I am not trying to convince you of anything; I just want to know what your immediate reaction is in your mind when I say it. The statement will be, "You have a drinking problem." Please remember that I am not trying to argue or force anything on you. Just tell me what thoughts go through your mind when I say it. Is this okay?

The client, presumably, gives consent. The therapist then repeats the statement with deep conviction and says, "Okay, what happened there?"

In many cases, the typical self-talk reported is something akin to: "My drinking is under control," "I don't have a problem," "I am doing just fine," "Nobody understands," or "I don't want to think about this." Defiant statements mixed with obscenities are also common. Such self-statements are designed to reduce awareness of the problem or issue. Awareness can be increased by focusing on these statements, examining their function in reducing awareness, and then disputing them in the cognitive behavioral fashion. Self-monitoring can be recommended so that clients can observe the operation of these thoughts in everyday life. If the therapist attempts to convince the client that there is a problem, however, the exercise can degrade into an argument.

Localizing Feelings as Sensations in the Body

Many difficult clients are unable to effectively communicate about, or differentiate among, nuanced feelings. Indeed, many such clients feel almost harassed by therapists who insist on working with feelings. According to Loevinger (1976) and other developmentalists, it is much easier for clients in lower developmental stages to identify sensations than emotions and feelings.

Often, clients can identify feelings by pointing to the location in the body where they feel tensions associated with the problem, as seen in Gendlin's (1981) focusing technique. It can be highly effective in enabling clients to eventually identify and verbalize feelings. For example, Joe, firefighter in his late 20s, sought therapy to resolve his shyness around women. When it became apparent that he had great difficulty identifying feelings, his therapist asked, "Joe, as you talk to me about your shyness, do you feel any sensations or tensions in your body?" Joe immediately pointed to his chest just under the sternum and said, "Yeah, I get really tight right here, and it's like I can't say anything."

Other clients report a feeling of tightness or heaviness in the pit of the stomach or in the chest or throat. Although a client may not be up to saying he is sad, he might have no trouble saying that he feels "choked up" in the throat. Once the area of the body is identified, the client can physically outline with the index finger how large the area is in which the sensation is felt. The sensation can then be used in self-monitoring rather than focusing on a feeling of sadness or fear that may still be too vague. From there, it is a natural progression to eventually identify actual emotions, although even then, they may only be felt and articulated in a primitive form.

Role-Plays of Others

Role-playing is part of many theories and schools of therapy and probably originated in the psychodrama school in the first decade of the 20th century (see Moreno, 1946). The adaptation of this old therapy technique is designed to facilitate the basic psychological act of stepping back or self-distancing. Role-plays can be highly effective with difficult clients when they are willing to engage in the procedure. However, many difficult clients dislike role-plays and will not engage until a relationship is well-established.

Awareness of a situation or problem can sometimes be enhanced by having a client do role-plays of people who know them well, such as current or former friends, current or former spouses or romantic partners, and family members. A trusted person is usually the best choice. Speaking as the person who cares about and knows the client well, the client becomes aware of how others view them. This technique can reveal aspects of self or behavior that have not been previously considered in therapy.

The role-play approach is particularly helpful for clients who demonstrate self-centeredness to the point of not knowing what effect they have on those around them. Following the role-play, the therapist can play the role of the trusted person and have the client respond to the earlier statements and observations given when the client played that same role.

The Empty Chair

The empty chair technique can be used as an alternative to role-plays. Typically listed in the category of experiential techniques, it is powerful in building awareness with some clients. It is another old technique that probably originated with psychodrama in the early part of the 20th century, although it is commonly associated with gestalt therapy. Unfortunately, many difficult clients will eschew this approach, steadfastly asserting that they will not talk to "a chair with nothing in it." Nevertheless, other clients will respond to this technique remarkably well in the context of a therapeutic relationship. It is one of those techniques that is best framed as an experiment (Polster & Polster, 1973).

Four modalities of roles qualify as candidates for "sitting" in the empty chair. The first is people currently available and accessible in a client's life. The second is people who have died or are otherwise no longer available. The third modality is subpersonalities or different parts of the self that have not been given a voice. The fourth modality is the client and consists of the current self, the past self (as in childhood), and the future self.

When doing the empty chair, it is important for the client to physically move into the other chair, assuming the identity that has been projected in it and communicating from that perspective. The interactive process continues until increased awareness results. The technique can result in the resolution of inner conflicts, reconciling unresolved issues with persons both dead and alive, and enhanced empathy for others.

Self-Monitoring

Behavioral and existential therapies use forms of self-monitoring to heighten awareness. Many difficult clients are not interested in homework assignments and will not do them. However, the therapist can issue a challenge to them to use awareness gained from a previous therapy session to apply in a self-monitoring context. When a client is only asked to observe themselves, the likelihood of compliance as a measured rate of homework completion increases (Kazantzis et al., 2014).

For example, Peter, a passive-aggressive client in his late 40s, was sarcastic, bitter, and defiant toward authority figures, especially in the workplace. He almost immediately displayed similar behaviors toward his therapist. Even though many of his complaints about his superiors were partially valid, his hostility made his interactions with them difficult.

During a role-play of a work situation, Peter was made aware of the intensity of his hostility toward authority. The therapist repeated the statement, "I need this by Friday," to him in the same condescending manner as his supervisor and processed it between repetitions. Before this role-play, Peter had firmly denied feeling any anger and resentment toward his supervisor, but he found it emerging through this process. Consequently, the therapist asked Peter to observe and monitor his feelings when in the general vicinity of his boss.

Peter soon reported that he had not suspected how much resentment he showed toward even the most benign directives from people in authority positions. Issues that arose between him and the therapist were used as opportunities to study his transference reactions based on his childhood spent with a verbally abusive father. As with many difficult clients, giving Peter homework tasks other than self-monitoring would have been premature and, quite likely, rebuffed.

Establishing the "Observer" or "Wise Mind"

Another tool involves helping a difficult client establish the "observer," or what Linehan (1993) called the "wise mind." Her use of the technique was effective with borderline clients and is a step beyond self-monitoring. This technique awakens the *observing self* (Deikman, 1982; Golubickis et al., 2016), that center of consciousness that is aware of and observes one's own emotions and behaviors even while acting out or giving into needs or demands. It often is present during or just after times of crisis or obsessive–compulsive behaviors (Zerubavel & Messman-Moore, 2015). It is also present when one sees the truth of a particular situation, "knows" the right thing to do despite temptations to the contrary, or when making mistakes in life.

The first step of this approach is to educate the client, letting them know that virtually every person has this capacity and that it is present and can be accessed at almost any moment. The second step is to point out a time when the client was cognizant or "used the observer" in various situations. The third step is to actively access the observer in the therapy session so that its manifestation is by choice, not circumstance. Homework assignments can then be issued in which the client uses the observer in various situations in their current environment. If a client learns this skill, the confronting and awareness precursors can be greatly enhanced.

The Use of Paradox

There are times when instructing a person to continue their lack of awareness can bring about awareness. For example, a 15-year-old girl in treatment for cocaine use was perceived as compulsively manufacturing lies by a treatment team and her fellow group members. She would not, however, admit to having such a problem and repeatedly and loudly declared that she was being unfairly accused. After some discussion, her therapist contracted with her the paradoxical directive that she was not to tell the truth in group. The therapist explained to her that she had to lie about her past, her beliefs, her behaviors, her family, and so forth. After she agreed to try this experiment, her fellow group members were also (necessarily) informed and were glad to help by going along with whatever she said, even asking her questions that required further lying on her part.

The intent of this intervention was for her to achieve an initial awareness of telling lies by consciously and constantly differentiating truth from falsehood, as required by the intervention. In other words, to be a successful liar, she also had to know what was true. Eventually, she asked the therapist if she could start telling the truth because she was "getting tired of lying." She articulated no specific insight, but after six of these group sessions, she reported that her lying was indeed a problem. Subsequently, it was much easier for her to address it as part of treatment, and her mother enthusiastically reported improvement in following up on the intervention's success. It was also a classic example of how insight can both follow and precede behavior change (see Arkowitz, 1989).

Setting and Contrasting Contexts

A problem will seem so only within particular contexts (Bateson, 1979; L. S. Brown, 2018). For instance, alcohol use does not seem a problem at all in the context of the bar and its inebriated inhabitants. In the context of family or workplace, however, alcohol use is usually seen as profoundly problematic. Similarly, some people may justify behaviors in a business context that are questionable in other contexts, such as friendships. If directed toward friends, businesslike behaviors and attitudes may be seen as cold or even cruel. Another obvious comparison arises when contrasting the killing of human beings in the context of war versus the context of murder. Both involve killing, yet the former is socially sanctioned (Shaw, 2015).

A client may come to understand that a problem, issue, or concern is acceptable in a particular context but does not transfer to others. The therapist's task in this strategy is to describe the contexts and then make the dialectical switch. By pointing out that the problem behavior is acceptable and fine in one context, the therapist can then switch the context so the negative aspects of that behavior stand in stark contrast. This approach often results in increased awareness, accompanied by a marked increase in cognitive dissonance.

One way to utilize contrasting contexts involves running groups with substance-using teenagers who insist they do not have a problem. For example, the group leader has members take turns naming the three most important things in their lives. Typically, the teens name friends, family, freedom, and love as the most important. The group leader then asks the group members to explain how using drugs and alcohol affects each one of those important aspects of their lives. This contrasting of contexts draws out many dysfunctional beliefs and behaviors and makes for spirited, animated group sessions and interesting insights. It can be done individually as well.

Acting-Out Theater

Acting-out theater is an awareness approach for groups and is not unlike what might be done in psychodrama. The technique involves designating a stage that the group can observe as an audience. One group member portrays another member's negative attitudes or acting out behaviors without saying who it is. The group's challenge is to guess which member is the one whose behavior is being portrayed. Group members must be reasonably familiar with the behaviors and attitudes of their fellows, or the approach is likely to fail. This method is especially effective with children and adolescents in both inpatient and outpatient settings where there is sufficient contact between members. One of the most interesting aspects of this technique is observing how the person being portrayed protests as the other group members loudly assert that the portrayal was indeed accurate. It has considerable potential to build awareness in clients.

Handling Intentional Unawareness

Some difficult clients deliberately reduce or diminish awareness in order to maintain a problem behavior. Such clients are unlikely to change without addressing this deliberate act. Clients whose presenting problems arise directly from treating others poorly or without compassion or empathy are often unwilling to admit they are unfeeling or insensitive. Many have deliberately dulled their awareness so they can remain convinced that they are good, decent people. These clients directly cause their presenting problems but typically blame them on others. In many clients who are harming those around them, a carefully considered choice seems to take place just outside of their awareness: Never inspect or evaluate harmful behaviors or attitudes. People who make this choice can thus be antisocial without the criminal elements that would normally qualify them for a personality disorder diagnosis.

People who have made this choice believe, usually without being aware of the belief, that if they are not aware of harming others, their selfish behaviors can continue unchecked. They deliberately and even passionately keep their continuous harmful behaviors out of awareness. We have found that many such clients will not improve until this mechanism is exposed or until they admit that their selfishness or self-centeredness is harming others. The executive who believes that he does what is best for the business or company and that he has to be "brutally honest" and direct with employees is one such example. Another is the harsh father who believes that he must be "stern" with his children and wife so he can keep them "disciplined," when in fact he is abusing them. The employee who embezzles property or company funds while rationalizing and complaining about management and how badly she is mistreated at work is another. Such people are unlikely to change because they are dedicated to remaining oblivious.

Getting a client to be cognizant of harmful or insensitive behaviors is difficult in part because the ignorance is intentional. A helpful strategy for reversing this ignorance is the use of paradox. A client can be told that, for 1 day per week, they are to be "deliberately unaware." The therapeutic task is to avoid observing how those around them—family, friends, coworkers, employers, and employees—respond to their actions. In some cases, this will actually spark awareness. In other cases, the therapist can directly challenge the client, courteously and empathically, about whether or not they really want to know how they are affecting others.

Empathy as a Remedy

In the CHANGES model, empathy is viewed not only as a necessary characteristic for an effective therapist but as a mark of mental health and well-being for people in general. Cautela (1996) observed that developing empathy in clients should be a routine aspect of therapy. He referred to the insensitivity of people who regularly harm others as *empathy immunization* (p. 341). Perhaps *empathy inurement* is more apt. Many clients who harm others lack empathy. These clients do not necessarily meet the criteria for antisocial or narcissistic personality disorders, and many have no criminal involvement, but they are similarly cold, callous, and unempathic. They are found in many walks of life, but that empathy deficit is a shared characteristic.

The idea of social interest or community feeling, Adler's most important concept (Adler, 1979; Watts & Bluvshtein, 2020), is based on the idea that a healthy person is one who is sensitive to and identifies with others, extending ultimately to all of humanity. The concept is built around empathy (see Adler, 1956; Buechner, 2023). Because they do not feel the pain of others, people lacking in empathy find it easier to perpetrate selfish acts on those around them. Nonempathic people may be so self-absorbed and limited in the awareness of others that they may be deeply and continuously upsetting those around them without a clue they are doing so. Such a person's road to change is built on becoming aware of how they contribute to so many of their problems. Rehabilitating empathy is one approach to such clients (Hart et al., 2018; Simard et al., 2023).

Perhaps the best approach for helping a person see how they affect others is the feedback received in group therapy. Yalom (1995) indicated that of all the therapeutic factors provided by group therapy, *interpersonal input* was the most important and provided the greatest therapeutic benefit. The feedback provided by group members concerning how unempathetic members affect them is invaluable, and the effective group therapist will take advantage of this at every opportunity. Such feedback can also occur in family and couples therapy. Although it can also be done in individual therapy, it lacks the dramatic impact of having one's insensitivity exposed by a group of peers.

Building Tolerance of Confusion

Another clinical observation of difficult clients lacking in the awareness precursor is that some seem to have a low tolerance for confusion, which inhibits or shuts down the development of awareness. These people can withdraw from or avoid any sort of complexity, disarray, or disorganization, and in that act of withdrawal, they abandon awareness. When the thoughts and events in their minds are in disarray, they are unwilling to explore the mess. For these people, it is helpful to outline, diagram, or draw problem situations, reactions, impulses, and anything else that may be excessively complex or confusing.

Examining Maladaptive Beliefs About Awareness

Several maladaptive beliefs interfere with cultivating awareness. If these can be isolated, identified, and successfully disputed, there may be fewer obstacles that prevent the client from developing awareness. These beliefs are so fundamental that clients cannot be expected to mention them, except perhaps in blurting one out unwittingly. The therapist would need to present each belief to a client for comment to see if they agree with the statement. In addition, the belief should be stated using language familiar to the client. Disputation and replacement are the best means for handling these beliefs. The following statements indicate maladaptive beliefs about awareness:

- "To be aware is to feel pain."
- "Awareness only makes pain more intense."
- "If I am not aware of something, it can't hurt me."
- "Awareness interferes with my fun."
- "If there is no awareness, there is no suffering."
- "Awareness is a risk and a liability."
- "Awareness only reveals how bad I am."
- "Awareness reveals how empty I am."
- "To be aware is to know that I am unlovable."
- "Awareness exposes all my faults."
- "Awareness will make me feel ashamed or guilty."

A CLOSING NOTE ON AWARENESS

Psychotherapy hardly functions without client awareness. Awareness is at the heart of all effective therapies that facilitate therapeutic change, even serving to bind theoretically opposed practices such as existential and behavioral therapies. Therapists can build awareness by calling almost any phenomenon into play for a client to consider or contemplate. At the same time, one of the hallmark challenges of therapy with difficult clients is figuring out how to activate client awareness of a problem when that client has no idea the problem exists. Upon realizing a problem, most clients become motivated to address it. However, if you don't see a problem, what is there to fix?

This is nowhere truer than in the field of drug and alcohol rehabilitation counseling. The techniques in this chapter and the addiction-focused Chapter 15 in this volume are designed to help therapists grow client awareness of problems, as well as the various thoughts, feelings, and beliefs that connect to those problems. The road from obliviousness to awareness is challenging for therapists and clients alike. However, when a client realizes they can actively contemplate nearly anything without having to be ensnared or entrapped by it, a feeling of empowerment emerges that can truly be powerful.

7

N: Necessity for Change

If necessity is the mother of invention, then it is also surely the mother of therapeutic change. A sense of necessity arises when one assesses a situation and determines that certain circumstances, feelings, thoughts, or conditions should not or must not be allowed to proceed further. When a client reaches this point, necessity for change can become a driving force in their life. Although therapeutic change can be a wonderful experience, it is not something that people seek out as a recreational diversion as they do with shopping or sporting events. Therapeutic change almost invariably requires some degree of sacrifice and disruption of routine, as well as an often uncomfortable degree of uncertainty and mystery. Before contemplating therapy, many clients must first consider it necessary. Without that motivational force, difficult clients are particularly unlikely to seriously pursue meaningful change beyond trifling with it or giving it mere lip service.

However, it must be noted that this precursor alone does not have sufficient power to produce change (Hanna, 1995). As a necessary yet insufficient condition for change, a client can have an abundance of necessity and a tremendous amount of urgency yet never accomplish therapeutic change when the other precursors are missing. A recognition of necessity may bring a person to seek therapy and indeed to seek help of almost any type, from fixing a muffler to getting one's computer repaired. However, simply having or recognizing the need is no guarantee that change will occur. It is only an admission or recognition that change is needed. There are six other precursors that work interdependently and in conjunction with necessity. At the same time, therapeutic change is unlikely without the presence of this precursor.

Case examples have been disguised to protect client confidentiality.

https://doi.org/10.1037/0000451-008
Therapeutic Change With Difficult Clients: Precursors and Techniques in the CHANGES Model, Second Edition, by B. D. Wilkinson and F. J. Hanna

HOW A SENSE OF NECESSITY LEADS TO THERAPEUTIC CHANGE

The emergence of a sense of necessity in life is a remarkable phenomenon. People often recall its precise moment of emergence with great clarity, including where it arose and how they responded to it, many years after an incident (Bellaert et al., 2022; Kemp, 2013). A recognition of necessity is more than mere motivation: It is a driving force for personal change and a major factor in many of the great political reforms throughout history (Goshe, 2019; Townshend, 1987).

A sense of necessity is thus not merely an intellectual matter of priorities or values. It has a definite affective component in the form of a felt urgency about the need for change. It also involves recognizing the importance of replacing a set of circumstances with different ones. There is a palpable feeling that the current conditions in one's inner life (e.g., sadness or anxiety) or outer life (e.g., intimidation or threat) are in some way unacceptable if left unattended. The awareness of necessity comes from assessing a situation, whether of emotion, mind, or environment, and declaring that it must be altered or ceased. A feeling of necessity is observed in the pressure felt by a child to get acceptable grades at school or a man reckoning with the need to change his behaviors to save his marriage. Other obvious examples are the desire to rid oneself of depression or the recognition that one's binge drinking must cease.

When someone recognizes that change is necessary and that things must not continue as they are, a remarkable reorganization of the person's perceptions and values takes place. This realignment orients priorities and actions toward the immediate activation of change. The way to change may not be clear, and the means of change may be obscure, but the person is indelibly certain that change must take place sooner rather than later.

When a sense of necessity arises in such a moment, something profound and deeply meaningful takes place. A cognizance dawns that something is desperately wrong and needs to be set to right. This is accompanied by a feeling of urgency, and sometimes even desperation, that indicates change must occur. Part of this feeling of "wrongness" can be viewed as a response to *cognitive dissonance* (Festinger, 1957), which arises as a feeling of discomfort or anxiety when two mutually exclusive or incompatible beliefs or perceptions are present in a person. The discomfort motivates the person to seek a reduction in the level of discomfort. Although such seeking behaviors do not always lead to a sustained change orientation, cognitive dissonance is closely tied to the complex process of therapeutic change (Axsom, 1989; Harmon-Jones, 2019).

When a client displays little or no awareness of necessity, cognitive dissonance is the therapist's best friend. As seen later in this chapter, there are ways to activate cognitive dissonance and, with it, a carefully nurtured sense of necessity. When dissonance arises, the goal is to inspire clients to actively reduce the discomfort via attitude or behavioral change rather than engage in dissonance reduction strategies, such as distraction, forgetting, trivialization, rationalization, or outright denial (McGrath, 2017). Some people deal with cognitive dissonance by seeking to resolve it, whereas others find creative ways to avoid it, particularly when the level of discomfort is insufficient to disturb maladaptive beliefs or attitudes about how life, relationships, and oneself ought to be.

SIGNIFICANT MOMENTS OF CHANGE INVOLVING A SENSE OF NECESSITY

A sense of necessity helps people act. For instance, a 33-year-old battered spouse initially questioned whether leaving her husband was the best decision. She felt there was a necessity for change, but it was not particularly strong. However, when she grasped the damage caused to her children by witnessing their mother being assaulted, her recognition of the necessity for change was sufficiently strengthened, such that she sought out a women's shelter. The woman did not yet value her own well-being enough to consider change necessary, but she considered the welfare of her children to be of the utmost importance. Preserving their safety made all risks tolerable, the threat of suffering notwithstanding.

In another example, a 41-year-old recovering alcoholic informed his therapist that a sense of necessity was crucial on the most important day of his life: The day he decided to seek recovery. Having used drugs and alcohol almost daily for 15 years, he awoke one morning with a broken tooth, stitches in his face, and no recollection of the previous night. His son recounted how he had chased some neighborhood kids who called him "a drunk," slipped while climbing a fence, and fell face-first onto the concrete. As his sons spoke, he felt deep shame and did not want to believe it. He even poured a drink to try to curb the shameful feelings, but something was different. For the first time in his life, he said, "I thought about killing myself and not hurting these people [his family] anymore." The realization that he was hurting his family activated a sense that his belligerent behaviors must end. He reoriented his life toward avoiding alcohol and drugs, put himself into treatment, and regularly attended Alcoholics Anonymous.

CLINICAL MARKERS: HOW TO RECOGNIZE A SENSE OF NECESSITY

Sometimes the easiest way to gauge the presence or absence of necessity is simply to ask the client. Some difficult clients are willing to answer this question honestly and forthrightly, but others obviously may not. If the direct question does not produce satisfactory results or if the client is manipulative or dishonest, therapists can look for certain behavioral markers in clients' nonverbal and verbal communications.

Nonverbal cues can be apparent from the very beginning of therapy, even during an initial telephone conversation. A client who feels a sense of necessity may have a tone of urgency in their voice or demeanor regardless of the problem described. This urgency might take the form of an intense determination or a plea for help. Certain emotions and feelings can also be clinical indicators. The most obvious is a fear that if change does not occur, some tragedy will ensue. In some people, the fear manifests as a frantic preoccupation with the need for change to take place. In other cases, the person broods or mopes. Apprehension, foreboding, or agitation may also manifest with the awareness of necessity for change. Anxiety, of course, is typical, especially when accompanied by cognitive dissonance.

A client with the necessity precursor tends to be alert and attentive during sessions and actively listens to what the therapist says. Such a client may seek clarification of a question or statement by the therapist and often makes intense eye contact, although people of some cultures avoid eye contact, as do many motivated children and adolescents. Posture can be indicative but is unreliable, as some clients have a high level of the necessity precursor but are also suffering from depression or fatigue that delimits their engagement. Additionally, clients with a high sense of necessity will generally attend sessions on time, but therapists must remain cognizant of the fact that childcare needs can be a hindrance for even the most motivated clients.

The clearest indicator of a client's acceptance of necessity is the importance they ascribe, either directly or indirectly, to change. Of course, this assumes that the client is being honest and is not scheming or being manipulative, as in the case of clients attempting to graduate (i.e., escape) from substance use treatment programs. Dishonesty aside, clients are often quite happy to inform a curious therapist about their awareness of necessity for change, despite being difficult in other ways.

If a person believes that change is important or that action needs to be taken when things go awry, this is an indicator that the person will likely assess a specific situation as in need of correction or change. Whether the client's locus of control is internal or external does not affect this precursor; it matters not whether the person considers the problem as being caused by the environment or by their own doing. Thus, a client with a high sense of necessity may still blame another person or institution for their problems. While such a belief may indicate a lack of other precursors, such as awareness and the readiness for anxiety or difficulty, it does not impact their necessity precursor. In fact, knowing what triggered a sense of necessity is technically irrelevant for therapists and clients alike. What matters is that it has been activated.

HOW TO DETECT THE ABSENCE OF A SENSE OF NECESSITY

When a sense of necessity is fully absent, change appears to be entirely unnecessary or a waste of effort and time. Some clients who adamantly deny a need to change have worked hard to get things the way they are in their lives and are not about to allow some therapist to wreak havoc with their carefully ordered, tightly knit system of thought and behavior. This stance can be particularly true for both criminals and executives. Some clients may appear listless, inattentive, or lackadaisical and will be late for or skip sessions altogether. Even if the client's living conditions or problems seem intolerable to the therapist, the client will appear resigned and apathetic, perhaps stating, "It's no big deal," or "There's no need to get excited." The client may make a statement that indicates a core belief is inhibiting this precursor, for instance, "Nothing really matters anyway," and will find little need to form the all-important emotionally charged bond with a therapist (Laska et al., 2014).

Alternatively, some clients low in necessity may vacillate between engagement, ambivalence, and disengagement. A lack of sustained and focused motivation to change is the most obvious indicator of a low awareness of necessity. Although such clients will usually show up for therapy, there is a feeling of tedium in session as they wait for the therapist to change their lives as though with a magic wand. They may put off or avoid completing homework assignments, even if they suggested some degree of interest during the session. In a similar vein, some court-ordered clients will appear engaged and compliant, but their sense of necessity is directed toward graduating from treatment programs and reclaiming their freedom rather than changing their problematic behaviors.

People who have experienced abuse and suffering often equate it with change that is negative and destructive. Consequently, they may unconsciously associate the prospect of any kind of change, positive or negative, with that same pain or historical trauma. Having had enough of change, they will not consider it a worthy pursuit. Others feel undeserving of anything better in their lives and may feel guilt or regret about things they have done. They may erroneously believe that getting better could be dangerous to the people around them, and the only solution is to remain publicly innocuous yet personally miserable—a twisted proof of their goodness. Finally, other clients appear uninterested in change because they have not envisioned its benefits. Such clients often battle hopelessness, becoming so discouraged with life that they believe enacting positive changes will set them up for more disappointment. They have learned that change is threatening and that the familiarity of misery is far better than the uncertainty of change.

TECHNIQUES: INSTILLING NECESSITY

Some therapists like to set goals for therapy with a client in the first or second session. The general wisdom for setting these goals is that the client and the therapist agree on their worthiness and importance. Unfortunately, without a sense of necessity, goal setting is often premature and unlikely to have its desired effect. Any goals initially set with a difficult client may not be genuine or realistic for that client, as they may be going through the motions. While there are tremendous variations in presentation, pattern, and temperament among difficult clients, a fairly reliable commonality is that difficult clients are typically low in this precursor. As a result, a more fruitful approach in the beginning stages of therapy with such clients is to instill an awareness of necessity, increase motivation, and get the client oriented in the general direction of change.

Rate the Necessity for Change From 1 to 10

Once a behavior or feeling that needs change is decided upon, the therapist can ask where, on a scale from 1 to 10 (with 10 representing the most important and urgent thing in one's life and 1 the least important), the client would rate the importance of personal change or solving the presenting problem. The response will indicate the level of urgency the client feels about the problem. This quick, simple rating helps determine how important therapy is to the client and provides a clue to their degree of motivation. If someone else says the client has a problem—for example, a judge or a spouse—they should rate the problem in the same way.

If the client gives a low rating, which is to be expected, the therapist can ask what it would take to get the rating up to, say, 7 on the scale. Do not imply that it should be 7; only ask what would have to happen to get it there. Answers to this question might be, "If I knew I was hurting someone," or "If I thought I would get in trouble." Such answers provide insights into what motivates the client and what they consider important. The next step is to connect the problem to those evaluations of importance, so as to increase the level of necessity.

Find Out if Change Is Important to the Client

For some clients, rating something on a scale of 1–10 is not particularly interesting or appealing. The problem may be too vague, or the person may blame someone else for causing the problem or issue and want the blamed person to solve it. Rating may also seem too much like a game the therapist is making them play, and the client may not be interested in what looks like "jumping through a hoop."

If the client is involuntary or has no presenting problem or issue, it can help if the therapist suggests a few possible examples to determine the kinds of change the client may be interested in. These suggestions can be as mundane as getting in better physical shape or as abstract as being better able to solve problems or make friends. Once a client hints at a desirable change, the therapist can ask if it would be nice to have that change actually happen. If a change is regarded as desirable, the therapist can ask if it is a little important, highly important, or urgent. This is a more casual alternative to the 10-point scale and takes a little more time. In any case, the desired change should not be dismissed, as it can serve as a stepping stone in the direction of change activation. Thus, therapy should be reoriented to help bring about the desired change.

Find Something Important to the Client and Align It With Therapy

In cases of a trace or nonexistent level of necessity, a client might deny any need to work on a problem and display outright apathy about resolving it. If a therapist were to point out a particularly negative problem or situation, the client might shrug and say, "So what?" A classic problem in psychotherapy is how to motivate such a client. For such clients, going directly after change is asking too much. It is much better to find out what is important to the client in their overall worldview. Reflecting meanings can help here (see Chapter 3, this volume). The therapist can then instill a sense of necessity by aligning therapy to whatever is most important to the client.

The Story of Carl

For example, Carl was a difficult client who was suspicious of therapy and lacking in verbal and articulation skills. He sat with his arms crossed and slouched far back in his chair. Carl was 36 years old and had two children with his wife, Ginger. He had worked in an automobile textile factory for 21 years. He claimed to have problems with his marriage. It was clear for the first half hour of the first session that Carl was rigid and unbending in his thinking and convinced he did not have a problem. He was especially low in the necessity and willingness precursors. The dialogue begins with addressing the metalogue:

THERAPIST:	Tell me if I'm wrong, but we have been talking for a while now, and it seems you don't care much for any of this therapy stuff?
CLIENT:	Yeah, you're right about that.
THERAPIST:	I see. So here we are, doing something that you really don't care about, and it's all supposed to be about you anyway. That must be a pretty strange position to be in.
CLIENT:	Right again. No offense, but this doesn't interest me much.
THERAPIST:	Yeah … Let me get this straight. You originally said you are here to save your marriage, but really you're just here because your wife demanded it. You really don't expect anything to actually happen.
CLIENT:	Well, I guess. She said that I really needed it, so here I am talking to you.
THERAPIST:	But you really don't expect much to change.
CLIENT:	(looking at the therapist intently but briefly) To be honest, no, I don't.
THERAPIST:	So, as far as you see it, you think you're pretty much okay.

CLIENT:	Yeah. I mean, I ain't perfect, but she makes a big deal about lots of things that ain't important.
THERAPIST:	Like what?
CLIENT:	Like I said, it ain't important.
THERAPIST:	You don't feel like talking about it.
CLIENT:	You got it. (adds a smug smile)
THERAPIST:	Okay. I get the message. But it's part of my job to ask questions. And we have to fill up the time somehow. Do you mind if I ask you a question now and then? You obviously know you don't have to answer anything if you don't feel like it.
CLIENT:	(with a wave of his hand) Go ahead.
THERAPIST:	You seem to be a guy who is pretty sure of himself. There must be something wrong in your life, or you wouldn't be here talking to somebody like me. I have to think that if you didn't care about your marriage, you wouldn't be here at all. Am I wrong?
CLIENT:	No. You ain't wrong there.
THERAPIST:	So, the marriage is important to you. (Client nods.) My guess is you think your wife is the one with the problems, and she's the one that should be in here.
CLIENT:	Yep.
THERAPIST:	Okay. But before we get into all that, can I ask you a question, Carl? (Client nods.) How important is it for you to save your marriage? A little? A lot? Give me an idea.
CLIENT:	I guess it's pretty important. I don't want to get divorced. I don't want to go through all that bullsh— again.
THERAPIST:	So, you've done it before, and it was pretty rough.
CLIENT:	Yeah.
THERAPIST:	Carl, I'll make you a deal. Tell me what you think. You and I will work on saving your marriage. I can see you went through a pretty rough time before, and you don't want to get divorced again. I might be able to help. Is it worth giving it a shot?
CLIENT:	(nodding slowly and deliberately) Okay.

Carl's interest was sparked, and with it, an alignment of purposes arose between client and therapist. What was important to him was now connected to and aligned with therapy.

The Story of Nick

Another example of this approach was in the case of Nick, a 22-year-old client who said that having sex was the most important thing in his life. He had had a few relationships and dozens of one-night stands and said that sex made him feel "great." He was in therapy because of a problem with alcohol but was not interested in working on that at all, despite his employer recommending it. When asked if he ever felt empty after any of those one-night stands, Nick genuinely and openly laughed at the therapist. From his perspective, he had good reason. He was already so empty that sex was one of the few things that could occupy the void in his life. In his narcissism and lack of empathy, he was aware of little else other than his own needs.

Cautiously, the therapist advanced the idea that therapy could help him understand women better. For the first time, his interest was kindled. He had no idea, of course, that the therapist's intent was to help him acquire empathy for women as opposed to exploiting them. He eventually admitted that many women thought he was, in his words, "a jerk," and the therapist helped him to see why. This single inroad led to working on many of Nick's issues, including his alcohol use.

Addressing and Using Subpersonalities

An approach that is often successful in motivating indifferent and apathetic clients has to do with addressing subpersonalities. This approach is based on century-old ideas in psychotherapy that assume that the human personality comprises many separate parts, each containing different attitudes, purposes, and interests. It is not at all the same as multiple personality or dissociative identity disorder. This phenomenon has been described in various ways across the writings of Jung (1934/1969), Assagioli (1965), and James (1890/1981). While the concept of subpersonalities is central to internal family system therapy (Schwartz & Sweezy, 2019), it also plays a role in various transpersonal and humanistic therapies. One of the most effective ways of dealing with apathy is acknowledging and accepting its presence, building empathy, and avoiding power struggles. From there, using a subpersonality can be helpful. The following story illustrates the technique.

The Story of Tracey

Tracey was a 17-year-old high school senior who displayed a majority of the characteristics of borderline personality disorder. She engaged in self-mutilation (cutting and scratching designs into her wrists and forearms with various sharp implements) and reported that it made her feel better. She often stated that life was too depressing to be worth living. She had a history of sexual abuse perpetrated by an uncle and was promiscuous with boys who were clearly interested only in using her. She regularly abused drugs and alcohol and occasionally engaged in binging and purging. She was extremely vigilant for the slightest sign of a lack of caring or presence by the therapist and engaged in intense emotional outbursts at such times. A phrase she used several times to describe her perceived lack of affect was that she felt "empty inside," and it was clear she had little or no sense of self, being almost totally dependent on others for any sense of identity. At the time of the critical session, Tracey was failing three subjects in school.

There were a host of issues on which to focus with Tracey. Unfortunately, she was deeply apathetic about doing anything for herself. Whenever it was suggested to her that she do something for herself or that she might take better care of herself, she merely shrugged her shoulders and said, "Whatever." When asked if she was concerned that her boyfriends might be taking advantage of her desire to be liked, she admitted that she thought this was true and that she hated men, but she showed no awareness of the necessity for change. The "whatever" response appeared again when Tracey was asked if she cared about her failing grades and again when she was asked if she ever worried about what was going to happen to her. This did not appear to be a game or power struggle on her part. It was as though her necessity for change was frozen or paralyzed, as if something vital and dynamic in her personality was missing—a characteristic often seen in personality disorders.

When the critical session occurred, she had had 15 previous therapy sessions. By this time, a fairly strong relationship had been established with a reasonable amount of trust. After seeing no change but recognizing the pain this client routinely experienced, the therapist decided to use a different approach. Being met by indifference and apparent apathy at every turn, the therapist decided to believe this girl was not as dedicated to being as miserable as she appeared. Her wall of apathy was still imposed on the therapist, who struggled to find a way to get around, past, or through it. The therapist decided to try the subpersonality approach.

The therapist said, "Tracey, from what you have told me, it seems like you know things are not quite right in your life and could be much better, but you don't seem to really want to change anything. Is that right?" Tracey smiled and said, "Yeah, I guess so." "Well, can I ask you another question? And if it's okay, I would really like you to think about this one before you answer." She looked at the therapist a bit suspiciously but then agreed. The therapist continued. "Tell me, Tracey, is there a part of you, some tiny little part of you, that worries about what is going to happen to you?" Hesitantly, she asked, "What do you mean?" The therapist replied, "Maybe it's a little voice in the back of your mind or some part of you that you don't pay any attention to, but I wonder if there is that part of yourself that is worried about what is going on in your life."

She looked at the therapist, unsure of this new territory, and said, "Yeah, there are times when I hear a little voice that says things like 'You shouldn't do that' or 'You have to study,' things like that." The therapist was cautiously enthusiastic; it seemed some progress might be occurring. Even her tone was different. "How much of the total you is that part that cares?" Many clients can give percentages—for example, 20% or the like—but this was not her style. She was noncommittal. The therapist took out a piece of paper, drew a circle, and said, "Pretend this circle is like a pie that represents all of your personality. Can you draw a slice of it that shows me how big that part of you is that cares about what will happen to you?"

She drew a wedge that represented 25% of the total. This was, surprisingly, quite a bit, as many difficult clients draw 10% or less, although other clients judged as difficult can estimate up to 40%. "Can I talk to that part of you, Tracey?" She thought about it briefly and said, willingly, "Sure." Sensing that a therapeutic window was opening, the therapist immediately asked this newly identified part of Tracey, "I understand that you are worried about what's going to happen to you; is that true?" She looked at the therapist steadily, but her face seemed a touch softer than before. "I am very worried. I think I do a lot of things that are wrong and get myself into trouble. And like, I know better, but I don't stop it."

"Like, what do you do that's wrong?" Tracey paused and said, "Like what I do with boys, for one thing, and I drink too much and smoke too much weed." This was a brand-new side of Tracey coming out now. "Is it like your life is out of your control?" She looked down, seemingly sad as she agreed, "Yeah." Once again, the therapist tried to see if she was interested in change. "Would you be interested in changing the things that get you in trouble and get more control over your life?" Tracey paused for a moment, looked up at the therapist, and said, "Yeah."

"How about if we work together on this in counseling?" She nodded, and the therapist, gathering momentum, forged ahead. "Help me understand something, Tracey. Remember the pie?" She nodded again. "If the part of you that wants to change is 25% of the whole pie, is it fair to say that the other 75% of you is out of your control?" Tracey said softly, "I never thought about it like that, but yeah, I guess that's about right." The stage was finally set. "How much control would you like to have?" She thought about it for a while, then took the pen and paper and drew another pie circle. This time, she shaded in about 75%. "That's how much," she said, looking intently at the therapist. "So, you want 75% control instead of the 25% control over yourself that you have now?" She looked at the therapist almost longingly and asked, "Can I do that?" The therapist replied, "It is definitely possible, and we can give it our best shot. Are you willing to give it a try?" Tracey looked like she was preparing for a fight. Finally, she said, "Yes."

For the first time, Tracey was a motivated client with a sense of necessity for change. The apathetic Tracey would often emerge, but it was now identified as such. When it did happen, it was relatively easy to access the part of her that she eventually came to call "the real me," which grew in size relative to the rest of the pie. As far as the precursors were concerned, she was now on the rails toward change and was responsive to established therapy approaches. Although she never achieved change in leaps and bounds, she did manage to make steady progress.

The Use of Cognitive Dissonance

Therapists have long known that cognitive dissonance can lead to change (Festinger, 1957; Harmon-Jones, 2019). It begins with the presentation of incongruent, inconsistent, or contradictory information concerning the self, beliefs, behaviors, or lifestyle. This produces anxiety, which is followed by a desire to resolve the incongruency and anxiety. This desire is closely related to a sense of necessity. There are many ways to produce cognitive dissonance; some are innocuous and simple, whereas others are provocative and require more skill and finesse.

Are You Getting What You Want?

An established method of producing cognitive dissonance can be borrowed from reality therapy (Glasser, 1965). It is a three-stage process that begins with asking a client the general question, "What do you want in your life?" This may or may not be related to the presenting problem, if there is one named at all. The answer to this question should not be superficial, such as getting a Ferrari or winning the lottery. For this approach to work, it is important to concentrate on getting a proper reply from the client, that is, one that is somehow related to cognition, affect, behavior, or relationships. A client might say they want happiness, love, work, or more friends.

Once this is established, the second step is to find out what the person is doing in their life relative to the want or desire. For example, a 15-year-old young man may say he wants more friends. Some exploration reveals that he is angry at many people, including teachers, family members, and peers. Further inquiry reveals he is suspicious, untrusting, critical, and abrasive toward those around him and given to temper outbursts as well. It is not surprising that he lacks friends when what he is doing is alienating and antagonizing people.

With this information, the final question is posed to the client in this way: "You have told me how you interact with people—saying mean things and losing your temper. Is what you are doing getting you more friends? Is it working for you?" When the client admits that it is not working, the therapist can ask if the client is willing to explore different ways of making friends that may be more efficient than what he has already tried. On the other hand, if the client is hesitant to say that it is not working, it can be effective to present the problem in a single sentence and wait for a response: "Explain to me how you can make friends by driving people away from you." Assuming that the client really does want to make friends, this approach can be effective in many cases. Once again, producing cognitive dissonance produces discomfort or anxiety, which allows the therapist to point out a well-established way to alleviate that anxiety: therapy.

What Would Happen if Nothing Changed?

Another way of producing cognitive dissonance is by asking a client what would happen if nothing changed, that is, if the client continued to do little or nothing about the issue or problem. This approach assumes the client has at least trace levels of awareness that there is an undesirable situation in their life. The question is whether the problem would stay the same or get worse. Typically, a difficult client will assert that a problem stays the same if unattended. However, if a therapist can establish a pattern of decline or progressive worsening of the problem over time, this can lead to an increase in dissonance and, thus, a sense of necessity for change. For example, if a client consistently blames others for problems that are mostly due to their own actions, ask if the blaming has served to resolve the problem. One can also ask if the blaming makes the client feel better, and if so, how much and for how long. The answer is usually something on the order of "Not so much, and not so long as I'd like."

Spitting in the Client's Soup

A technique called *spitting in the client's soup* is a way of increasing anxiety levels in the interest of change. Adler (see Dinkmeyer et al., 1987) originated this version of raising anxiety levels and gave it its name. This technique is especially useful for clients who boast about disorderly or destructive behavior. There are many situations worthy of this dynamic confrontation technique. Obvious examples include when clients report destroying a coworker's reputation, enticing a friend's spouse into having an affair, or loving competition to the point of always trying to outdo friends or family members.

Spitting in the client's soup requires a considerable amount of skill to be done smoothly, using a dispassionate, casual, and somewhat aloof demeanor while remaining empathic and compassionate. To be successful, the therapist's voice must be free of even the slightest inflections or intonations that hint at resentment, impatience, condemnation, or moral judgment. Because many difficult clients are extremely sensitive to being judged as a bad or wicked person, the therapist's voice must remain steady, curious, and caring. If the slightest trace of the therapist's personal issues becomes evident, many clients will pick up on it and immediately initiate a power struggle. It is also important to remember that the client is never discouraged from, or told not to engage in, the questionable behavior. The purpose is to make a behavior unattractive but not interfere with free choice. The following illustrates this technique.

The Story of Jason

Jason was a 27-year-old factory worker presenting with depression about his marriage and life in general. In the first session, it was clear that Jason was only toying with therapy and minimizing his problem. His rating for the necessity precursor was 1. In the third session, he disclosed that he had cheated on his wife with a number of women, both before and since he had been married. When asked to be more specific, he reported with great certainty that his many transgressions were necessary to his self-confidence and that it was the only thing that could get him out of his depression. He was convinced that his affairs had nothing to do with the difficulties in his marriage, and he maintained that the failing marriage was all his wife's fault.

CLIENT:	Look, I'm good at hooking up. Women love me. My wife doesn't love me like that anymore, so I've got to get mine. If you're good at something, you got to get it. I mean, it makes me feel good, you know what I mean? I love sex more than anything.
THERAPIST:	So, having these affairs is important to you, almost like a lifesaver for your ego.
CLIENT:	(pausing) Exactly ... I guess.
THERAPIST:	Just curious, Jason; do these women know you're married?
CLIENT:	Of course not.
THERAPIST:	What would they say if they knew?
CLIENT:	They wouldn't like it, so I don't tell them. C'mon, man! How do you expect me to hook up if I say I'm married?
THERAPIST:	So, all these women that you seduce are just like your wife. They want loyalty and faithfulness just like she does.
CLIENT:	Yeah (smiling), they're all the same, you know. They want me to be faithful and take care of 'em and all that. What they don't know won't hurt 'em.
THERAPIST:	I see. Am I right to say that the pleasures in your life depend on hurting people?
CLIENT:	(visibly stiffens at the statement) Well, I wouldn't say it like that. I make women feel real good, you know.
THERAPIST:	Jason, I believe that you're a good person who doesn't want to hurt anybody.
CLIENT:	Yeah, that's right. I am.
THERAPIST:	But I'm also tempted to believe that feeling good is so important to you that you're willing to hurt some nice, decent people just so you can feel good yourself.
CLIENT:	(long pause) Nah, man.
THERAPIST:	Can I say something else, and you tell me what you think?
CLIENT:	Yeah, you're going to tell me anyway.
THERAPIST:	If I was mean and uncaring toward the feelings of people who cared about me the way you are toward your wife and these other women, I'd be depressed, same as you.
CLIENT:	(shaking head) But it's the only thing that makes me happy.

THERAPIST:	I'm not telling you to stop, Jason. I'm wondering if the one thing that makes you happy in one way makes you really unhappy in a bigger way.

THERAPIST: I'm not telling you to stop, Jason. I'm wondering if the one thing that makes you happy in one way makes you really unhappy in a bigger way.

CLIENT: (mixed anger and sadness) What, so you're saying I have to stop having sex?

THERAPIST: No, not at all. It's kind of like a man who's stuck on a diet of beef jerky. He has a need for a good steak, but he doesn't know there's such a thing. He knows there has to be something better, but all he ever gets is beef jerky. That might be the case with you. Maybe you never learned how close relationships can make you even happier than sex and that sex in a close relationship can be particularly good.

CLIENT: But hooking up makes me feel better *now*. I don't know what to do about my wife.

THERAPIST: I understand what you're saying, but the question is whether the effort might be worthwhile. If all you know is beef jerky, then you've never had the real pleasure of trying a porterhouse or filet mignon. It could be worth the extra effort.

CLIENT: (with a tone of protest) So, you're saying I need to try to fix things with my wife.

THERAPIST: I'm only asking if any of this makes sense to you, and if so, whether you're willing to try something different and see if it helps with your depression. I'd also like your permission to find out some of your beliefs about women and relationships. These attitudes might be part of your depression. Are you willing to give it a try?

CLIENT: Yeah. I mean, I see what you're saying. We can try it.

With this approach, the therapist instilled a sense of necessity in Jason by spitting in his soup and using a metaphor relevant to his situation. He was more willing to discuss his depression and no longer minimized the affairs to the same degree. The remainder of that session, and the next several, were spent discussing the notion of viable and satisfying relationships and how not having them in one's life can lead to depression. Jason's beliefs about women were examined and linked to his depression and failing marriage. Eventually, he engaged in couples therapy with his wife.

Identify Secondary Gains or Cross-Purposes

For many clients, therapeutic change is in direct conflict and at cross-purposes with other goals. A sense of necessity for change will not emerge if there is a greater necessity to remain the same. The problem, disorder, or issue is retained because it serves a purpose that the client deems important, usually referred to as *secondary gain*. Take, for example, the case of a person who receives worker's compensation for a painful back injury. The person is referred to a clinic that includes therapy for the emotional and psychological aspects of managing the pain. Some of these clients are highly difficult to work with because any decrease in pain threatens their eventual financial settlement. Thus, the client will resist any decrease in perceived pain to eventually gain financial reward, usually through a lawsuit.

Another example of secondary gain is in the case of a client with explosive anger outbursts. Such a client typically recognizes how quickly others comply just to avoid confrontation. Thus, it pays to hold on to and use the angry attitude to maintain control over others. Malingering, or illness used to gain attention and care from others, is an established example of secondary gain.

It is often tricky to determine what purpose the problem, disorder, or issue serves, and many clients find it difficult to identify and discuss secondary gain. It is sometimes up to the therapist to suggest it as such. When identified, it is often helpful and rewarding to weigh the benefits of change against the benefits associated with the secondary gain. It also helps to rate the benefits of change and of remaining the same, and when possible, to find a solution that will bring the benefits of both. If a client sees the irrationality of maintaining a disorder or problem, an awareness of necessity will likely arise that can motivate the person toward change.

Recognizing the Client's Need for Power or Control

Some difficult clients believe that change is tantamount to an admission of defeat and a loss of pride. This belief interferes dramatically with the necessity precursor. Such clients may compete with the therapist to prove they are fundamentally smart and savvy.

There is not necessarily a power struggle here, but there is a double bind. On the one hand, to admit to the need for change brings about a feeling of being stupid and wrong. On the other, to deny the need for change leads to feelings of hopelessness and apathy. It is extremely important for such clients to see any move toward change as their own idea and as brought about under their own power. If a therapist has any need to be acknowledged for great therapeutic ideas or interventions, there will be a higher chance of failure with this type of client. Such clients often take pride in the way they have lived their lives and in the way they have survived hard times. It is difficult for them to admit to making mistakes. The bottom line is they must feel like the final decision to change was their own brilliant, self-determined choice—and so it is.

Giving Voice to Loneliness

Loneliness is a common feature of anxiety and depression that has become increasingly prevalent (Haidt, 2024). There is an aspect of loneliness that can be painful, and some clients are responsive to the idea of loneliness as a kind of hurt due to separation. At some stage, the client who admits to being lonely might be ready for this approach. Some are ready sooner, and some not at all, but it can be worth a try. The prospect of easing the pain of loneliness can be used to motivate some clients to become involved in therapy by increasing a sense of necessity.

Story of Jeannie

Jeannie was a 17-year-old girl in treatment for a meth addiction. She had few or no friends by her own admission, and fellow clients in her treatment program for teens had rejected her due to their belief that she was constantly lying and "fronting" (i.e., putting on a false veneer to impress people). Jeannie was hostile toward peers and defiant toward treatment program personnel.

Nonetheless, her therapist had established a reasonably close therapeutic relationship that allowed for some honest self-disclosure on Jeannie's part. A significant self-disclosure was reporting to the therapist that she was lonely and that although she wanted friends, she didn't know how to make them. She said meth took away all of her negative feelings and made her feel good and believe in herself. But, upon questioning, she admitted that after the meth wore off, her loneliness was much more intense, which in turn, increased her desire to use again at the earliest opportunity.

The therapist asked her if she felt the loneliness somewhere in her body, and Jeannie nodded. The therapist asked her to name the part of the body where she felt it and then point to it. Jeannie pointed at the center of her chest and said, "Here, in my chest." The therapist asked her to outline the area with her index finger and asked, "Does it hurt?" Jeannie nodded again. The therapist asked her to look inside her chest and report what was in there. Jeannie replied, "Nothing." Next, the therapist highlighted that Jeannie had said there was loneliness and hurt there, to which Jeannie reluctantly responded, "It's kind of nothing, but it also feels lonely and hurtful."

At this stage, the therapist, having set up the key question, asked, "If that feeling of loneliness weren't there, would you use meth as much as you do?" Jeannie shook her head. The therapist then stated, "If you could make almost all of that loneliness feeling go away without the drug, would you do it?" Jeannie paused for some time, staring at the floor, and said, "Well, yeah. Can you do that?" The therapist carefully explained that reducing that feeling is the purpose of counseling, and if she agreed, they could make that their goal. Jeannie agreed, and in the following twice-weekly sessions over 60 days, a variety of cognitive and experiential techniques were applied to the point where Jeannie reported a 70% reduction in the loneliness and hurt and a corresponding greatly reduced degree of craving for meth.

Use Feeling Good as a Motivating Force

It is amazing what people will do to reduce suffering. It is one of the major reinforcers in all of life. Going to therapy is just one of the things that people will do to reduce suffering and bring desirable feelings into their lives. Taking illegal drugs is another. One of the hidden promises of therapy has to do with holding out the possibility of feeling good. In itself, it is a rather crude entice-ment, but it can be persuasive to clients who think in hedonistic terms. If a client can be convinced that therapy may make them feel better, a sense of necessity may well emerge out of dark emotions and bitter attitudes. No promises should be made, of course, but it is certainly fair to mention feeling good as a possible outcome.

Examining Maladaptive Beliefs About Change Itself

Maladaptive beliefs inhibit the necessity precursor for most clients, particularly those who have never verbalized such beliefs. Knowing this, it is sometimes helpful to infer the belief and submit it to the client, awaiting their comment. For example, a therapist could say, "I sometimes get the sense from you that, deep down, you believe that nobody ever gets any better, so why bother. Is this true for you?" Once identified and disputed in classical cognitive therapy fashion, the doors to change, including second-order change, can be opened. Examples of maladaptive beliefs that can inhibit or prevent a sense of necessity are

- "I don't care about anything."
- "I'm fine the way I am."
- "I don't care what happens to me."
- "If I change, I'll feel terrible."
- "I don't deserve anything good, so why even think about it?"
- "Only fools think they can better themselves."
- "There is nothing worth trying for in this world."
- "Nobody ever really gets better, so why bother?"
- "If the problem were to change, it would only get worse."
- "If I changed, it would only mean that [a specific disliked person] was right."
- "Everybody is screwed up, so why should I be any different?"

A CLOSING NOTE ON A SENSE OF NECESSITY

The ancient philosopher Epictetus (ca. 130/1944) held that the recognition of necessity was a guide for human action and a key to human freedom. A sense of necessity may lead a person to seek freedom from many limiting circumstances, although a certain amount of inspiration is necessary. For example, no one in their right mind would put their hand in a fire if prompted. However, if an infant were seen to be wandering into flames, most people would consider it necessary to risk the flames to save the child. Because therapy often involves dealing with painful memories, confusing thoughts, and intimidating situations, people will not generally contemplate such unpleasant things without an awareness of necessity. People tend to avoid pain unless there is some perceived necessity to face it. Therefore, it is often incumbent upon the therapist to learn ways to identify, lean into, and grow a sense of necessity for change with difficult clients.

8

G: Grit, or Willingness to Experience Anxiety or Difficulty

Psychological grit as a personality tendency denotes "perseverance and passion for long-term goals" (Duckworth et al., 2007, p. 1087) and is generally associated with measures of goal-oriented achievement (Lam & Zhou, 2022). Within the precursors model, *grit*, or *the willingness to experience anxiety* or *difficulty*, can be defined as an openness to allowing change processes to occur, accompanied by a preparedness to feel the anxieties, emotions, and difficulties that routinely manifest as a result. This precursor therefore involves a meta-cognitive capacity to tolerate and even welcome emotional pain, confusion, or intimidation. It denotes surrendering to the change process, as grit metaphorically requires rolling up one's sleeves, gritting one's teeth, and preparing to get one's hands dirty. There is also an element of courage in facing the anxiety and difficulty that often comes with both the process and therapeutic results of change.

When this precursor is established, the client acknowledges anxiety rather than evading or shunning it. Further, the client acknowledges the difficulty that comes with change and is willing to tolerate it so that change can take place. Alternatively, grit is often a missing ingredient when therapists are puzzled by unchanging clients. Many difficult clients want change to occur without having to endure anxiety or difficulty along the way. As such, consideration of this factor can aid therapists in understanding why certain difficult clients appear unable to make any lasting progress toward change and in providing suitable approaches and techniques that can help.

Case examples have been disguised to protect client confidentiality.

https://doi.org/10.1037/0000451-009
Therapeutic Change With Difficult Clients: Precursors and Techniques in the CHANGES Model, Second Edition, by B. D. Wilkinson and F. J. Hanna

Grit is the diametric opposite of *defensiveness*, which is usually defined as the effort to avoid anxiety due to some kind of threat. Openness to experience, as opposed to defensiveness, has long been associated with successful outcomes in literature reviews (Hill et al., 2022; Lynch et al., 2015; Orlinsky et al., 1994). If the person is not ready to meet the difficulties inherent in the change process, they will likely balk at any movement in that direction. Frank (1961) originally pointed out that a common factor of any successful therapy involves the client becoming emotionally aroused. This precursor is also related to the "corrective emotional experience" that interpersonal therapists tend to emphasize as a central aspect of change (see Teyber & Teyber, 2014).

ANXIETY OFTEN ACCOMPANIES CHANGE

Introducing change into a rigid mindset often requires some confusion and disorder. The same is true for a mindset that is chaotic and disjointed. Both types of client are likely to resist change, even though they may be in desperate need. Therapeutic change appears to such clients as confusion and disorder, when it is actually a process of establishing a higher degree of order and function and is a natural part of the improvement process.

For example, when one does spring cleaning, disorder manifests in displacing furniture and household items while sweeping and dusting. If the disorder is resisted, the improvement cannot take place or is significantly hindered. Cleaning sometimes initially requires making a mess. Similarly, to an out-of-shape, unconditioned body, the early part of a physical exercise program looks more like pain and stress rather than muscle toning and cardiovascular health.

Likewise, when one's habitual thoughts and behaviors need altering, some mental confusion and disorder are inevitable and often produce anxiety. A mindset filled with dysfunctional beliefs and painful memories is in delicate balance. When one is not secure in the first place, the mere thought of altering one's beliefs or dredging up memories can produce a sense of unease or difficulty that reverberates throughout the entire mental framework. If one fights this process, change does not occur. Thus, in the real world, if a therapist, judge, spouse, probation officer, or teacher requires or recommends a change in thinking or behavior, some people perceive such a recommendation as an insult or attack. This anxiety can arise as a factor in clinical practice. If a client can be educated to recognize and be willing to experience such anxiety and disorder, they will likely be more amenable to the change process.

PHILOSOPHICAL ROOTS

This precursor has some interesting philosophical grounding. Heidegger (1927/1962) was probably the first to describe it and note its importance for change. One of the most important philosophers of the 20th century, Heidegger wrote the classic, deeply insightful book *Being and Time*. Much of this book was highly psychological in nature, and he defined and noted the importance of achieving authenticity as a human being and outlined how to achieve it. Heidegger (1927/1962) used the term *resoluteness* to describe being "ready for anxiety" (p. 343) and emerging from a sense of "lostness" (p. 345) toward authenticity. He said that to be resolute, one has to follow one's own growth path, which often requires going against the grain of empty habits as well as social pressures and demands. He used the term *fallen* to indicate a person who has given in to societal and personal inclinations toward avoidance and disingenuousness. Resoluteness involves recognizing those inclinations and pressures, refusing to be carried away by them, and choosing instead to move steadfastly toward being authentic. "Resoluteness" would be quite acceptable as the name for this precursor if it were slightly more descriptive.

OWNING THE PROBLEM

It has often been noted in the psychotherapy literature that a client will begin to make progress when they "own" the problem and stop complaining about it or blaming others for it. A person owns the problem when they acknowledge and accept that it is real, that it must be addressed, and that it is their own responsibility to do so. *Responsibility* can be defined as the willingness to take charge, control, or command of any memory, thought, image, problem, behavior, relationship, or feeling. When a person takes responsibility for a problem or issue, they are far more likely to see the issue through to its resolution Acceptance of a problem or issue is central to 12-step programs, with the Alcoholics Anonymous (2012) literature citing acceptance as a powerful influence on abstinence and recovery.

When a client has a sense of necessity but is not willing to experience anxiety or difficulty, the client will typically want the therapist to do most of the work. It is like knowing that the house is in dire need of cleaning but not being willing to go to all the trouble to clean it. Such a client will dump rather than describe their issues and problems. *Dumping* is characterized by exaggerating the problem's severity, a desire to be rescued from the problem, and very little willingness to own the problem or issue. Such clients are avoidant of important or key issues and prefer to keep things at a superficial level. They may claim that therapy is not helping and blame the therapist for the lack of change. Deep down, these clients are experiencing pain and discomfort and want therapy to provide the magic wand to make it all go away. They may even mistakenly believe that therapy is designed and intended to enable them to avoid or eschew pain and discomfort.

HOW GRIT LEADS TO CHANGE

As a willingness or readiness to experience anxiety or difficulty, grit involves surrendering to the process of change itself. The person lets go of established routines and habitual behaviors or thought patterns and is open to the possibility of forever altering them. But the key contribution to change is delving headlong into the unknown. With therapeutic change—and especially second-order change—awareness of the unknown causes no small amount of anxiety.

Thus, the willingness to admit oneself into the disarray that comes with the disruption of established and settled mindsets and behaviors is an essential act in the change process. For change to occur, a client must be willing to "give up or modify clinging to the past" (Strupp, 1988, p. 78) and welcome the new or unfamiliar. Negative feelings and anxieties must be acknowledged as they arise. Over time, the client learns to assimilate and integrate problem experiences under new headings or schema, so what was once disordered becomes understandable, no longer rejected but recognized, acknowledged, and accepted (Tedeschi & Moore, 2021).

The psychodynamic term "working through" has become a household expression. Many things can be worked through, and it is grit that facilitates the process. The presence of this precursor readies the person to reduce hesitance, break through self-imposed limits, and take command of the uncomfortable emotions that result. This precursor does not cause these acts, which will become clear when we examine the precursor of effort or will. However, just as will can lead one to take such "risky" actions as going white-water rafting or riding a giant roller-coaster, the willingness to experience anxiety or difficulty also involves engaging in risk.

When this precursor is abundant, it can produce a sense of adventure that makes the change endeavor not only possible but pleasurable. Even when a client is examining the effects of, for example, experiences of failure, physical abuse, or destructive behaviors, this precursor provides the opportunity for exploration and discovery that often marks the chief difference between cooperative and difficult clients. The latter have to be coaxed and persuaded to engage in the process. The former often have to be held back and paced.

For instance, a suicidal, highly rigid client was referred by a hospital after discharge from its psychiatric unit. When she arrived, she said to her therapist, "I know I need to change, so tell me what to do. I'll do it." Her necessity precursor was high, but her willingness to experience anxiety was low. She was rigid and avoidant, often telling the therapist that she did not want to discuss certain topics. At such times, the therapist had to remind the client of her initial willingness to "do anything." In effect, the therapist consistently asked her to surrender to the process, which brought the client back to the task at hand and eventually paved the way for systematic desensitization work related to her panic attacks. Such a case highlights how a client's awareness of necessity can be effectively used to establish a willingness or readiness for anxiety or difficulty.

The discussion so far on grit as a willingness to experience anxiety or difficulty has described the change process from the perspective of inner experience. Worldly or environmental perspectives must also be tolerated. For example, a passive, submissive client had a considerable degree of anxiety when she contemplated confronting a friend who was ridiculing her. The anxiety was so paralyzing that it completely inhibited the client from acting to stop the ridicule. Yet, if she did not manage her anxiety and cope with this problem, the situation might have continued indefinitely. The willingness to experience anxiety often opens the door for the confronting precursor.

Another example is a woman who was compulsively shopping, running up credit card bills to the point of bankruptcy. Since compulsive shopping is usually accompanied by the secondary gain of fun and anxiety reduction, the mere thought of imposing some discipline on spending was an action that flooded the client with mixed feelings. Those feelings included anxiety and shame about spending too much and an unwillingness to lose the fun and satisfaction of spending money. She began to feel emptiness and despair at the thought of no more shopping. For change to manifest, she needed to tolerate those feelings of anxiety, shame, and emptiness and to manage them so that self-regulation and self-management could take effect.

SIGNIFICANT MOMENTS OF CHANGE INVOLVING GRIT

Vanessa, a 32-year-old woman, and one of her two children were being severely emotionally and sometimes physically abused by her husband. In great fear for years, she finally decided that she must leave him and did so unannounced during the day while he was at work. She moved herself and her children to a town 600 miles away without his knowledge.

He traced her and followed her to that city, and he repeatedly threatened by telephone to shoot and kill her with one of his many firearms. He called her regularly to inform her of her daily activities and tell her that she was in the crosshairs of his rifle. He also followed her to her job and falsely reported to her employer by telephone that he was an FBI agent and that she was about to be arrested for selling drugs, and requested their cooperation. He had flowers sent to her place of employment charged to her own credit card. He also stole her car and vandalized the cars of two friends who were visiting her at the time. Finally, she contacted the FBI, who recorded some of his death threats, and he fled and had not been in contact with her for more than 10 years.

According to Vanessa, this man had her immobilized until she realized that death was the source of her fears. She realized that she had to be willing to face death itself to escape this man. As she put it, "I was pushed to the brink in facing my fears." She described herself as having been a person who worried a lot, and she reported that she had since become "very low key" and had learned to "live in the present." Through such processes as enduring the situation, not reacting in the way her husband expected, working with the police and the FBI, and informing her employer of the situation, she acquired "inner control" as she withstood the threats and phone calls. She said, "I'm not the same person. I learned to survive. [The experience] altered the way I am today. Because of that horribleness, I'm a better person." She reported that this was the most valuable experience of her life in terms of lessons learned and coming to terms with death.

CLINICAL MARKERS: HOW TO RECOGNIZE GRIT

Although grit is likely the most difficult of the precursors to gauge or clinically assess, there are some signs that can discern its presence. Like a sense of necessity, this precursor can be detected by asking clients to assess its presence in themselves. Once the client has described the nature of the desired change, the therapist can ask a simple question such as, "Are you willing to go through the difficulty necessary to make this change?" If the client is not being manipulative or attempting to deceive the therapist, chances are the therapist will get an answer that can help with the assessment. Many clients are able and willing to inform a therapist about their willingness to experience turbulent affect or painful memories.

One of this precursor's most obvious behavioral manifestations is an eagerness to "dive in" to the problem or issue. The client will display a markedly high level of tolerance of pain or discomfort as if they know that one "has to get through this" and that this is what has to be done. Such clients are active and cooperative during sessions and convey to the therapist that they are willing to suffer through tough issues without backing off. In many respects, these clients will appear courageous, their resoluteness often evoking the admiration and respect of their therapists.

Intrinsic to the mindset of this precursor is the belief that problems are solved by holding one's ground and not avoiding or running away. Clients with this precursor believe that positive change is worth the sacrifice and difficulty that comes with it. Conversely, the belief that anxiety and discomfort are always to be avoided directly negates the operation of this precursor. Another cognitive aspect of this precursor is the belief that opening oneself to the unknown can have positive results. A client who is willing to experience anxiety or difficulty is more likely to explore the unknown by probing the recesses of the mind or testing new behaviors in new environments.

A person high in this precursor generally believes that taking risks is a valuable and important part of living life and achieving one's goals. Such a person believes the old saying "nothing ventured, nothing gained" and lives by it from a psychological perspective. In terms of anxiety, a person with an ample amount of this precursor believes that it is not intimidating or intolerable but something that is a source of new lessons to be learned and new self-knowledge to be gained. At its most optimum levels, a person views anxiety not as a threat but as a challenge that holds the promise of a reward of insight and enhanced understanding.

One of the most important affective markers is a mastery of fear. The client may be intimidated by the prospect of change and may even express outright fear of it, but the fear is not so intimidating that it inhibits the act of enduring discomfort. Another way this precursor might manifest amid difficult therapeutic moments is as perseverance. The client will persist in the task at hand regardless of the anxiety aroused by the prospect of becoming aware of painful issues or problems.

Ideally, a person with a willingness or readiness to experience anxiety or difficulty is also able to express emotion in a way that results in catharsis. The person is aware of various feeling states and is close to the inner source of emotions and feelings. This precursor also allows a person to explore emotions directly as an activity in itself and not only as a means of isolating thoughts and behaviors. Some people may be more willing to explore certain emotions at the expense of others.

HOW TO DETECT THE ABSENCE OF GRIT

When the willingness or readiness to experience anxiety or difficulty is absent, the client may believe that therapy is too difficult or that the therapist, however reasonable, is too demanding. Such a client may be inclined to miss or be late for sessions, not so much because a sense of necessity is lacking but because they wish to avoid the inherent difficulties connected with change. Thus, avoidance is a prominent and observable feature when this precursor is lacking.

An absence of grit can drain change potential from the therapeutic encounter. Just because a client is willing to talk about a problem does not mean they are willing to experience the anxiety or difficulty associated with it. Some clients approach problems with an emotional detachment that shields them from, or filters out, the hurt and pain connected with an issue so they can talk about it with some composure. Specifically, when the talk is not "curing," the person often seems remote, even if they may be intellectually active and engaged in the analysis of the problem. The remoteness comes from a hesitance to experience the emotions or feelings aroused by the issue. Such emotional self-distancing from a problem is often accompanied by a distancing from the therapist (Kross & Ayduk, 2017). A solid relationship is crucial to closing this distance.

In the case of substance use treatment programs, some clients learn the proper treatment language and use it to tell therapists and counselors exactly what they want to hear. Such clients' ostensibly honest and heartfelt testimony is mere lip service designed to manipulate the staff into granting early, undeserved graduation. In such cases, a pivotal missing ingredient is assessment of the willingness to experience anxiety or difficulty.

Other difficult clients are willing to acknowledge that a so-called problem is there but insist that there is "no need to get into it." They will insist that the problem can be solved without much effort. A classic example is the alcoholic who says, "I can quit drinking any time I want." Such clients are not willing to admit how difficult abstinence is or to experience the anxieties and discomfort involved. Of course, it may also be true that the person does not know how difficult it may be, in which case the next precursor, awareness, comes into play.

When a willingness or readiness to experience anxiety or difficulty is missing, a client may become evasive with the therapist and may resist probing questions about troubled areas. The client may divert the therapist's questions toward "safer" topics on which to focus or elaborate. Often, the client is not aware of such diversions, but at other times, the client is aware, and questioning them about such diversions is perfectly acceptable and often productive. At other times, the client becomes annoyed or irritable and engages in rationalizations in the honest belief that the therapist is causing them needless pain and anxiety. This indicates a classic mindset or belief system that maintains that anything worth pursuing should not be uncomfortable or painful.

TECHNIQUES: ESTABLISHING GRIT

A client with a high sense of necessity but no willingness to experience anxiety or difficulty will probably want the therapist to do the work. This section describes how to help clients prepare for the work that only they can do. Some clients need preparation for therapy and change, much like athletes need to warm up and mentally prepare for meets, tournaments, and games. Therapy can involve something akin to hardship, and working through issues requires some degree of "getting in shape" to deal with it. Dealing with difficult people, marital turmoil, and emotional pain requires determination. In promoting and building grit, therapy comes close to resembling active coaching.

An effective therapist can inspire a client, through persuasion, to work through difficult, painful, anxiety-ridden problems. Through the empathic connection, therapists can promote this precursor without being coercive; surpassing the tolerance limits or threshold of anxiety can be harmful and discourages a person from further work in therapy. This chapter catalogs techniques and strategies that can inspire a person to recognize and be willing to tolerate and experience the anxiety and difficulty that come with therapeutic change. The use of metaphors is a major approach to increasing this precursor.

Metaphors That Illustrate Grit

Many possible metaphors or reframes can help point out the importance of grit as a willingness to experience anxiety or difficulty in the therapeutic change process. All too often, difficult clients simply do not know that this precursor is helpful and can be enhanced. Some may see this precursor as threatening. Thus, education is often essential when seeking to activate grit as a willingness or readiness to experience anxiety or difficulty.

No Pain, No Gain: The Workout Metaphor

The workout metaphor essentially states that one gets out of therapy what one puts into it. In the world of physical conditioning, weight lifting, and bodybuilding, a common phrase is, "No pain, no gain." It is often advised that the muscles have to "burn" or be sufficiently stressed to grow and develop. Many clients can readily understand and relate to this perspective. One example was a 20-year-old bulimic woman who was regularly binging and purging. Like many people with this problem, she worked out furiously for 2–4 hours a day in an effort to lose weight. She knew and operated on the "no pain, no gain" principle.

However, when it came to looking at psychological issues, she was unwilling to tolerate anxiety to any marked degree. In fact, it was soon established that whenever she felt the anxiety or edge of her emotional pain, she was off to the gym or binging on junk food. She was able to recognize this pattern with relative ease. Her understanding of therapy and the therapeutic process shifted dramatically when it was explained to her that "no pain, no gain" also applied to therapy. The muscles burn in physical exercise, she was told, just like anxiety "burns" in mental therapy. In either case, the burn is important and necessary for growth, but it should not be overdone. In her case, the therapist promised not to deliberately ask her to confront painful memories or feelings unless she was willing and ready.

Workout Machines

Along these same lines, many people buy abdominal exercisers or various other workout machines, knowing they have to change some part of their body or health. Unfortunately, in so many cases, those machines are not used because many people are not willing to experience the difficulty that comes with actually exercising. As a result, the machines are bought with the best intentions but collect dust because of the person's lack of willingness to experience the discomfort that accompanies exercise. Similarly, people can pay for therapy and "have it around" for years, but they may not ever really use it to make changes in their lives. Thus, therapy gets wasted and "collects dust," just like those workout machines.

The Stuffed Closet

The stuffed closet is akin to the cleaning house metaphor. Clients who report that they do not like to think about their problems lack grit as a willingness to experience anxiety or difficulty. The problem can be likened to a closet that is packed full of "stuff": Every time the client wants to avoid something, they throw it into a mental closet. Eventually, the closet gets so full that the door will not close properly, and the client is constantly trying to cram the door shut. Eventually, the closet overflows and spills painful material into the rest of the house.

Alternately, the mind can be likened to a house with several rooms and closets. Some people stuff one mental room after another full of painful issues and difficult problems. They continue to ignore them until there are so many rooms full that the person has only a fraction of their mind left in which it is comfortable to live. Guests are also kept out of those rooms. Some people spend the bulk of their mental life keeping the doors to those rooms closed so they do not have to think about what is in there. Anxiety builds, and whatever peace of mind or contentedness the person may have had begins to fade progressively. As the metaphor goes, if a person were to take the time to sort out all the stuff, they would eventually be able to breathe easier and be more comfortable. The willingness to experience anxiety or difficulty has to do with being willing to go through and clean out all the junk and get the house in order.

Driving With the Brakes On

Another metaphor illustrates how some people want change to occur but inhibit themselves in various ways. A therapist can inform a client how research shows that experiencing emotions and anxiety is conducive to the change process. But being willing only to talk about things and not to actually experience the anxiety connected with those issues is rather like driving with the brakes on. The car might move along in jerky motions, or it might not move at all. Furthermore, after a while, the brakes begin to wear out from overuse. Similarly, a person who resists the pain while talking about it might go through years of therapy but may not ever arrive at any viable or lasting change, ending up exhausted after fighting the anxiety over the years.

Washing Hands With Gloves On

Talking about issues in therapy without ever getting into the experiential aspects is like washing one's hands while wearing gloves. The washing is good, but the hands never get clean. The problem never gets contacted or worked through because it is never really experienced. Eventually, it becomes time to take the gloves off.

To Properly Clean, You Have to Get Dirty

When one cleans, if the job is challenging, one is bound to come into contact with dirt and grime. The paradox is that cleaning up requires looking for, exposing, stirring up, and scrubbing away dirt and dust. To clean, you have to get dirty, and the same is often true in therapy. Therapy can be viewed as a cleansing of the mind, feelings, and behaviors. Things can get messy with emotions and beliefs, but that is part of any cleaning process. One can hire someone to clean the house and yard, but in therapy, only the person can do the work; no one else has direct access to another's mind, feelings, and behaviors.

Old Pipes and Dirty Water

For a person who is hesitant to touch or come into contact with what phenomenologically appears as messy—painful emotions and feelings—a metaphor of old, rusty pipes can be used. When the pipes have not been used for a long time and the faucet is turned on, the water will flow a dirty brown color, but if the water is allowed to flow, it will eventually turn clear and clean. The same is true for those "messy" emotions and feelings once they begin to be experienced, processed, and discussed.

It Takes Guts

The guts metaphor is ideally suited for many defiant adolescents who are suspicious of and ridicule the idea of counseling and therapy. With this metaphor, therapy is framed as an exercise in courage. Many difficult clients might respond to a statement like, "Anyone can ignore their thoughts and feelings, but it takes guts to be honest about them and not back off from what you are really about." A variation designed to increase this precursor with defiant, aggressive adolescents might be, "Anybody can go and punch someone that pisses them off, but it takes real guts to face up to your feelings of anger and hurt."

Identify the Internal Dialogue That Avoids Anxiety

This cognitive-behavioral strategy can effectively remove obstacles to being open to experience. If the therapist knows a possible issue for change, they can ask the client to just consider making the change in question, and then to describe any automatic thoughts or self-talk associated with the change. If the client is especially difficult, they can first be told, "Please do not make the change; I just want to ask you something related to it." Usually, the client will agree to this quasiparadoxical approach. Also, when clients are hesitant to experience anxiety or difficulty, they are prone to deflect questions and change topics. It is often essential to repeat questions and, if necessary, get prior permission to interrupt a client's rambling on other less disturbing topics.

For example, Tony, a man in his late 40s, admitted that he liked to fight with his wife, Sara, to get her agitated and upset. He knew this was mean and even cruel, but he said he enjoyed it and did not know why. Sara, meanwhile, was extremely angry with him and knew all too well that he enjoyed it. She told him she would not take this kind of treatment any longer. This client had not responded to any approach to changing this behavior, and the CHANGES assessment indicated a rating of 0 or 1 in the willingness precursor:

THERAPIST: I'm going to ask you only to think about changing your "agitating behavior" with your wife. Please don't change it or stop it. Once you are considering the change, I'll ask you a question or two about it. Is this okay with you?

CLIENT: Sure.

THERAPIST: Get the idea of supporting your wife's peace of mind and happiness, and tell me when you have it. (Client nods.)

THERAPIST: What do you feel like at this moment as you think about it?

CLIENT: It's okay with me.

THERAPIST: Didn't you just tell me that you like to get her agitated and upset?

CLIENT: Yeah, I guess I did, but it's not like I don't want her to be happy.

THERAPIST: Of course. Do you ever start a fight with her when she's sad?

CLIENT: No.

THERAPIST: Do you ever start a fight with her when she is angry about something?

CLIENT: No.

THERAPIST:	Let me bounce something off you, and tell me if I am wrong. When Sara is happy, does it kind of bug you in a way? Does it sort of get under your skin, and you have this urge to mess with it?
CLIENT:	Well, yeah. It's like I get kind of mischievous. (smiling and looking for agreement)
THERAPIST:	I'm going to say something very direct to you, and I want your permission to do so. If you want me to sugarcoat it, I will.
CLIENT:	Go on, tell me straight.
THERAPIST:	It sounds like one of the roles you play in your marriage is to keep your wife from ever knowing happiness and joy. What do you think?
CLIENT:	You make me sound like a real ass.
THERAPIST:	I'm not saying that at all. I'm trying to understand your role in the marriage.
CLIENT:	(irritated) I work hard, long hours and do lots of overtime. I keep the house and yard together.
THERAPIST:	No doubt, and I bet you're good at what you do.
CLIENT:	Damn right.
THERAPIST:	Tony, I'm just trying to understand what's going on here between you and Sara, and pardon me for saying so, but it sounds like you don't want to answer me about not wanting her to be happy. Do you want me to repeat it?
CLIENT:	I know what you said. (pauses … silence) I feel kind of ashamed about it, you know.
THERAPIST:	Did that feeling of shame get in the way when I asked you earlier to tell me your thoughts about your wife and your marriage?
CLIENT:	But you don't know how much she bugs me. She's all the time acting like she knows everything and it drives me nuts. (Client continues in this vein for 2 or 3 minutes.)
THERAPIST:	Can this be one of those times when I can interrupt you?
CLIENT:	(mildly surprised) Yeah.
THERAPIST:	I noticed that when I brought up that feeling of shame, you started talking about Sara instead of your feelings. Do you find it uncomfortable to talk about that feeling of shame?

CLIENT:	(shifting in the chair) I don't know, whatever. Can we talk about something else?
THERAPIST:	Sure. For now, though, if you can give me a yes or no, it would help me understand where you're coming from. Do you not like to talk about those kinds of feelings?
CLIENT:	Yeah, I don't. It's like I just don't want to think about it.
THERAPIST:	And it's easier to complain about her?
CLIENT:	Maybe.
THERAPIST:	What do you think would happen if you got into that feeling of shame?
CLIENT:	I'd end up feeling down and depressed, and I don't feel like getting into all that.
THERAPIST:	So, you believe that if you ever come into contact with or get into your feelings, you'll end up getting depressed?
CLIENT:	Well, yeah, wouldn't you?

At this point, a dysfunctional core belief was isolated that obviously interfered with the therapeutic process and specifically the willingness precursor. Tony believed that contacting or experiencing his feelings would result in depression. The therapist disputed the belief and used the "old pipes and dirty water" metaphor to help Tony understand that contacting feelings is not a formula for depression but can be part of a way to alleviate his depression.

In addition, the therapist asked Tony if he had a habitual pattern of avoiding difficult feelings, as he had just displayed in therapy. He said that he did, indeed, all his life, and when asked, he said he thought this was what one "was supposed to do" with such feelings. The stuffed closet metaphor was then used to advantage with Tony to illustrate how he had stuffed so many aspects of his life into a mental closet that the door could no longer be locked shut, and "material" was seeping out from the cracks around the door. It took one session to establish this precursor with Tony, moving him from a rating of 0 to 2 on the scale. He was more open to emotional experiences after this and much less avoidant.

Typically, when clients are ready to experience anxiety or difficulty, they find therapy to be a much more tolerable and perhaps even rewarding endeavor. In Tony's case, he eventually explored his desire to prevent Sara from being happy. Therapy went relatively smoothly once he was willing to experience the anxiety that came with facing the incongruence between his self-image as a fun-loving, nice guy and his behavior of interfering with the happiness of the woman he married.

The Use of Paradox

Research findings on paradoxical techniques have shown them to be highly effective (Browning & Hull, 2021; Peluso & Freund, 2023). Paradox can help develop several of the precursors, including the willingness to experience anxiety or difficulty. For example, Cindy was a woman in her mid-40s who was extremely sensitive to emotional pain. She would consistently deflect attempts to discuss anything unpleasant or anxiety provoking. Her conversation seemed geared more toward making the therapist like her and think that she was acceptable as a human being than it was toward alleviating her presenting problem of depression.

The therapist attempted to validate and reassure her of her value and intelligence in many ways. After the initial relationship was formed, the therapist explained to her that therapy sometimes required difficult topics to be addressed and discussed. She said she knew this but that it was "really hard" for her. The therapist asked her what was so hard about doing so. She said, "I don't want to hurt anymore." Using the old pipes and dirty water metaphor helped a bit, but she was still extremely sensitive to any further pain, even though she was intellectually aware that she would eventually need to deal with it. Sensing her fragility in this regard, it was clear that to expose her to painful emotions at this point in therapy would be premature. The therapist decided to introduce a paradoxical technique:

THERAPIST: Cindy, I understand that you don't want to hurt anymore, and that's why you don't want to talk about anything uncomfortable.

CLIENT: It's so hard, and I just don't have the energy anymore.

THERAPIST: What would you prefer to talk about?

CLIENT: You mean, anything?

THERAPIST: Yes.

CLIENT: I like to talk about the novels I read. I also like to talk about stores and sales.

THERAPIST: Would you like to try an experiment?

CLIENT: What is it?

THERAPIST: Let's talk about any of the things you mentioned but with one added ingredient.

CLIENT: What's that?

THERAPIST: How about if you talk about what you find enjoyable and, during the entire time, deliberately avoid discussing anything painful or uncomfortable. Are you willing to try it?

CLIENT: Sure.

THERAPIST: Please remember, you can stop this at any time if you want.

Cindy was soon talking about books, and then about friends and neighbors and a variety of other topics. This went on for 10 minutes, with the therapist acknowledging, reflecting, and asking an occasional question. At two points in the conversation, the therapist interjected a question verifying that Cindy was still deliberately avoiding anything painful or uncomfortable. She said that she was.

THERAPIST: Okay, Cindy, you have been telling me about all kinds of things for about 10 minutes now. Did you notice anything while you were deliberately not talking about anything painful or uncomfortable?

CLIENT: Yes (speaking softly). It's the same thing that I do all the time anyway. I've been through so much in my life that it seems whenever I talk about anything, I'm trying to not think about the bad things that have happened to me. (begins to cry) I don't know if I can ever feel better.

THERAPIST: So, what you are saying is that your emotional hurt is so close to the surface that it's always there to some degree, even when you try to forget about it.

CLIENT: (softly crying) Yes. It's always been like that. A lot of the things I enjoy doing I'm really doing because I'm trying to forget about the bad things that have happened to me.

THERAPIST: Has it worked for you?

CLIENT: What do you mean?

THERAPIST: Have you been able to forget about the bad things by avoiding them in your actions and behaviors?

CLIENT: Not really.

THERAPIST: Would you be willing to try a different approach? Therapy exists so that feelings of hurt and pain can be diminished to the point of not having them on your mind all the time.

CLIENT: I guess I knew that.

THERAPIST: True, but it didn't seem you were willing to give it a try. Am I wrong here?

CLIENT: No. It's just that it's so hard.

THERAPIST: What if we only go a little bit at a time, and you tell me when it's getting too intense and then I'll back off as soon as you tell me.

CLIENT: That would be okay. I just don't want to cry all the time. I've done so much of that, and I'm afraid it's what you want me to do.

THERAPIST: I think it's cruel to ask a person to go swimming in all their pain if they can end up drowning in it. What I'm asking you to do is to go wading little by little, toes and ankles first, until you feel comfortable in the water.

CLIENT: You know there's a lot that has happened to me ...

Therapy was conducted very carefully at first, checking with Cindy to see if she was feeling overwhelmed at any time. Eventually, she disclosed several traumatic experiences and was able to work through these to her satisfaction. In this case, the paradoxical injunction to avoid anything painful showed her that it was what she was already doing. Cindy further realized that she had been fighting and resisting painful memories and emotions throughout her life. She eventually reported that she had become so accustomed to keeping those feelings at bay that the thought of not doing so was intimidating and disorienting.

Taking Ownership and Stopping Blame

In many ways, owning the problem is the opposite of blaming, or compulsively attributing responsibility for a problem to another or others. Difficult clients typically blame others for their problems and issues. Getting a difficult client to take ownership of a problem can be demanding work, but when successful, it is rewarding for all concerned.

A key to bringing about a sense of ownership is, of course, to help a person see that they have some influence over the problem. Even if the person is truly blameless or not at all responsible for what happened, as in cases of sexual abuse, the person is still responsible for how they think about that problem (see Frankl, 1992). A person's attitude toward a situation or problem can still come under their control. Blaming, and its close associate, hating, is often the result of a decision.

Following his experience at Auschwitz, Frankl (1992) learned a lesson that therapists can present to clients. He said that although he had no control over what the Nazis did to him and the other people there, he did have control over his attitude toward what they did to him and others. This story and lesson can be used to advantage with people who blame, complain, or detach from events that have affected them. Recommending his book can be helpful, if the client will read it.

The following list of questions and statements may be useful to those who habitually complain or blame others for a problem or a particular issue:

- How is this problem controlling you?
- Has complaining about the problem helped any?
- Do you feel better when blaming [a person or situation] for the problem?
- Has blaming [the person or situation] helped to ease the difficulty?
- Perhaps you don't give yourself enough credit for your own influence.
- Have you set this problem up so that you would be helpless over it?
- Have you set yourself up to be weighed down by this problem?

- Is having someone to blame important to you?
- How has this problem robbed you of your freedom?
- Is this problem worth giving up your freedom for?
- Sure, you didn't cause the problem, but can you control your reaction to it?

Some of these questions are highly confrontative, whereas others are designed to induce processing. Each is meant to be used appropriately to match different clients' situations at different times. All are questions that many difficult clients will seek to avoid, and therefore, they need to be pursued. If asked curiously and openly, each has the potential to open a therapeutic window. The questions or statements, and variations of the same, will need to be repeated in many instances to achieve some depth of processing. Processing these questions and statements can help a client understand that blaming involves the avoidance of anxiety that comes with responsibility (see Yalom, 1980).

Blaming inhibits the ability to respond by placing all control in the hands of the blamed person. This lack of ownership of a problem or issue often comes from never having accepted the problem and its associated thoughts and feelings. As such, acceptance of undesirable thoughts and feelings can be a powerful change factor (Hofmann & Asmundson, 2008). The goal is for a client to learn that blame brings neither solutions nor joy, whereas responsibility can bring both. Generally, *responsibility* is the willingness to take charge of the circumstances that make up the problem. Clients can be taught that "responsibility" is not a word that weighs 500 pounds and sits on one's shoulders. It can be described as the ability to respond, or "response-ability."

The Control or Freedom Challenge

Therapists can use a specific technique to help clients stop blaming others as a means of avoiding anxiety or difficulty. The technique focuses on a mechanism used by difficult clients of all ages. An example might be the sixth grader who says, "He made me do it," and another the domestic violence perpetrator who says, "If she didn't make me angry, I wouldn't have hit her." The proper response to these statements is to indicate somehow that the client themselves has given up control of their life to the person being blamed. This is not at all the same as indicating to a client that they lack self-control, which is a familiar song to these clients that will usually end up being uneventful.

The therapist must point out that the person has given up control over behaviors and thoughts to the person who is being blamed, as this is, in most cases, a more accurate representation (see Hanna & Hunt, 1999). For example, when a sophomore in high school says, "Joey made me do it," the response could be, "So Joey now controls your life?" Similarly, when an abusive husband says, "She nagged and nagged and got me so mad I just hit her," a proper response could be, "So you have no control over your emotions and behaviors?"

Such statements can be followed up by saying, "It's too bad you don't have any freedom." This is a provocative statement, and therapists must recognize it as such and be aware of the consequence of increased anxiety. Another statement might be, "It's too bad you no longer have any say over your life." The therapist can then offer to help the client get their life back.

This approach is especially effective with defiant and conduct-disordered adolescents (Hanna & Hunt, 1999). Because it is provocative, this technique usually evokes self-righteous protest and even defiance by clients prone to blaming others. The therapist responds to the increased anxiety levels by saying, "I mean you no disrespect. I'm only wondering if you know that you give up your life and your freedom to other people every time you blame them." After the anxiety level reduces a bit, the therapist can say something on the order of, "Tell me if I'm wrong, but it seems like [the person] is controlling your emotions and behaviors with their words and attitudes. Do you have any freedom left, or have you given it all away?" At this point, the therapist can again offer to help the person take back that freedom. This is initially done by having the client observe and reflect on times when they blindly acted out in response to stressful situations. For this technique to work, the therapist must be compassionate as well as dispassionate in using it.

Once again, the therapeutic strategy is to show that whenever people blame others for their own actions, they have given their self-control or freedom away to the person blamed, and even their thoughts are now controlled by the blamed person. This approach is especially effective if the person blamed is someone the client dislikes, does not respect, or is competing against in some way. It brings about considerable cognitive dissonance and will often influence a client to be willing to experience anxiety or difficulty in seeking to regain freedom or control over behaviors. The technique is a classic example of a difficult situation that produces a moment of great therapeutic potential. It is unwise to use the term "freedom" with children under 14 years of age, as they do not seem to respond to it. Using the term "control" is much better with that age group.

Self-Monitoring the Waxing and Waning of Anxiety

The behavioral technique of self-monitoring (Korotitsch & Nelson-Gray, 1999; Meichenbaum, 1977) can be used to show some difficult clients that they have a low tolerance for anxiety and resort to avoidant behaviors rather than face it. The technique involves pointing out moments in which a client shrinks from, deflects, or otherwise avoids anxiety. Many defiant adolescents have a low tolerance for anxiety, even though they may assert that they can handle any kind of confrontation or difficult situation. Highlighting the low tolerance is best done in vivo, during the session, with the therapist asking permission to do so.

For example, Marie was a teenager who seldom studied, being more interested in entertainment of various kinds. She was, nevertheless, highly sensitive about her low grades and would get irritated or annoyed at the mere mention of them. Her therapist used this, in combination with a strategy for increasing the client's necessity precursor, as an opportunity for her to learn about anxiety:

THERAPIST:	Have you noticed that some people can deal with things without getting upset, and they just seem to be very cool and not let things get to them?
CLIENT:	Yeah.
THERAPIST:	Would you want to be more like that?
CLIENT:	(protesting) I am like that. Don't you think I am?
THERAPIST:	In many ways, you are. But you also know that many people know exactly what to say to get you annoyed and irritated, right?
CLIENT:	Yeah, I guess.
THERAPIST:	How would you like to get less annoyed and irritated and be more on top of things?
CLIENT:	I can do that?
THERAPIST:	Yes. Can I explain to you about a thing called anxiety?
CLIENT:	I guess so.
THERAPIST:	Anxiety is an agitated feeling that we all get when something happens that we don't want to happen or we feel sensitive about. It's like an itch you can't scratch.
CLIENT:	Yeah, so?
THERAPIST:	Well, I'm going to deliberately say something about your grades, but I don't mean what I say; I just want you to watch the feeling you get. Is that okay with you?
CLIENT:	So now you are going to tell me to get good grades, too?
THERAPIST:	Do you have that agitated feeling right now, Marie? The itch you can't scratch?
CLIENT:	(protesting) I thought you said that you didn't care about my grades.
THERAPIST:	I said that I cared more about you than your grades. But this is not about grades. Can I go on?
CLIENT:	Whatever. I'm just so tired of people bothering me about my grades.
THERAPIST:	I understand. Marie, have you noticed that any time someone mentions your grades, like right now, you get irritated with them and say things like "Whatever," or "I don't care," or "Leave me alone"?
CLIENT:	Yeah.

THERAPIST:	Well, I'm going to say it deliberately again so that you can watch the feeling rather than give in to it and get all irritated and angry. Is it okay if I do that?
CLIENT:	Okay.
THERAPIST:	(playing the role with a stern voice) Marie, your grades are terrible, and you can do a lot better. What happened when I said that?
CLIENT:	I wanted to strangle you.
THERAPIST:	Fair enough. But what did you feel the moment I said that?
CLIENT:	I felt like I was going crazy ... like I can't stand it.
THERAPIST:	Right. That "can't stand it" feeling is the anxiety I'm talking about. How often do you feel that feeling?
CLIENT:	A lot.
THERAPIST:	If that didn't bother you so much, would your life be different?
CLIENT:	Well, yeah, a lot different.
THERAPIST:	How?
CLIENT:	I wouldn't, like, be going off on people and yelling at them to leave me alone all the time.
THERAPIST:	Would you like to learn how to handle that anxiety feeling so it doesn't bother you as much? You can, you know. And it might help you to feel better.
CLIENT:	Uh, yeah. What do I do?

The therapist then explained to Marie the idea of self-monitoring. In this case, it involved watching her anxiety levels at school, at home, and with her friends. She was told to watch what she did whenever she felt it and to "look, don't think." She did this quite well and soon was paying attention to her anxiety responses with relatively little effort. Once she was willing to experience the anxiety, she began to use the stress management techniques she had previously ignored. Her progress in therapy was enhanced as well. With difficult clients, merely speaking of anxiety usually will not communicate the point, but demonstrating it to a client can do so effectively. Unfortunately, the anxiety sometimes needs to be induced in the session.

Examining Maladaptive Beliefs About Anxiety, Difficulty, and Pain

There are several maladaptive beliefs that can interfere with establishing grit as a willingness to experience anxiety or difficulty. If these beliefs can be identified and disputed, therapy is likely to progress more quickly. It may be helpful to recall that many maladaptive beliefs related to anxiety and pain avoidance involve implicit learning (Cleeremans, 2019; Hartmann, 2019) and may have been formed preverbally. Thus, when seeking to isolate such a belief, the exact wording is not as important as the concept underlying the belief itself. Some beliefs related to this precursor include

- Experiencing emotional pain is self-torture.
- Experiencing emotional pain makes me weak.
- Experiencing anxiety drains my energy.
- Anything unpleasant is a sign of impending pain.
- Only fools immerse themselves in emotions.
- To open oneself up to emotional pain threatens the integrity of the self.
- If I begin to feel, I will begin to fall apart.
- There is always a way to avoid anything difficult.
- I can avoid anything.
- If I have no feelings, I have no pain.

A CLOSING NOTE ON GRIT

It is important to recognize that the grit precursor only manifests when the client willingly and intentionally experiences anxiety and difficulty. Simply having anxiety or finding oneself in difficult circumstances is insufficient. As mentioned earlier in this chapter, grit aligns with the workout motto of "no pain, no gain." When a person engages in weightlifting, running, or other forms of exercise, they willingly endure strain on the body because doing so increases strength, endurance, and resiliency. Transformative change demands a willingness to endure hardship and discomfort, whether in the gym or in a therapy session. People vary widely in their capacity for grit, but those clients who demonstrate the greatest capacity for psychological discomfort are often well suited to the challenge of therapeutic change. Helping clients grow this precursor can also have a far-reaching effect in life, as clients learn that anxiety and negative feelings will reduce in intensity, or even subside altogether, when willingly experienced. The strategies and techniques in this chapter provide a solid foundation for growing grit as a necessary internal capacity for change.

9

E: Effort, or Will to Change

Effort or will toward change seems quite simple on the surface, but its implications run deep to illuminate the complex relationship between perceived engagement in therapy and therapeutic change. Talk therapy can often be a verbal, passive, cerebral experience in which too little action takes place. It is common for the therapeutic relationship to become exceedingly comfortable, with conversations flowing freely in a pleasurable and meaningful way. It is extremely easy to talk to most therapists and counselors, so much so that the talking and sharing itself displaces the overarching goal of therapeutic change. Such therapy becomes a soothing opiate whereby a client engages in a close relationship with a therapist who seeks to nurture, reassure, and console.

Of course, some benefits can certainly arise from the pleasure of a listening ear and the catharsis that accompanies it. But talking is usually not enough to instantiate meaningful change in life. For most clients to stabilize and improve, they must actively and effortfully change their conditions of mind, behavior, and environment. A client may be aware that their house is a mess and actively talk about their frustrations with a dirty home in session, but such discussions are pointless if they do not exert the effort to physically clean their house. Thus, it is usually not enough to be aware of, open to, or to confront a problem. In so many cases, there is no substitute for effortful action, and therapeutic change may not occur without this crucial ingredient.

According to the CHANGES model, *effort* is the deliberate and self-determined exertion of physical or mental energy or resources toward therapeutic change in the form of self-improvement or positive alterations to one's environment. It is observed when one executes the psychological and behavioral tasks necessary to reach the goal of change and marks the transition between contemplation and

---

Case examples have been disguised to protect client confidentiality.

https://doi.org/10.1037/0000451-010
Therapeutic Change With Difficult Clients: Precursors and Techniques in the CHANGES Model, Second Edition, by B. D. Wilkinson and F. J. Hanna

action (Krebs et al., 2019). In the CHANGES model, effort or will is how the hard work of change is accomplished.

How much effort a person expends seems to depend on the presence of other precursors, even as effort itself can sometimes activate other precursors. Confronting is often enhanced when exerting effort toward resolving a problem or situation, but without confronting, effort might never be engaged at all. Hope also has a strong influence on effort. If a person can see no realistic, desirable outcome for an expenditure of effort, they are not likely to attempt it (Bandura, 1977). A therapist attempting to increase the effort precursor cannot lose sight of the importance of hope. Alternatively, a sufficient degree of a sense of necessity can be enough to spring a person into effort and action, even when neither hope nor self-efficacy is present.

THE NATURE OF THE WILL

When a difficult client who makes little or no progress toward change seems unable to act, it may be wise to recognize this as an affliction of the will, just as Rank (1936) noted. In fact, Rank recommended that clients strengthen their will as part of therapy and said in no uncertain terms that this personal quality was a core capacity of healthy human beings. Low (1952) also observed that the will, as the human quality that moves beyond instincts and drives, is the key to mental health. Similarly, Assagioli (1973) saw the will as the primary, active element in reaching higher stages of development. These early scholars were convinced that the will should be rehabilitated and restored in clients as a routine part of therapy. We do not believe, as they did, that an entire therapy should be built around the will. Nevertheless, it should not be overlooked as a point of rehabilitation in certain difficult clients, especially when a client simply won't act.

The idea of the will is a crucial yet seldom discussed and rarely appreciated aspect of effort (Robinson, 1990). It is conceptually ambiguous, to be sure, but just because a concept is ambiguous does not mean it should be ignored, especially if it has utility. Although the will is complex and even confounding, this is no excuse to avoid it. Effort toward change is seldom, if ever, engaged without some act of will. Commitment is a good example of the will in action, which serves as a major behavioral process in the transtheoretical mode of change (Prochaska et al., 1994). Glasser (1965) was one of the first to point out the importance of commitment to change on the part of a client as crucial to bringing about the effort needed to carry a plan through to its fruition.

Many clients are aware of a specific problem and the need to find a solution, and they can also be confronting and willing to experience anxiety or difficulty. But in spite of the presence of those precursors, they seem unable to garner sufficient momentum toward action, as though they are metaphorically chained or harnessed. Explorations into the phenomenology of agency have surged in the field of consciousness studies (see Bayne, 2008; Mylopoulos & Shepherd, 2020) and may provide valuable insight into how reticence arises as a pathology of agentive experience, perhaps in terms of the relation between directive mental causation and intentionality. It may be simpler to frame deficits in effort to more pragmatic neuroscientific causes, such as insufficient effort justification and the relative neurobiological cost of energy expenditure (Inzlicht et al., 2018). In any case, the issue of sustained effort or will is of central concern to therapeutic change practices, and understanding the complex nature of agentic effort should be prioritized in the field.

HOW EFFORT OR WILL LEADS TO THERAPEUTIC CHANGE

How does change come about through effort or will? To answer this question, it is helpful to first outline two essential modalities in which effort or will initiates change: control and maneuvering. In both modalities, change is implemented directly and with immediacy. Each takes place in three distinct though related contexts—the mind, the body, and the environment. Finally, we look briefly at how the efficient use of in-session time reflects a therapist's prioritization of effort in the therapeutic change process.

Will as Effortful Control of Thoughts and Images

Researchers generally tend to discuss will in terms of self-control (Duckworth et al., 2018), with some distinguishing between forms of self-control, such as resolve and suppression (Ainslie, 2021). However, will can also be understood as a sense of ownership over one's actions. This aligns with the classic definition set forth by the 18th-century English philosopher Hume (1739/1978), who said that "[will is] *the internal impression we feel and are conscious of,* when we knowingly give rise to any new motion of our body, or new perception of our mind" (p. 399, italics in original). If we substitute effort in this definition, it does not lose its descriptive power. That is, perhaps, why James (1890/1981) noted how effort and will are intimately related—so much so that he viewed them as essentially equivalent.

Control in this context refers to the psychological act of directly influencing the content and operations of the mind. Maladaptive beliefs are discarded and replaced with new, more reasonable beliefs. This can take place immediately, as in some cases, or it can be a psychological act that is repeated continuously until the original maladaptive belief is pushed to the background of the mind or deprived of its power. For example, if a client has the belief "I will not trust anyone," the act of will or effort replaces this notion with a more rational "I can trust some people but not just anyone."

The act of replacing the old belief may have a larger role to play in bringing about change than the content of the new belief. For example, a client learned that his idea of the perfect woman was one who is beautiful, intelligent, self-willed, and proud, and yet he also expected this imagined woman to be submissive, needful of direction, and willing to sacrifice her desires and goals for his own. Such a bundle of self-evidently contradictory traits cannot exist except within one's imagination. In the act of change, whereby effort and will were engaged, the client directly altered this flawed image in his mind, and this act was just as important as the image that was put in its place.

In the case of the will directly affecting the body, an obvious example is a client who is unhealthy and overweight and finds it necessary to establish a workout routine. If this client actively engages the will to get up and jog, do aerobics, climb stairs, or whatever the exercise may be, then change will surely result from such effortful engagement of the will.

In the case of directly affecting the world or environment, an example is a client who is troubled by the unethical actions of the company she works for. The act of will is engaged when she commits to finding a new job and exerts the effort toward quitting the old one. If the will is not engaged, the person can be aware of the need and confront the problem itself but will talk about the need to quit for years with no result.

Maneuvering Around Problem Areas

Maneuvering involves therapeutic action around or away from issues or problems that are beyond one's control. For example, a therapist may ask a depressed client if they "know where to find an area of pain" in their minds. The therapist then asks with curiosity whether the client can "go there" if they so wish. We have found that many people can do this with little trouble. If they know how to "go there," they also know precisely how to maneuver away from troubling regions of pain.

The body can also be maneuvered to avoid problem areas and difficulties. For example, a person insulted in a public meeting may need to engage the will to "hold their tongue," which is one way of maneuvering around a potentially difficult situation in which saying something at that moment may be ill advised. This simple lesson is often helpful for defiant teenagers.

Similarly, in maneuvering around worldly or environmental dangers, a recovering alcohol abuser who is driving by one of their old bar hangouts and experiences a powerful urge to stop for a drink may need a deliberate act of will to keep the car going in a direction away from the bar and the possibility of relapse.

Effort and the Efficient Use of Time

Effort must be integrated into a client's everyday life before substantial change can manifest. One way of looking at this is to consider that there are approximately 112 waking hours in a week. Depending on the treatment arrangement, a client sees a therapist for only one of those hours, or perhaps more if the person is hospitalized or in an outpatient format where therapy is conducted several times a week. The small number of therapy hours is often insufficient if the lessons from therapy are not converted or integrated into the client's everyday living. Effort toward change needs to be implemented by the client throughout the week for in-session lessons to merge with worldly experience. When effort is directed toward therapeutic tasks throughout the week, therapy time becomes more meaningful, productive, and valued by the client.

Therapists should also be cognizant of how many minutes per session are intentionally and meaningfully devoted to change. Session time is wasted if the precursors are not actively engaged, and client progress can sometimes be gauged by this measure. A 50-minute session with a difficult client may have only five truly productive minutes in which the therapeutic change process is actually engaged. The other 45 minutes of session time might be spent in denial, avoidance, manipulation, or any form of circuitous communication and evasive actions. However, when a client puts in substantial effort with a therapist who emphasizes change, in-session productivity radically increases as a result of efficient focus on important therapeutic change factors.

SIGNIFICANT MOMENTS OF CHANGE INVOLVING EFFORT OR WILL

Mary's experience of significant change occurred when she found out she was pregnant. The man had told her that he had had a vasectomy, and thus the pregnancy was a shock. Putting that and other information together, Mary recognized that the man she was involved with was a pathological liar. Her first duty was to attend to the pregnancy, as she had decided that she did not want the baby. The doctor did an abortion under a medical D&C and performed a tubal ligation at her request. It was while she was being taken to the operating room that she realized, "I was on my way to taking control of my life." She also realized that "fate wasn't dealing me a hand. I was responsible for my life—I did have control . . . I have choices." Having attended to these matters, she faced him at home, spoke her mind without reservation, and removed him from her life. After telling her story, she looked at the therapist and said that before that experience, "I always felt things happened *to* me." That insight was a major factor in the long-term stability of her change.

Another story of change happened to a social worker named Ellen. She recounted considerable test anxiety as an undergraduate, with symptoms such as stomachaches and even vomiting before exams. She worked on her test anxiety with a therapist, hoping the results would influence what she called her "general anxiety." She engaged in cognitive-behavioral therapy that included desensitization, meditation twice a day, and countering each arising "negative self-statement with two positive ones." After 12 weeks of treatment, she was relaxing on the deck of her apartment and suddenly experienced a flood of memories and repressed feelings and emotions. She said, "I think of it as a dam bursting or a wall crumbling," as memories of childhood sexual abuse rose into her immediate awareness. These memories were associated with "anger, guilt, hurt, and pain," and she described the experience as simultaneously "exciting and scary."

Looking back on her realization, she said, "Up until that point, I thought people could do things to me and that I had no control over it." She also thought that "people and situations just happened to me, that I couldn't make things happen myself ... everything felt accidental." Later, she was reading about locus of control and realized, "I could wake up tomorrow and my life didn't have to be accidental; it could be intentional." Ellen's anxiety dramatically improved thereafter, and she reported knowing that she had handled the problem after successfully passing comprehensive exams for her master's degree.

CLINICAL MARKERS: HOW TO RECOGNIZE EFFORT OR WILL TOWARD CHANGE

The client with a high level of effort or will is relatively easy to identify, although one should avoid mistaking a manic or hyperactive client for one exhibiting effort to change. Clients with this precursor tend to display high energy and in some cases even eagerness to complete therapeutic tasks and homework assignments. Such clients seek out and ask for therapeutic exercises and activities they can perform on their own and then proceed to carry them out to completion with attention to beneficial change. They are eager to try new techniques, from role-playing to the empty chair, from paradox to journaling negative self-talk and disputing dysfunctional cognitions. They impress their therapists with their willingness to actually "do therapy" in the purest sense. In short, they take action to change.

In therapy sessions, these clients exert effort to actively help the therapist do a more thorough job. Such clients are movers and shakers where therapeutic change is concerned. They display an experimental attitude toward change with the stated intent of improving their lives, reaching their goals, or being of benefit to others. They are not hesitant to take action to correct difficult situations in their lives, such as getting out of debt, improving a relationship with a spouse, or disciplining a defiant teenager. Energy and actions taken toward change are chief markers, but the overlap with confronting should be obvious as well, although the two should not be confused.

When a client is endowed with this precursor, the therapist will sense an abundant determination to solve problems, accompanied by engagement of the body in action on the environment. Thus, such a client will actively transfer in-session learning experiences to understanding outside activities and situations. These clients may be interested in learning not only about their own issues but also about the process and nature of therapy itself. When they are hesitant to act, they will be curious about the nature of the hesitance, realizing that this is an issue in itself.

These clients can easily alter thoughts, change beliefs, and reorganize entire patterns of attitudes. They are also able to construct or deconstruct images or illusions to accomplish therapeutic tasks. For instance, a 30-year-old client named Marcus was puzzled by difficulties in his relationship with his fiancée. He realized after six intense, active sessions that he had harbored a false image of his fiancée functioning as his therapist. When he saw that he had a faulty or misguided image of a nurturing woman, in a matter of minutes, he reorganized his beliefs about women in this regard and told his therapist that he dissolved the image on the spot. In doing so, he realized that he had been difficult to get along with and that he had been demanding too much from women in his life. He reported that he had somehow grown up thinking that a woman should be his "emotional servant." In a whirlwind of insight and activity, he changed his mental attitude and patched up the relationship with his now overjoyed fiancée. This is effort at its height, attaining change remarkably quickly, deeply, and with great facility.

As one client who had a high level of this precursor once said, "I don't need a reason to be happy. I can just go ahead and force myself to feel that way whenever I want to." The apparent fact is that feelings do not have to be binding, and one can act to directly alter feelings (see James, 1890/1981) as well as behavior and cognitions.

HOW TO DETECT THE ABSENCE OF EFFORT OR WILL TOWARD CHANGE

A client lacking in effort or will consistently takes the path of least resistance and gives up easily on projects. Such a client seems to lack energy for therapeutic tasks, procrastinating and making excuses. Such clients may talk about procrastination as being a problem in itself, perhaps openly shrugging their shoulders and saying something like, "I know it is something I need to do, but I just don't seem to get around to doing it." Other clients will devote only a limited amount of energy to working in therapy and may make it appear like they are expending great amounts. This can be the case even though their abilities are considerable. Therapists may consider three particular styles of difficulty in this regard: the passive–compliant client, the falsely compliant client, and the ambivalent and conflicted client.

The Passive–Compliant Client

Some clients display a puzzling style to which therapists should be alert. The "passive–compliant" client is ostensibly compliant but is so passive that real action is outside their current capacity. This client initially seems to be anything but difficult, coming across as admirable and compliant. Such clients are highly cooperative in session and willing to discuss and disclose even the most intimate details about their lives. They appear to have many of the other precursors, such as the willingness to experience anxiety or difficulty, high awareness, a sense of necessity, and are even confronting the problem. They are willing to examine thoughts and beliefs. However, when the client is asked to carry out a therapeutic task or actually change anything, they will find excuses to avoid direct manipulation of mind or world.

Such clients may flatter the therapist or come up with amazingly creative diversions to avoid effort. A client once told her therapist that she could not do her homework assignment because the therapist was "so great that all she could do was think about our sessions and how much she learned from them." She said this during their 20th session while her life was coming down around her. Another client told his therapist that he was so fond of his old, maladaptive beliefs that "it would be a shame to lose them." This admission came following weeks of in-session work to identify, modify, and replace certain maladaptive beliefs. The client had been so compliant in sessions that the therapist genuinely believed the client had effectively replaced the beliefs many weeks earlier.

The Falsely Compliant Client

The falsely compliant client will return to the therapist and report with great authority, "I did what you said, and it didn't work." Usually, the therapist never gave direct advice and never told the client to do anything that would make anything "work." Such clients are attempting to manipulate the therapist, avoid actual effort, and prove that their situation is impossible. They rarely do the tasks assigned, and what they do usually leads to negative consequences. For such clients, effort expended has a way of making the problem even worse.

For example, a male client was given a homework assignment designed to deal with his tendency to get angry at his children. At the next session, he tells the therapist that it did not work and that he lost his temper, but he confessed several sessions later that he never attempted the assignment. In another case, a particularly difficult client in his mid-30s was convinced that his father hated him and was seeking to ruin his life. The therapist asked him, while gathering information, if he had ever talked to his mother or siblings about it. Rather than seeing this as a question, he took it as a "direct order." He came back and told the therapist, "I did what you said, and it was a waste of time." Eventually, he confessed that he had talked to his mother but only about whether she loved him. Then he told his father that the therapist said he was "neurotic," a term the therapist never used. His efforts were not consistent with the precursor of effort toward change.

Such falsely compliant clients may not be ready for homework assignments that require interpersonal skills. It may be more important to first establish other precursors before sending the client off to do tasks in their environment. For these clients, tasks should be confined to the realm of mind in the form of cognitive rehearsals and role-plays until the precursors increase and stabilize. Tasks assigned should be realistic, concrete, and clear.

The Ambivalent and Conflicted Client

Another client who is unlikely to be able to effect change experiences a massive infiltration of counter-intentions in the mind. An example is the drug user desperately seeking a way to get clean but is so in love with the drug that they cannot act on any intention to abstain. This person wants to keep using far more than they want to quit, but both intentions are there, nevertheless. If this is the case, the person is stymied, and real effort toward change will not be expended.

TECHNIQUES: INCREASING EFFORT

Effort is fundamental and essential for change. Even when it spontaneously arises out of insight and the resulting change appears "effortless," the client may have expended great amounts of energy. Where there is great interest, great effort appears effortless. Whenever possible, a sound approach is to increase the client's interest in the task, thereby increasing the degree of effort expended toward change. This section lists ways to encourage the client to expend effort in doing homework assignments and to increase the client's interest in exerting effort. These are methods to inspire a person to get off their fence, couch, or behind, as the case may be.

Metaphors That Illustrate Effort

Like so many other precursors, the idea of exerting effort lends itself well to the use of apt therapeutic metaphors. Many clichés also apply, such as "Nothing ventured, nothing gained" and "You don't know unless you try." The following additional metaphors may help clients understand the importance of effort or will.

The Finger Technique

We have found that some clients who do not understand that the act of will moves a person into action can be helped with a bit of psychoeducation. The finger technique is a thought experiment that illustrates the act of will through a simple demonstration. It is especially helpful with procrastinating clients, and the therapist should demonstrate it first and then ask the client to try it. Ideally, the client does the exercise along with the therapist.

The technique begins with the therapist holding up an index finger. The therapist explains to the client that exerting effort begins with an act of will. Holding the finger up, the therapist shows different ways of bending it. The therapist first explains that they are thinking about bending the finger. Of course, the finger does not move. Next, the therapist shouts at the finger to bend, and still, it does not move. The therapist begs and pleads with the finger to move, with no effect. The therapist then says in a procrastinating way, "Don't worry, I am going to bend it tomorrow." The finger does not move. The therapist says they are forming a mental image of bending it, and the finger almost moves, but not really. Finally, the therapist actually exerts the will to move the finger, explaining that this is the only thing that will get it to move and that the act of will accomplishes the task. It can be explained that virtually all human actions that are not on some automatic or autonomic routine are executed in this way.

The therapist asks the client to bend their finger several times and to closely observe the act of will that brings the motion about. Performing this simple act of willing, a person can often come to understand what procrastination is and what it takes to engage effort toward a task. If the will is not exerted, effort is not expended. Once the exercise has been done, if a client does not do a homework assignment, the therapist can use the metaphor by saying, "So you didn't move the finger?" In this way, the client will readily understand the metaphor as it relates to therapeutic goals and tasks and to the fundamental act of achievement and accomplishment.

The House Cleaning Metaphor

The house cleaning metaphor is appropriate for some clients in communicating the importance of effort. The person's mind or life can be likened to a house in need of cleaning. One can be acutely aware of how dirty the house is and even confront every detail of the dirt and grime, but it will not get cleaned by awareness or confronting. It will also not get cleaned by talking about how much it needs to be cleaned. At some point, a person has to sweep the carpets, do the dishes, scrub the floors, and disinfect the bathroom. That is the effort precursor, in essence. If a person is not willing to go through the actions, the house accumulates more and more dirt until it becomes unhealthy. The same is true for the effort needed to change the conditions of one's mind, behavior, or environment.

Acknowledging Freedom of Choice

From a slightly different perspective on will, studies have demonstrated that many selection tasks are more efficiently completed by those who perceive they have freedom of choice in approaching those tasks (Barlas et al., 2017; Barlas & Obhi, 2013). Therefore, it is unsurprising that clients are more likely to complete homework assignments, for instance, when provided options and their power of choice is validated (Kazantzis & Lampropoulos, 2002). In cases of antisocial personality disorder, therapy is more effective when the free choice of these clients is emphasized (Kierulff, 1988; McRae, 2013). Many young people with a criminal record will do nearly anything to gratify their desires and passions, regardless of law or convention (DeLisi et al., 2018; Shoemaker, 2018). In fact, the goal of "getting one over on" the law or societal conventions is the challenge that often guides their choices. Rather than attempt to inhibit this distorted way of being, it occasionally helps to demonstrate the paradox that while freedom is indeed precious, exercising it unwisely can lead to a loss of that same freedom.

Clarifying the Goal

Many clients display a lack of effort when it is not clear to them what exactly it is they are trying to achieve. Often, this occurs due to busy therapists inadvertently assuming that a client understands why they have recommended a particular task. To a lesser extent, there are times when a client knows the goal but does not have a sufficiently detailed image or conception of it. People tend to demonstrate increased effort to change when they believe that the task has value (Klug & Maier, 2015) and, as previously noted, the expenditure of effort is of their own choice (Barlas et al., 2017). When difficult clients clearly see how the task relates to the "What's-in-it-for-me" question, compliance is likely to result. Thus, the client must believe they are exerting the effort by free choice toward a realistic, clear, and desirable outcome or result.

Self-Observation

Some difficult clients simply will not complete homework assignments. For these clients, the most appropriate form of assigned work is self-observation or self-monitoring, which can be done in and out of therapy. Rather than issuing a homework assignment, the therapist can ask the client to not actually change anything but only to watch or be aware of a particular behavior or situation in everyday life and report on it in the next session. While this paradoxical approach is suitable for building awareness, it is also a good preparation for exerting effort and energy toward change. A client can also do role-plays in which they are not expected to do anything other than observe what happens in terms of behavior, self-talk, or emotions. Once the client has done some self-observation, it is possible for them to engage in tasks requiring specific acts. Resistance to self-observation could mean the client decided to dull or diminish their awareness, and that is the issue that needs to be addressed.

Assigning Graduated Tasks

Some clients are not up to performing complex tasks, and it is easy to overestimate what they are capable of doing. In such cases, graduated tasks increase the likelihood that a client will follow through with a homework assignment. There is a threefold requisite to assigning graduated tasks. First, the therapist should check with the client to establish that the task is realistic. Second, the therapist should ensure the client is interested, understands the rationale, and agrees it is necessary. Finally, the therapist should assign only those tasks that the client is capable of performing successfully because to do otherwise is to set the client up for failure, which could lead to premature termination. Once simple tasks are done successfully, the client can move on to those that are more difficult or challenging.

Empathic Validation

Clients who are not in therapy of their own volition are unlikely to exert effort toward change. They may even string the therapist along, making excuses or only pretending to be cooperative as a means to graduate from a treatment program. Of course, these clients are likely to lack a sense of necessity.

Empathic validation communicates a therapist's complete acceptance and understanding of the client's current goals or attitudes toward therapy. Rather than push a therapeutic agenda and a series of corresponding activities, it is more important for the therapist to deal with clients exactly where they are at in terms of how they are feeling and thinking about treatment itself. These clients need the freedom to admit (and the therapist to acknowledge) that they do not care about therapy, the therapist, or any related program. The therapist must make it clear that they completely understand and acknowledge that the client probably feels that their rights to freedom as a citizen are being violated. This acknowledgment will bring involuntary clients closer to a viable relationship and encourage a willingness to self-disclose to a therapist. No one will exert much effort toward a goal without it resonating with some sense of meaning or purpose.

Subpersonality Approach to Effort: Mode 1

Once empathic validation has helped establish a therapeutic relationship, a subpersonality approach (see Chapter 9, this volume) may be used to address a part of the unwilling client that does want to work toward change but has yet gone unacknowledged. The therapist can ask the client if there is a part of themselves that does indeed want to work toward change. Although this might take some discussion, most clients will eventually admit they do. The therapist can ask to talk to that part. Once a subpersonality has been identified, it can be directly addressed, with the permission of the client, so as to give it voice. Thus, from their own mouth, the client "hears" their own inclinations toward change. The subpersonality of the person that was uninterested in change can eventually be disidentified with and treated as being well intended but ultimately detrimental to the person's well-being.

Subpersonality Approach to Effort: Mode 2

Some clients say they do want to exert effort toward change, but they never get around to it. Many of these difficult clients appear to have a strong sense of lethargy. They might report that they wanted to change, but it seemed too difficult. Sometimes, this is related to a lack of grit, or willingness to experience anxiety or difficulty, but in other cases, the willingness precursor may be adequately present, yet effort is still rated at trace or nonexistent. For such clients, the subpersonality approach can be of occasional service. In this application, a subpersonality may be actively but silently opposing intentions or goals.

To address this brand of lethargy, the therapist can ask whether the client wants to complete the task. If the client replies in the affirmative, the therapist can validate the client and suggest that there is probably a good reason why they did not carry out the homework assignment. The therapist can ask if the client is willing to explore this possibility and ask any of the following subpersonality questions as appropriate:

Is there a part of you that ...

- ... does not want to do anything to change?
- ... does not want to do anything in therapy?

- ... does not want to do the homework assignment?
- ... is stopping you from completing the task?
- ... believes something bad will happen if you do this?
- ... feels nervous or hesitant about the task?

Next, the therapist asks to talk to that part of the client. In carrying on an empathic dialogue with the subpersonality, much information is gained that can then be addressed using other techniques offered in this chapter. Several approaches can follow. For example, the empty chair can be used, or perhaps a role-play in which the therapist plays the client or the subpersonality so that an ensuing dialogue leads to some integration of the lethargic self. The technique aims to increase expended effort by reducing the lethargy produced by being at cross-purposes with different aspects of the self. When the client's counter-effort reduces, more energy is available to devote to effort toward therapy goals without the previous inhibition or hesitancy.

Mapping Intentions

Once again, if the client genuinely states a desire for change but is not doing anything to achieve it, it is often helpful to recognize that there might be a good reason. At one level, the client may truly want change, but at another, less conscious level, change is threatening. It is often the case that a client "knows" change to be a liability and unconsciously works to sabotage all efforts even while consciously attempting it. A diagram of intentions oriented around and in relation to a therapeutic goal can reveal why effort is stalled.

The therapeutic task with such clients is to understand what the intentions and purposes are in the client's mind and to map or diagram them in terms of intentions and counter-intentions, or purposes and counter-purposes. The therapist records on the map both intentions that are conducive to achieving the goal and intentions that directly counter it.

This technique is not the same as listing the pros and cons of a particular activity or goal, which, in our experience, is largely unproductive. The mapping intentions approach is different because it lists active intentions rather than reasons. A counter-intention is not listed in negative terms and judged as a "con" but is recorded as a purpose in and of itself that simply runs in a different direction. In the mapping process, it is important to state each intention in an active context, avoiding terms such as "not." "don't," "should," or "must." After all, a counter-intention is nothing more than a conflicting intention. The intention "to travel the world" is an intention, but it can be a counter-intention when juxtaposed with "to get a doctorate." Each is active and each typically excludes or denies the other, at least in terms of time periods.

Naming each intention properly is also important, and the client must agree that the wording is accurate. After the intentions and counter-intentions are mapped, the therapist asks the client to examine each intention to determine if it should be supported, altered, suspended, or eliminated. The goal is to allow the person to see the patterns of intention and to be released from them so that effort can be freed up to pursue change.

For example, Carla, a woman in her mid-30s, was in great distress over the verbal abuse her husband heaped on her and her two children. He was a charming fellow who was often apologetic after a particularly cruel outburst. Carla had decided to leave him. She set a task for herself of calling a lawyer to initiate divorce proceedings, but she could not bring herself to act. Her progress in therapy was stalled, and she was low in the precursors of effort and confronting.

With the help of the therapist, she mapped her intentions and counter-intentions. Her intentions were to be happy, protect her children, be free, and grow as a person. Her counter-intentions to the goal of seeking a divorce were to have financial security, help her husband, be true to her marriage, show her children that marriage can work, and prove to her parents and friends that she had good judgment in men.

In therapy, each intention and counter-intention, as revealed and identified, was newly evaluated, with Carla deciding whether to support, alter, suspend, or eliminate each. She supported all of her intentions. With her counter-intentions, she chose to temporarily suspend her goal of having financial security, knowing that she would be facing hardship through the divorce. She also suspended (with considerable relief) her goal to be true to her marriage and eliminated her intention to prove to her parents and friends that she had good judgment in men. As a result, she finally went into motion and acted by filing the divorce proceedings.

Facilitating the Decision to Change

Therapeutic change often comes from a specific decision and manifests as a firm commitment. Many factors combine to culminate in a pervasive, integral decision. Unfortunately, we know no easy way to facilitate such a stalwart decision; many precursors seem to weave together in such cases. It seems that confronting and a sense of necessity are especially involved. At times, a client can be asked, straightforwardly, whether they have made an active decision to change. If no change has been forthcoming, the client will likely admit that they have not made such a decision. Last, the therapist can ask the client what it would take to make such a decision. They can also ask the client, in the tradition of the Adlerian "as if," to go ahead and pretend to make the decision, to try it on for size and see if it "feels right." This can sometimes influence a decision and a commitment.

Identifying and Disputing Automatic Thoughts or Negative Self-Talk

This approach consists of asking a person to perform a therapeutic task, preferably in the session, and then having them immediately watch for and report any opposing, contrary, or negating thoughts that arise. Such automatic thoughts can sabotage effort. For example, Michael, a client in his early 20s, had a female employer who was verbally abusive but veiled her hostility with biting jokes and laughter. Michael found it extremely difficult to ask his employer if she would stop and could not bring himself to do even graduated tasks. However, he was willing to do role-plays.

To discover possible automatic thoughts, the therapist and client agreed to set up a role-play in which Michael was to address the therapist, who was playing the role of his verbally abusive employer. The variation was that instead of going through with the role-play and being concerned with what to say to his boss, Michael was to report any opposing thoughts in the way of doubts, criticisms of self, negative expectations, and distorted images associated with speaking to her boss. Once these were addressed and disputed, Michael found it much easier to do realistic role-plays and eventually confronted his employer in an assertive and nonaccusatory manner. In their meeting, he informed her that even though she meant no harm, telling him that he was "dumb" and "silly" was hurtful and did not help him perform better on the job. What was more helpful, he told her, was when he was given details and instructions on how to do better. He was pleasantly surprised when his employer quietly but deliberately agreed to his request.

Attending to the Metalogue

It is easy to hand out homework assignments to difficult clients, and it is just as easy for clients to listen and show (or feign) interest. The question is whether a client will execute the assignments and make self-initiated actions toward change. In many of these cases, a cognitive approach may be enhanced by attending to the metalogue between client and therapist. The client may be engaged in a metalogue that is inhibiting therapeutic progress. For example, many difficult clients will say that as soon as their therapist suggested a task to be completed outside of therapy, they immediately responded with an unvoiced statement such as, "Yeah, right," "I don't care about this," or simply, "No way." Clients may be only dimly aware of this response until asked. Curiously, a client can simultaneously engage in such self-talk while externally agreeing to do the assigned tasks.

Addressing and vocalizing the metalogue can reduce interference with the effort precursor. Once the metalogue is identified and articulated, it can be handily treated by using the subpersonality approach, mapping intentions, or finding maladaptive beliefs. As long as the metalogue is not addressed, however, the therapist runs the risk of the client's continued ambivalence and lack of cooperation, both within and outside of therapy sessions.

Examining Maladaptive Beliefs About the Effort to Change

When effort is not occurring, a host of maladaptive beliefs may be inhibiting a person from moving toward change. When maladaptive beliefs are disputed, the person may spring into motion and make an effort toward therapeutic tasks and goals. While some maladaptive beliefs emphasize a tendency toward dispositional passivity, others indicate fears about the consequences of, or inability to enact, change. The following are possible maladaptive beliefs that may inhibit effort and exertion of the will:

• Being happy means doing as little as possible and just enjoying myself.
• I don't deserve to get better and won't do anything toward it.
• I've hurt too many people to deserve to devote effort to myself.
• I screw everything up anyway, so why try?
• I can't be trusted to succeed.
• Becoming effective will only make me capable of hurting people more.
• I know that if I try, I'll fail.
• I'm afraid of making more mistakes.
• I feel guilty if I try to help myself.
• Someone else should do the work for me.
• I'm waiting for someone to rescue me from all this.
• God will take care of me.

A CLOSING NOTE ON EFFORT

Effort or will toward change is a precursor that leads to multifaceted, multilevel transformation and ties together many of the other precursors. When effortful control is operative, there is a sense in which one's thinking, feeling, and behavior are seemingly driven by a deep wellspring of desire and determination. Some clients find such effortful control simple to tap into, but many difficult clients struggle in this area of action as if the will itself has been rendered immobile. When effort or will to change is inactive in therapy, it becomes the responsibility of the therapist to implement basic strategies and techniques that might help clients move toward self-directed action to change.

10

S: Social Support for Change

Social support is the condition in which a person receives physical, emotional, attentional, and other resources from other human beings. A person has social support when they are surrounded by a network of friends or family who feel positively about them, are empathic, and are willing to help. The ideal social support network consists of people who are available and willing to invite, receive, and accept emotional disclosures. Social support also includes a person's perception that the community or environment is conducive and actively contributing to their well-being. It gratifies the primary needs of acceptance and belonging in human relationships.

Social support is a powerful reinforcer in both positive and negative ways. In effect, this precursor is like fire in that it can be used positively or negatively to produce constructive or destructive results. It is important to consult with the client to determine whether a social support is beneficial and constructive or deleterious and dysfunctional. For example, many adolescent offenders will note that their peers have supported them in committing criminal acts. The supportive statements sound something like this: "It's okay, you can do it. We were scared too at first, but don't worry. You get used to it and don't even think about it after a while." This message could as easily be about getting good grades as committing a crime. In the armed forces, the same message is given to soldiers coming to grips with the fact that they may be called on to kill.

Likewise, social support can exist in varying grades of quality. Even in its lowest grades, it may be seen as precious, and its influence should not be underestimated. Probably the best perspective on understanding this phenomenon is Yalom's (1995) therapeutic factors of group therapy, which include universality, group cohesiveness, and catharsis. Such therapeutic factors can

---

Case examples have been disguised to protect client confidentiality.

https://doi.org/10.1037/0000451-011

Therapeutic Change With Difficult Clients: Precursors and Techniques in the CHANGES Model, Second Edition, by B. D. Wilkinson and F. J. Hanna

occasionally be found in street gangs, however twisted these may be. For instance, a gang member named Lollo once showed up for a session at an outpatient substance use treatment center with a severe hangover and a large bruise on his forehead. He had a devastatingly sad family history, having long witnessed his mother being sexually abused by his uncle, who also physically abused him.

The therapist inquired about the injury, but Lollo defiantly replied, "Yeah, I was drunk, so what?" and insisted the therapist would "never get it." The therapist said that although he might not understand, perhaps Lollo could teach him something. Lollo idly shrugged but explained how he had been drinking with fellow gang members the previous night when the gang leader, whom Lollo deeply admired, told him in an emotional outburst that they would always be friends. He then threw an empty beer bottle, hitting Lollo in the forehead and leaving the bruise while yelling that he loved him like a little brother. For Lollo, this distorted declaration of affection and care was precious and gave him an immense sense of belonging and acceptance. It is not surprising that he thought the therapist would not understand, and it is also evident that even low-grade social supports that prevent positive change can invoke a feeling of belonging and care.

A multitude of theorists, ranging from Adler and Maslow, to Bowen and Satir, to Johnson and Hayes, have noted the need for belonging and acceptance by fellow human beings. Social support is just another term for this primary human need. Recommending it is stating the blatantly obvious, rather like saying that eating nutritious foods is a good idea. In the same sense that certain vitamins can cure rickets and scurvy, social support can alleviate loneliness and a sense of abandonment. It meets the need for companionship, warmth, intimacy, and communication, all of which give meaning to life (Yalom, 1980, 1989). It may be that the service provided by support groups such as Alcoholics Anonymous (2012) is valuable because it replaces negative social support with a social support system oriented toward positive change.

HOW SOCIAL SUPPORT LEADS TO THERAPEUTIC CHANGE

Common factors researchers have long identified perceived social support as an active ingredient in therapeutic change (Wampold & Ulvenes, 2019), and it has also been identified as a source of spontaneous self-improvement (Lambert, 1992). It can be a major influence on recovery from depression (Woods et al., 2021) and a protective factor against suicidal ideation (Arenson et al., 2021). Various meta-analyses identify social support interventions as critical in improving mental health outcomes among survivors of intimate partner violence (Ogbe et al., 2020) as well as posttraumatic stress disorder among both civilian (Wang et al., 2021) and military (Blais et al., 2021) populations. It has been positively correlated with effective pain management among cancer patients (Warth et al., 2020). Preliminary research on the everyday use of chatbots indicates that artificial agents may be perceived as warmly supportive companions that reduce loneliness (Bendig et al., 2022; Ta et al., 2020), while companion animals produce even more pronounced results (Brooks et al., 2018).

According to the CHANGES model, the primary contribution of social support for change seems to be its interaction with the other precursors as a potentiating agent. Its presence makes the other precursors more powerful. The social support precursor affects nearly every aspect of a person's life, including physiological health. Like hope and a sense of necessity, it is seldom, if ever, a sufficient condition for change by itself, but it enhances the power of all the other precursors in both subtle and direct ways. It can be a source that inspires motivation and engagement, although we have found that in some cases of extraordinary human resourcefulness, it did not seem to be necessary at all. Even in those same cases, however, it probably would have been helpful.

Social support has a resounding influence on hope (Martínez-Martí & Ruch, 2017). Change seems easier to envision when the encouragement of loved ones and friends is present to convince a person to contemplate new possibilities. When one has little hope for oneself, knowing that trusted family and friends are convinced of a bright future can bring about a contagion of hope. Effort can be enhanced in kind, as one approaches tasks and goals with more conviction. When a person is filled with self-doubt, the confidence of family and friends can induce the exertion of effort. Similarly, social support makes anxiety or difficulty easier to tolerate. When one knows that people are there to help one get through the ordeals of life, the sheer difficulty of it can be much reduced.

Social support can also help establish a sense of necessity by informing a person of the importance of a particular change. For example, if a client expresses little or no interest in change, the advice, counsel, or concern of a friend or friends may convince them that things are not acceptable as they are and that a change is needed. Awareness may also become enhanced in this way. A verbally abusive husband may listen to a friend saying, "You are being too rough with your wife," but resist the same statement by a mother-in-law or therapist. Finally, in terms of confronting the problem, a safe and socially supportive environment is needed to look at threatening beliefs, mistakes, memories, or feelings. A person who feels secure is more likely to steadily and deeply confront problems (see Hanna & Puhakka, 1991).

SIGNIFICANT MOMENTS OF CHANGE INVOLVING SOCIAL SUPPORT

Alicia was a licensed psychologist in her mid-30s, and her second-order change experience took place 8 years prior to the following therapeutic encounter. She explained to her therapist how, 8 years earlier, she was planning to get married when her fiancée died from a chronic heart ailment. "I went nuts," she said, "and I started cutting myself." She revealed her arms, which still bore the extensive scars from her self-mutilation. She explained that she became "really depressed" and started to lose control of her life. "This stuff was always there" in the background, she reported; this tragedy had just brought it to the foreground.

She went for therapy at her university counseling center, but it was ineffective, and she eventually dropped out of school altogether.

She tried to overdose on sleeping pills soon thereafter. She was hospitalized in critical condition. As a psychiatric ward inpatient, she eventually found a particularly helpful therapist. With this therapist, she said, "There was some hope," and the road to her recovery began. Long after her release from the hospital, however, she was still very angry and resentful. That summer, Alicia worked with kids at a Christian camp "just to give something" to people. She was also in a therapy group and was getting a lot of "positive affirmations" and support to return to school. However, her therapist moved out of town, and after about 2 months, Alicia "started getting scared again."

By this time, she had entered another university and found her way to its counseling center. The therapist there proved to be extremely helpful and disclosed that she had once had similar problems. In Alicia's work with the new therapist, she learned more about her relationship with her mother and her mother's influence on her life. "I learned that I really did need her love and that she really did love me." This was an important insight for Alicia. At one stage, all of this had built to a climax, and the "therapist let me cry." This experience was the crux of change for her. It was a "letting go of anger, frustration, hurt, watching it all wash away. I learned to listen with a different heart. That was a major changing point," she said. She came to see that she could "get the things [she] needed from other people, and it's okay."

After this experience, she "became less angry" and "related to people differently." She learned to "phrase things differently." She added that she learned "that you have to take control of your life and not let life control you." She also said, "The experience reaffirmed my faith in God." During the ensuing years, she reported no acts of self-harm. This example is typical of the excellent social support for change available through effective therapy.

CLINICAL MARKERS: HOW TO RECOGNIZE SOCIAL SUPPORT FOR CHANGE

The therapist can assess the presence of social support from information provided by the client and the nature and tone of the conversation about it. There are many signs and indicators of the presence of social support. Perhaps the easiest and most direct method is to ask the client if they feel supported by friends and family and to what degree. Therapists can also ask if clients know of a network of friends who are supportive and helpful to each other, whether they are a part of that network, and, if they are, how much. It also helps to examine the client's conversation for descriptions of relationships and interactions with others.

To determine the quality of support in those relationships, one can gauge the degree of perceived empathy by asking if the client feels those people truly understand them and, if so, how much. Trust is another element that can be assessed when gauging the quality of those relationships. It helps to ask a client if they actually trust anyone and, if they do, to name those people. When trust and empathy are present, the relationship will tend to be especially valued by a client, and levels of ambivalence or hostility toward the person will be low. In addition, those people described by the client should be spoken of as accessible and available in times of need.

Common references to the support of family and friends are an obvious indicator, especially when the person takes comfort in and works to maintain and develop those relationships. It is also helpful to assess religious or community involvements in terms of social support to see if they are characterized by empathy and encouragement and are not critical, demeaning, or disempowering. Some difficult clients may be members of religious groups with cultlike features that invoke deep suspicion of therapy and try to sabotage any apparent progress (Goldberg, 2017).

A client rich in social support may also demonstrate relationship skills with the therapist; this is a vital sign of the client's interaction skills. A client with this kind of skill will make the therapist feel supported in attempting to help the client. Needless to say, this type of client is especially appreciated by a therapist. In terms of the therapeutic relationship, however, it is important to ask the client for their assessment of how empathic or trustworthy the therapist may be, as research clearly shows that client assessments of therapist empathy tend to be more accurate than self-assessments by therapists themselves.

HOW TO DETECT THE ABSENCE OF SOCIAL SUPPORT FOR CHANGE

A primary problem with difficult clients is often a profound lack of social support, especially for positive change. Many have destroyed the possibility of positive social support through manipulation and harmful acts toward others. We have known some difficult clients who did not change even with the help of the most compassionate and skilled therapists and well-meaning family and friends. A common example is the case of some chronic alcohol users who continue their self-destructive behaviors despite a network of caring friends, family, and therapists. By the time some clients have discovered a sense of necessity for change, they are profoundly alone.

A lack of social support is frequently quite obvious in therapy. In the absence of social support, a client may complain about feeling "all alone" or having "no one to talk to." There may be direct references to "not having anyone to rely upon," such as the single mother working multiple jobs without family or friends who can lend a hand for childcare needs. Depressed clients are also likely to report that they are without close friends or family who understand them (Arslan, 2019; Franck et al., 2016). When stated as a global declaration, the complaint that "there are so few understanding people in the world," or the related belief that life itself is unjust, should be explored in the context of lifelong changes and patterns of social support (Stauffer, 2015; Ucar et al., 2019).

Many people lacking social support are likely to perceive their families with either open hostility or deep ambivalence. They are likely to see their families as a source of anxiety, emotional hurt, depression, abuse, or ridicule. They may accuse their mother or father of having ruined their lives. They describe brothers and sisters as distant or having so little in common with the client that there is no point in maintaining the relationship. All this may be true, but this does not diminish the glaring fact that the person sadly lacks a vital source of social support.

Assessing social support in people with personality disorders is more complex. Many narcissistic clients will boast about possessing a wide network of friends and admirers. They may boldly assert their popularity and appeal to others. The need for admiration on the part of this client is a clue to the nature of their relationships. Such clients do not describe so-called supportive people as those to whom they might make vulnerable self-disclosures about shame, guilt, or mistakes made in life and will abruptly cut off relationships with critical people. With gentle but pointed questioning, such a client may admit that no one "really cares" and claim all people are out for their own gain.

Other difficult clients will see interpersonal support as a liability and will avoid it as a potential source of pain. This is often true of borderline clients, who may interpret any gesture of help as a cause for suspicion of eventual betrayal. Many difficult clients have issues of abandonment and engulfment. Gaining social support is both a need and an admission of weakness and while they actively seek it, they may simultaneously despise the fact that they need it. Many borderline clients are unconsciously convinced that they are so worthless and undeserving that anyone who likes them must be a fool or stupid or both, and they treat potential friends with mixed neediness and contempt. Thus, to help, a therapist must be willing to be seen as an object of contempt and derision, at least for a while. The end result, of course, is that a person with borderline traits may tolerate the idea of improvement. In addition, they often punish those who try to help.

Antisocial clients also tend to believe that needing the help of others is a sign of weakness and will manipulate those who try to help, perhaps by taking advantage of them in terms of money, sexual favors, gaining status or connections, or the like. Social support systems for these clients, if they can be considered that at all, are usually extremely low grade and are characterized by internal dishonesty, cheating, and betrayal. The underlying belief is that one can expect others to help only when they are ultimately manipulating the situation for their own gain. Alternatively, a client with schizoid personality disorder will be unlikely to complain about a lack of friends and will probably prefer to be alone in their private world.

In conclusion, when a person lacks social support, it is easier to minimize or explain away problems. Change will be viewed as an individual struggle requiring more effort than necessary, and experiencing anxiety or difficulty will look rather like torture, to be endured all alone. Further, the awareness of a problem may not crystallize with the clarity that comes with trusted feedback, and the problem may not seem quite so imminent or real to the point where confronting may actually be necessary or helpful. Clients without social support will also be inclined to give up hope more easily, lamenting that the future is an essentially lonely undertaking. Finally, clients will respond to therapy when they experience their therapists as having positive expectations for them (W. R. Miller & Rollnick, 2012), which is a vital aspect of social support generated by the therapist.

TECHNIQUES: GROWING SOCIAL SUPPORT

Helping clients develop social support consists of three separate but related modalities. The first modality is to minimize contact with people who are harmful, abusive, negative, exploitative, or otherwise oppressive to the client. If uncorrected or undeterred, such people can discourage the presence of the precursors of change just as surely as a good therapist can encourage them. In general, of course, it is usually futile to attempt to change people who are not supportive.

The second modality for increasing social support is to increase the presence of people who encourage the precursors of change. These people are generally empathic and helpful and serve as sources of understanding, trust, and active support. Increasing this kind of social support involves teaching a client social and communication skills.

The third modality is important for some clients who have lost valuable friendships. Therapy can help clients rebuild once-supportive relationships that have deteriorated. This goal is often unrealistic, of course. Many clients with personality disorders or alcohol or drug use problems tend to exploit people who trust them and make a habit of wasting relationships. It is common for them to regret having done so, and therapy can sometimes help clients recover those friendships. However, it can be delicate work because of the intense emotions and feelings, including betrayal, on both sides.

A Cautionary Note

Therapists should use caution in teaching skills that facilitate social support, such as reflection of feelings and other communication microskills, to clients who will use them in harmful ways. For example, sex offenders and criminal offenders may use advanced social support skills to victimize and exploit others, taking targets into their confidence only to betray them. The clinician must use careful judgment to ensure irresponsible clients do not use newly learned social skills to deceive, betray, or hurt the people around them. In our experience, empathy and responsibility need to be rehabilitated in such clients before they can be trusted with skills that engender the trust of others.

Teaching Clients to Recognize Empathy in Others

Many clients get themselves into trouble by trusting or becoming attached to people who are harmful and exploitative. This often happens in romantic relationships; a person marries or otherwise becomes attached to a partner who is not empathic. A battering husband may indeed love his wife, just as an abusive father may care for his children. However, these men have little or no intact empathy for the people they love. Love and empathy are not the same.

Clients can benefit from learning to recognize the presence of empathy in others. The telltale sign is whether the client feels understood by the other person, as if the person understands the client "from the inside out." Many clients need to be taught to recognize this fundamental phenomenon because they are simply not familiar with it.

Recognizing empathy is a skill that can be used throughout one's life. Teaching a client to recognize empathy or the lack of it in another person and to avoid confiding in nonempathic people can help them avoid many difficult situations and be able to recognize a vital aspect of healthy friendships. Perhaps the best standard of measurement for empathy is the therapeutic relationship. Clients can use it as a model, especially those who lack empathic relationships in other areas of their lives and have no way to compare the quality of relationships.

Identifying Sources of Social Support for Change

Once able to recognize empathy, the therapist should help the client identify sources of social support in their environment. In determining whether to discourage or increase a continued association, the therapist can explore with the client the value of reciprocal relationships and the presence of empathy in the person or group. It also helps to assess whether the person or group contributes to the presence of the precursors of change. Social skills training can be used to strengthen and reinforce positive relationships.

The Concentric-Circle Technique

Lazarus's (1989b) concentric-circle technique is an excellent means of gauging the closeness of the therapeutic relationship and the level of the client's self-disclosure to the therapist. It involves drawing five embedded, or concentric, circles on a full piece of paper. The inner circle represents closeness and trustworthiness, with each outer circle representing a degree of distance. The client is asked to write down the names of important people in their lives within an appropriate concentric circle, according to how much they trust that person. As part of developing social support, this technique can be used to gauge client closeness to people in their environment. Once this is done, the client can discuss whether the person in question contributes to their social support toward change, or whether the person is harmful to it, or even merely tangential.

The technique is useful in several ways. If a client has a habit of taking people into their confidence who then betray or abandon the client, the technique can be used as a tool to help delineate and establish boundaries. In other words, clients who have such boundary difficulties can begin to establish criteria for allowing a person entrance to each inner circle. For clients who have experienced pain from unwisely disclosing personal information to inappropriate people, this technique helps to determine who is a worthy candidate for this precious trust. If a client associates pain with allowing a person into the two innermost circles, this indicates that they need to be more perceptive and discreet. Another use for this technique is to count the number of people the client has allowed into the two inner circles. The therapist can ask the client how it feels to have so many people with intimate knowledge of them.

At the opposite polarity, some clients have allowed and plan to allow no one into the two innermost circles. This has consequences and a set of corresponding feelings. People who have shut out virtually everyone from emotional intimacy may feel alienated, lonely, sad, or resentful. The approach would be, once again, to determine what it would take to allow someone into those two inner circles. A client's criteria may be quite irrational, from too rigid on the one hand to too demanding on the other. A therapist can help clients formulate more realistic beliefs to ease the negative feelings associated with being disengaged from one's fellow human beings.

Identifying People Who Are Opposed to Therapeutic Change

Curiously, in almost every difficult client's life, there are people who oppose the client's therapeutic change. In such cases, beneficial change runs at cross-purposes to that person's intentions for the client. Some people need the client to remain exactly the way they are. Dysfunctional families tend to resist the improvement of one of its members because family systems naturally seek consistency, or homeostasis. Virtually all therapists have encountered these challenging situations. Many difficult clients swear that the people who are most harmful to them are also the most important people in their lives. Thus, helping clients identify these people's harmful or negative influences is often a major therapeutic task. This can include addressing the impact of influencers across social media platforms who may have an outsized influence on client's lives.

The therapist should assess, perhaps directly by asking the client, whether people in the client's life encourage therapeutic change. The client must be able to answer specific questions. For example, do the people in question tend to quell the sense of necessity, discourage confronting, or destroy hope? Do they seek to undermine efforts toward change? In the case of enabling, does a caring family member or spouse actively discourage the willingness to experience anxiety? Such questions can be formulated easily enough, and the therapist can present the evidence to the client for their consideration. The therapist can also ask some clients how they feel about themselves or their lives in the presence of the person to get a kind of visceral assessment. Another approach to facilitate insight is to ask what the person wants the client to believe about them. The overall goal is to help a client be able to gauge who is not supportive of their growth; in this way, a difficult client can recognize the consequences of associating with specific people and either avoid or directly address this source of needless anxiety and trouble.

Recovering Lost Sources of Social Support

Many clients live with the hidden regret of having lost relationships with close friends or family members who once provided social support. The relationship may have been lost due to the client's acting out, betrayal, manipulations, or dishonesty. Clients can feel considerable shame and guilt at the mere thought of these lost relationships. The client may try to convince themselves that the relationship was unimportant or that the other person was at fault. Many clients also use the excuse that the person in question "never really understood" them, so there is no loss when, in fact, such people may have understood a bit too well.

In some cases, social support can be rehabilitated with those relationships. In many other instances, the residual distrust is so great that the relationship is, for all practical purposes, beyond repair. Nevertheless, therapy can help determine how and why such relationships fell apart to begin with so the client can avoid making the same mistakes with new relationships. Help in recovering relationships is not recommended for clients who are criminal or extremely manipulative. In such cases, they may only again victimize people who were happy to be free of them. Protecting others from such clients is often the primary concern until they are no longer destructive in relationships.

Exploring Trust

For many difficult clients, the issue of trust is surrounded by irrational beliefs and righteous indignation. These clients must learn that trust has to be earned and that it is not a birthright. Many clients exploit and betray others, only to later complain that no one trusts them, as if they have been deeply wronged. Such blaming behavior can be addressed by setting up scenarios, role-plays, role reversals, and dialogue in which such clients can experience the effects of their manipulations. The purpose is to produce empathy in the client toward those who no longer trust them. In a role-play, the therapist can assume the role of the client, displaying the same behaviors that led to a loss of trust, followed by a role reversal. Responses and feelings can then be explored, which may lead to understanding how the relationship broke down.

Standard Social Skills Techniques

Standard therapy techniques and approaches can help clients develop social support networks. These are described in introductory textbooks on counseling and psychotherapy and are not described in detail here. Each is valuable in teaching clients how to find, build, and maintain supportive relationships based on empathy and caring.

Group Therapy

Group therapy provides a context and format conducive to developing social support. A well-run group can be tremendously powerful in teaching clients the power of empathy and compassion. The amount of empathy generated in a group that has achieved the working stage is exponentially more powerful than that of a single therapist. In a group, a person can come to experience empathic, supportive friendships that if provided by an individual therapist would violate ethical codes on dual relationships.

For a group to achieve the working stage, its members need to have progressed through the early-stage disagreements, personality conflicts, and the like and proceed to provide high-quality help to each other (see Corey, 2017). This is a standard aspect of the group process. The group therapist is only minimally active at the working stage unless carrying out a specific set of therapeutic techniques. In this regard, group therapy has far more utility than individual therapy. Ideally, group and individual therapy are done concurrently. They need not interfere with each other, and each can enhance the progress of the other. Done well, it is a model of empathic relationships. An additional benefit of group therapy that is not found in individual therapy is the opportunity the client has to learn helping skills and apply them in a therapeutic setting (Yalom, 1995). Unfortunately, we have seen many group therapists who have not experienced a group at the working stage due to limited training or poor treatment planning by agencies.

Examining Maladaptive Beliefs About People and Relationships

Difficult clients can possess an amazing array of dysfunctional, maladaptive beliefs about people and relationships. These can profoundly influence the kinds of people with whom they associate and the relationships they form and keep. When firmly held, maladaptive beliefs about relationships and people can influence a client to become attached to exploitative and self-serving people. Such beliefs also influence clients to develop behaviors that will subvert, undermine, and eventually damage potentially valuable relationships.

Many dysfunctional, maladaptive beliefs seem sound at first glance but have a logical flaw in them that, when acted on, can sabotage relationships. Identifying, disputing, and changing maladaptive beliefs can have an amazing effect on a person's willingness to engage in intimate relationships and choose to enter healthy, stable relationships. As with other maladaptive beliefs, clients require therapist support in examining personal belief statements, such as the following:

- People are sources of anxiety and pain.
- I can't live without love.
- I'm only alive when others are paying attention to me.
- If I can please people, they'll like me.
- I need other people to tell me how to be and who I am.
- I must have a person to whom I can give up control of myself.
- A friend is someone who will rescue me from my problems.
- Even cruel attention from others is better than no attention at all.
- I'm secure only when others are around.
- Only fools would be interested in supporting me.
- The people stupid enough to support me cannot be trusted for that reason.
- Nobody ever really cares about anybody.

- People only care about themselves.
- The presence of others threatens my survival.
- People are tolerable only when they are under my control.
- If I stay away from the company of others, they cannot hurt me.
- I'm not as good as anyone else and thus deserve to be treated badly.
- If I'm in conflict with someone, it's better to end the relationship.
- If a relationship requires work, it's not worth keeping.
- If I run into difficulty with one person, I can always find someone else.

A CLOSING NOTE ON SOCIAL SUPPORT

Contributions of social support to therapeutic change have long been discussed in psychotherapy, although its centrality as a client-specific change factor varies across theoretical perspectives. In terms of the CHANGES model, social support seems to enhance the potency of other precursors insofar as support by others can serve as a reminder to confront an issue, increase necessity, sustain hope, and take consistent action. When social supports are not in place, it is incumbent upon the therapist to determine the nature of relationships in a client's life so as to facilitate engagement of high-quality supports and confront the deleterious effects of negative or interfering persons.

THE CHANGES ASSESSMENT

11

Rating Client Potential for Therapeutic Change

There are many active ingredients of change in addition to the seven precursors. Many therapy outcomes, such as finding meaning in life or a cathartic release of emotion, are also responsible for changes (Hanna & Ritchie, 1995). In other words, what looks like an effect of change processes can also become a cause in its own right, creating a snowball effect of more change. Kant (1787/1929) noted that each effect contains within it a seed of causality. This seems to be true in cases of therapeutic change. Certain variables can be both cause and effect. A profound insight, for example, is an effect brought about by multiple precursors, but the insight can have enormous additional effects on behaviors, feelings, and cognitions. However, insight and other variables are not listed as precursors because they are more of an effect than a cause.

In the case of second-order change, each change factor plays a role in combining, culminating, recombining, and subsiding in a kind of global chain reaction. There are so many cognitive, metacognitive, physiological, affective, behavioral, interpersonal, and environmental factors operative in therapeutic change that studying it is like tracking and gauging the motion and influence of all the emerging bubbles in a cauldron of boiling water. Nevertheless, the seven precursors do explain a significant portion of therapeutic change. Not completely, of course, but enough to provide a manageable and workable explanation that informs the work of therapy.

Thus, the CHANGES assessment (see Table 11.1) is not offered as some unequivocal representation of the change process. It is a pragmatic clinical tool for understanding and implementing change with difficult clients. The model is

---

Case examples have been disguised to protect client confidentiality.

https://doi.org/10.1037/0000451-012
Therapeutic Change With Difficult Clients: Precursors and Techniques in the CHANGES Model, Second Edition, by B. D. Wilkinson and F. J. Hanna

TABLE 11.1. Assessing for Active Client Precursors: The CHANGES Assessment Form

Precursor and relevant marker	None (0)	Trace (1)	Small (2)	Adequate (3)	Abundant (4)
C: Confronting the problem					
• Steadfastly faces problems					
• Sustained attention to issue					
H: Hope for change					
• Positive future outlook					
• Coping/humor intact					
A: Awareness					
• Able to identify problems					
• Identifies thoughts/feelings					
N: Sense of necessity					
• Expresses desire for change					
• Feels a sense of urgency					
G: Grit					
• Able to manage anxiety					
• Willing to take risks					
E: Effort or will to change					
• Eagerly practices skills					
• Cooperative; high energy					
S: Social support for change					
• Network of friends/family					
• Many confiding relations					

Total score: _____/28

Scoring guide[a]

0–6: Change unlikely. Educate client on change. Focus on precursors with lowest ratings.

7–14: Change limited or erratic. Educate client and focus on precursors with lowest ratings.

15–21: Change steady or noticeable. Use lowest rated precursors to stay on track.

22–28: Change occurs easily. Highly motivated client. Standard approaches work well.

[a] Scoring intended only as a general guide to a complex process. Some precursors may be more potent than others for individual clients and/or individual contexts.

insufficient to explain the vastly complex change process itself. However, the seven precursors of the CHANGES model, in their nonlinear, interactive interdependence, can certainly provide a skeletal outline that indicates the bones of change, even if it does not fully capture the finer points of flesh, fluids, tendons, and tissues.

EMPIRICAL VALIDATION OF THE ASSESSMENT

Each of the seven precursors enjoys empirical validation in the psychotherapy literature as a catalyst of change. The assessment form itself, although not empirically validated, is empirically informed. It may be a mistake to exclusively insist on empirically validated treatment approaches (Beutler, 2000; Beutler & Forrester, 2014). We might alternatively insist that therapy practices be empirically effective and clinically sensible. The CHANGES assessment is neither a psychometric evaluation nor a diagnostic instrument. Rather, it is a clinical guide for identifying the presence or absence of each of the seven change factors. It is a tool, a clinical heuristic, that reduces some of the mystery surrounding difficult clients and simultaneously indicates a path toward change.

The CHANGES assessment has been particularly useful in clinical practice in charting a course of approach to difficult clients. It has been used in various forms with many populations having difficulty with the change process or not responding to treatment. We have given the assessment form to more than 1,000 therapists and trainees to rate their most difficult clients. Almost without exception, those clinicians have reported that their clients were indeed lacking in the precursors of change, and they routinely reported that the assessment was helpful in the treatment planning process.

The CHANGES assessment has helped put together treatment programs for antisocial, borderline, and narcissistic clients, as well as adolescent criminal offenders, adolescent sex offenders, and alcohol and substance users in general. The assessment was also found to be helpful with adolescent female and male victims of sexual abuse and adults in general who were perceived or reported to be resistant to therapy. It appears to be transcultural in its capacity and relevance to describe human change across cultures.

USE OF THE CHANGES ASSESSMENT FORM

Fortunately, this assessment is among the most simple and user-friendly that a clinician is likely to learn or use. The form is helpful for individual practice, individual or group supervision, and consultations in which difficult clients are the focus of attention. The form can reveal a configuration or pattern among difficult clients in a way that also makes its use in group contexts valuable. As seen in Chapter 12 in this volume, precursor activation among difficult therapists can be rated, too.

The assessment need not be applied to clients already doing well in therapy because the precursors are already amply present in such clients. Applying the CHANGES model with these clients might deter progress away from change. The assessment is of greatest help in identifying precursors that need attention when a client makes slow or inconsistent progress toward change.

Rating the Precursors

The ratings for the assessment form are based on the clinical marker sections for each precursor in their respective chapters. These sections provide a guide to determining the presence or absence of a precursor for the purpose of rating it on this form.

Each precursor is rated from 0 to 4. At 0, there is no evidence of that particular precursor with the client in question. At 1, just a trace of the precursor shows itself only rarely, or perhaps a hint is given every now and then. A rating of 2 indicates an identifiable but small degree of presence of that precursor; it is not much, but it is also not as elusive as in the trace rating. With a precursor rated 2, the clinician knows there is at least something with which to work. At a rating of 3, the precursor is evident and readily apparent and, therefore, active in a person's approach to therapy, change, and resolution of problems. Precursors rated 4 are extremely evident, and therapists often find themselves spontaneously admiring these qualities in a client. Ratings of 4 are seldom found in difficult clients. Total scores range from 0 to 28, with higher scores representing greater levels of precursors for change.

We strongly recommend consulting with clients to ascertain the presence or absence of precursors. Clients seem to have no difficulty understanding the precursors. Difficult clients can be willing to assess the presence of their precursors and their own potential and ability to increase them. Of course, with highly manipulative or deceptive clients, caution is needed because the intentions of these clients are not always honest. Nevertheless, the client should be consulted whenever possible and appropriate. Consulting with clients has worked well in clinical settings and is often therapeutic in itself in terms of its educational function. Additionally, both trainees and experienced therapists seem to be able to rate difficult clients easily and accurately.

Do Not Include the Therapist in Rating Social Support for Change

The therapist is expected to provide social support for change, but including the therapist in the rating of this precursor will confound the actual score. The focus of the assessment in this context is the amount of support in the client's environment. The therapist is viewed more as an agent of social support than a source of it in the client's living environment. This point is debatable, of course, but social support scores seem more accurate when the therapist is not included.

Rate the Actual Presence of Precursors

Rate only the actual presence of precursors as manifested in the here and now and according to the current problem or issue. One could rate the person according to their general ability or potential for change, but this is misleading and should be avoided.

For instance, Darnell was a 32-year-old bisexual African American who identified as genderfluid. The therapist used the CHANGES assessment to rate their overall capacity for change, based upon the evidence that Darnell had instituted many changes in their life. As a result, it was assumed that Darnell had high levels of precursors, and Darnell confirmed as much when speaking in general terms. When the counselor asked, "How willing are you to experience anxiety or difficulty, or to put forth effort?" Darnell said, "Super willing. I face it every day and work hard every single day." Of course, this was true in many instances since Darnell was avidly working to support lesbian, gay, bisexual, transgender, queer/questioning, plus (others) community members as a resource coordinator for a nonprofit advocacy group.

Yet a capacity for grit, effort, awareness, or any other precursor says nothing about particular instances in which change is needed. While Darnell exhibited tremendous grit and effort in many areas of life, there were other areas in which it was absent. For one, Darnell sought out therapy because they had recently been diagnosed with Type 2 diabetes and a related lung dysfunction. They needed to build an exercise routine but had tremendous difficulty with motivation in this area. Their CHANGES assessment score for the issue of maintaining an exercise routine was

1. Confronting the problem 2
2. Hope for change 1
3. Awareness 3
4. Necessity for change 3
5. Grit, or readiness for difficulty 1
6. Effort or will toward change 0
7. Social support for change 2
Total score: 12

The score of 12 was low but also accurately indicated that change was limited or erratic, as it had proved to be in therapy. Darnell was aware of the problem and felt enough necessity to seek therapeutic support. They would also discuss the issue in therapy but would change the subject after a few minutes to discuss other topics. The therapist had noticed this avoidance pattern but followed Darnell into new areas of conversation based on the belief that they had the capacity for change but just needed validation and consistent support.

Through consultation, the therapist was encouraged to review the CHANGES assessment scores in session. It became apparent through that conversation that Darnell had lied to the therapist about doing any exercises because they were embarrassed and wanted the therapist to be proud of them. Throughout his entire life, Darnell had never exercised and did not have any friends or family who exercised. It was a very unfamiliar activity that also connected to childhood traumas in which Darnell had been made fun of by peers due to their weight. The avoidance of exercise was an avoidance of shame, and Darnell had to work with the therapist to disconnect these fused issues.

If you are interested in rating the client according to their overall ability for change, then, by all means, do so. This might indicate what expectations to have or what to aim for in a client's overall growth potential. However, when a client comes into therapy, it is important to rate the presenting problem and have the client help you complete the rating if appropriate.

With clients who are court referred to therapy against their wishes, therapists should rate each person not only according to the issue at hand but according to the perceived change ability as well. When rating perceived ability to change, it might help to ask if the person has ever made changes in their life relative to, for example, diet or exercise, anxiety, depression, relationship problems, or work issues.

SCORING: DETERMINING THE LIKELIHOOD OF CHANGE

The scoring of the CHANGES assessment is a general guide. Nothing is carved in stone. Since the assessment is a clinical guide and not a product of psychometrics, no claims can be made as to the precise accuracy of scoring. However, scoring in clinical practice has been remarkably sufficient as an indicator or predictor of therapeutic change. In our experience doing supervision, trainings, consultations, workshops, and lectures on this topic, there is remarkably high agreement among raters on the presence or absence of various precursors. In any case, being off by a point here or there on a precursor is insignificant since the real purpose of the scoring is to identify the configuration of precursors for each person and find which precursors need attention.

Another source of scoring ambiguity is that precursors can wax and wane from day to day, hour to hour, or session to session. If we were to determine that the precursors could be consistently ranked according to potency, the scoring would be weighted, with the more potent precursors getting a higher percentage of the overall score. However, the variable nature of presenting concerns and the overarching complexity of human beings makes this possibility unlikely.

The precursors can also be far more present with one therapist than with another, as seen in Chapter 12 in this volume. Nevertheless, with difficult clients—who typically receive very low ratings—the precursors are likely to be far less variable than with clients whose ratings are in the middle range and above. It is sometimes helpful to do a quick rating on the precursors with the same client from week to week or even from session to session. A client can be consistently low for the first five sessions and then go consistently higher as therapy continues. Change is a skill, and it is born of knowledge and work. The precursors will naturally emerge in greater magnitude as clients learn *how* to change, especially when its suits their purpose.

Change Unlikely

When a client has a total score of 0–6, change is unlikely any time in the immediate future. As long as the score remains this low, standard therapy approaches may be inappropriate with this client, who might be better served by focusing on growing the individual precursors. Clients who score this low should be informed—in an empowering way—about what it takes to change.

Insofar as no one completely understands the therapeutic change process, clients should not be expected to either. In some cases, psychoeducation on the precursors themselves can be helpful and important. Therapeutic change can also be presented as a skill to be learned. Education on the CHANGES model and the change process itself is generally more effective when a client demonstrates some sense of necessity for change. The sense of necessity can drive a client to learn more about what it would take to make things better. However, education about change and the precursors may be inappropriate for other clients, such as those with paranoid or antisocial personality disorders. For the latter, it is more important, initially at least, to go straight to work on implementing the absent precursors.

Change Limited or Erratic

A score of 7–14 indicates that change will take place at a rate that is slow and unnoticeable. The process will be limited, erratic, and fraught with setbacks but may also yield triumphs so small they might not be noticed at all by outside observers or even the therapist. However, these small changes can seem large to the client. Educating the client is important at this level as well.

It may be of great help for a client to understand why progress is not happening as quickly as they might like. After six sessions of working with a client who had been diagnosed with obsessive-compulsive personality disorder, the client complained to the therapist that he was not making progress. The client was relieved when the therapist explained the precursor of grit and noted how the client sometimes deftly avoided or redirected conversations in therapy when he became uncomfortable. Of course, it took a while for the client to realize the ramifications of this issue, but it was an important educational experience that he did confront after a couple more sessions.

It can also be helpful for clients to understand why changes are being made. Clear communication between therapist and client is paramount in specifying such intent. In addition, for clients who had lower scores earlier in the therapeutic process, increased scores may indicate it is time for further education on change. The idea of change as a skill may be more readily grasped when scores reach a more advanced level, especially when a high sense of necessity is present.

Change Steady and Noticeable

A score of 15–21 indicates the person will make changes at a rate that is steady and noticeable, both to the therapist and to others. There is little need for the precursors approach with many of these clients. Nevertheless, scoring can be used to determine which precursors are lowest. A person's rate of change can still be increased by focusing on the precursors with the lowest scores.

Change Highly Likely

When the total score is above 21, the client will likely achieve change with relative ease. Using the CHANGES model is unnecessary and perhaps a waste of time since the client may respond to almost any appropriate therapeutic tool, technique, or procedure. Similarly, any theoretical approach will tend to be effective as long as the therapeutic relationship is established and the interventions and in-session rituals used match the client's problem and needs. Client-centered, psychodynamic, or cognitive therapy, for example, can work equally well with a client at this level.

Clients with high scores can be very insightful and surprisingly sensitive to the therapist's approach. Therapists do not become preoccupied with or worry about these clients, simply because these people are likely to do well even on their own. In many cases, these people do not need therapy and are likely to improve with the right book or with a friend who listens. But when they do roll up their sleeves with an intention to change unwanted conditions, the therapeutic sparks fly.

EXAMPLES OF ASSESSMENTS

In Chapter 2 in this volume, we describe three difficult clients, Tommy, Joy, and Ricky, who did not achieve success in therapy. To illustrate the CHANGES assessment, these clients are revisited here, and their configuration of precursors is charted. For convenience, we briefly summarize each case before reviewing their ratings. Again, no diagnoses are mentioned in these examples, although therapists will recognize many of the symptoms. Diagnoses are omitted to focus on the precursors and avoid the stereotypes that can occur with dependence upon diagnoses for client characterizations. In addition to the case descriptions, further details that were gathered by the CHANGES assessment are provided.

Case Example 1: Tommy

Tommy was the charming and thoroughly self-centered man who claimed he could not stop his promiscuous behavior and who was both proud of it and ashamed about hurting his wife, Julie. He had been to three previous therapists and had fought with them all. His chief anxiety was the fear of going to hell for his immoral behavior. He was in therapy at the insistence of Julie, who had no idea of his sexual improprieties. His apparent interest in therapy amounted to an attempt to reduce his anxiety without changing his behaviors. He wanted a therapist who would tell him that he was fine, that he was a good person, and that he would not go to hell.

Therapy was at an impasse for Tommy. No progress was made after three sessions, nor did it seem likely. The therapist soon realized that Tommy came to therapy with a purpose quite contrary to anything that could be regarded as therapeutic. His precursor profile looked like this:

1. Sense of necessity (rating: 2): When asked directly, Tommy readily admitted that something had to change. He said he could not "go on like this" for much longer without "burning out." On the other hand, he continued all his problem behaviors with the same intensity.

2. Readiness for anxiety (rating: 0): Tommy was unwilling to feel the anxiety associated with his behaviors and attitudes. He evaded or deflected any questions that led to exploring fears, feelings, or difficulty. He insisted the therapist help him feel better.

3. Awareness (rating: 1): Despite all his contradictory statements, Tommy seemed to know he was feeling bad and that something was wrong but saw his behaviors as a problem only from a religious perspective. He insisted that his infidelity was natural for a man and unrelated to the tension between him and his wife. It was fine as long as she did not find out. He seemed to have little awareness that his behavior was out of his control. In addition, he had trouble identifying specific beliefs and feelings.

4. Confronting the problem (rating: 0): Tommy was doing nothing in terms of studying or contemplating the issues that brought him to therapy. He expected the therapist to tell him what he needed to know.

5. Effort or will toward change (rating: 1): Tommy was also doing nothing to resolve his problem other than going to therapy, which was a kind of effort in itself. Once in therapy, he showed little actual cooperation.

6. Hope for change (rating: 1): The therapist asked if Tommy ever had thoughts of "giving up" or if "life wasn't worth living." He said no but that sometimes he did not think he could ever be happy. He could not envision a positive outcome.

7. Social support for change (rating: 2): Tommy reported that his wife was supportive of him to get through his therapy, although she had no idea he was cheating on her. He also said that although most of his friends admired and encouraged his promiscuous behaviors, two had told him that he was making a mistake.

Tommy's CHANGES profile, which yielded a total score of 7, accurately showed that he was not likely to change, just as his therapy history had indicated. He was lowest on precursors 2 and 4, and 3, 5, and 6 were also low.

Case Example 2: Joy

Joy was the former showgirl from the Lake Tahoe region in Nevada. She was so involved with new age pursuits that she insisted on avoiding anything that was not "positive," which meant anything associated with the slightest pain or anxiety. She also claimed that she was clairvoyant and psychically gifted and that therapy might help her to clear the blocks that stood in the way of her becoming an occult "adept." She also believed that therapy could help her forget and cut herself off from any negative emotions and relationships in her past. Joy reached an impasse in her therapy after eight sessions, impatiently claiming to have derived no benefit, and she often lectured to her therapist on several new age principles.

In Joy's mindset, change was clearly desired but, because of the conditions she set, almost impossible to attain. For her, achieving change was like insisting that a fire be started with wet logs and then becoming upset because there was no combustion.

1. Sense of necessity (rating: 3): Joy made it clear that change was important and necessary for her to reach her goal of attaining a high state of being.

2. Readiness for anxiety (rating: 0): Joy would not consider or allow any anxiety into her consciousness and became visibly upset at the prospect of it. Although it was clear that she was consumed with anxiety, she insisted on staying "strong." She believed she had to remain "above" all negativity.

3. Awareness (rating: 1): Joy was not aware of the obvious deeper issues within which she was immersed, nor was she particularly adept at identifying beliefs and feelings. Any awareness of negativity was shunned.

4. Confronting the problem (rating: 0): Caught in a fixed belief system, she was not willing to explore the painful or confusing aspects of her life and clung instead to her belief in the self she would become. She believed that addressing and attending to difficult issues was a grave mistake.

5. Effort or will toward change (rating: 1): Joy meditated regularly and used it as a means to ease her anxiety, but as an escape rather than as a means of dealing with it. She showed little cooperation once in therapy itself.

6. Hope for change (rating: 2): Joy was expecting a future state of peace and attainment, but not without difficulty. That was realistic to her, but how to proceed was not.

7. Social support for change (rating: 1): Joy reported many superficial friendships but only one friend in whom she could confide. However, she often argued with her friend, who she felt did not really understand her potential.

Joy's CHANGES profile, with a total score of 8, presents an interesting configuration. She was relatively high in necessity for a difficult client. She also made some effort, but in this regard, her effort was not focused on psychotherapeutic change. She showed little or no cooperation in the therapy sessions themselves. That she had reached a therapeutic impasse is no surprise.

Case Example 3: Ricky

Ricky was the street gang member, a drug dealer to many children, and he had fathered at least three children with three different adolescent girls. Although he never exhibited any overt violence, he was adept at displaying nonverbal threats of intimidation. Ricky was also highly intelligent, manipulative, and spiteful toward the world and people in general.

Ricky did not disclose anything other than superficial information in 6 months of treatment. He viewed therapy as an intrusion into his personal life and therapists as tools of the police. For him, therapy was an attempt to make him weak and rob him of his freedom and virility. Therapists were avowed enemies, and therapy was a war that he could easily "win." Unfortunately, he was correct.

1. Sense of necessity (rating: 0): Ricky claimed to have had a great life until the police interfered. There was nothing wrong with him, and nothing needed to be changed. If anything needed to be changed, it was to get out of the treatment program.

2. Readiness for anxiety (rating: 0): Ricky was not willing to experience anxiety or difficulty in any way. He believed that drugs existed to relieve that sort of thing.

3. Awareness (rating: 0): Ricky gave no indication that he was aware of any problems. He was certainly intelligent, but not in identifying problems, feelings, or issues. He did not see his drug and alcohol use as a problem.

4. Confronting the problem (rating: 0): Ricky was not confronting any aspect of his life other than sex, drugs, and criminal activity.

5. Effort or will toward change (rating: 0): Ricky was not putting any energy into changing.

6. Hope for change (rating: 0): Ricky did not believe that he would live past the age of 21. He was certain he was going to die, having seen several members of his own and other gangs shot and killed. As far as he was concerned, the future held little or nothing for him.

7. Social support for change (rating: 2): Ricky reported that he cared for his mother and his 14-year-old sister and was extremely protective of them. Both loved him dearly and came to family counseling sessions, wanting to help. His gang members were also supportive.

Ricky's CHANGES profile presents an extraordinary therapeutic challenge. Therapeutic change is nowhere in sight with that configuration of precursors and a score of 2. Confronted by such difficult clients, therapists are likely to give up on the prospect of change, and a caseload of such clients is a recipe for burnout (J. J. Kim et al., 2018). This challenge clarifies how therapists have a unique configuration of precursors for each client, as we examine in Chapter 12 in this volume.

USING THE CHANGES ASSESSMENT WITH GROUPS AND FAMILIES

The CHANGES assessment is easily used in therapy with groups or families that are considered difficult or not exhibiting therapeutic change. In groups, it is helpful to rate each group member on the CHANGES assessment first and then to rate the group as a whole. Clinical impressions of groups indicate that many groups have a unique character of their own. Rating a group as an entity provides insights into the precursors needed to enhance the group process toward change.

Similarly, in family therapy, each family member can be rated to determine their configuration of precursors (Wilkinson & Hanna, 2018). As in the case of groups, Whitaker (see Simon, 1985) pointed out that a family system has a character and personality of its own. A difficult family can also be rated as a whole to determine which precursors are missing in the family system and need attention. Many of the techniques given in later chapters for implementing the precursors can be adapted for therapy with groups and families.

Even when not mentioned specifically, many of the techniques described have been adapted as appropriate for use in group and family settings.

USING THE CHANGES ASSESSMENT ACROSS VARIOUS DIAGNOSES

The CHANGES assessment outlines and elucidates the potential for therapeutic change across the wide range of disorders classified in the various incarnations of the *Diagnostic and Statistical Manual of Mental Disorders* (5th ed., text rev.; *DSM-5-TR*; American Psychiatric Association, 2022). It is applicable to people with depression, anxiety, and personality disorders, as well as substance use disorders. In terms of disorders with organic or congenital components, such as bipolar disorders, traumatic brain injury, or schizophrenia, the CHANGES model may still be applicable, but further evidence is needed to determine its efficacy with such populations.

The *DSM-5* defines a *personality disorder* as consisting, in part, of unchanging, dysfunctional personality traits (American Psychiatric Association, 2013). Thus, part of the essential definition of a personality disorder in general is precisely the lack of qualities and conditions described by the precursors. In one important sense, a personality disorder is a lack of therapeutic change characteristics. The CHANGES model seems to apply quite appropriately in work with clients who have received various personality disorder diagnoses, but each personality disorder has its own style. Although that style may differ from disorder to disorder and person to person, the different precursors apply to all at a fundamental level that lies well beyond personality traits and styles. For example, an antisocial client and a borderline client may both be low in the confronting precursor, and each will have their own style of avoiding confronting, but both are likely to improve if confronting is activated. A person with a personality disorder who also has ample presence of the precursors will tend to change faster than the person with the same personality disorder who is lacking in precursors. The therapist's task is to use strategies and techniques that will activate the precursors.

A FINAL NOTE ON RATING CLIENT POTENTIAL FOR CHANGE

It seems to be the case that clients with a high degree of precursor activation will find therapeutic change likely and welcome. Conversely, a client unlikely to move toward beneficial change lacks the critical mass that an adequate presence of precursors provides. The CHANGES assessment is a relatively simple clinical tool to determine precursor presence and level of activation, so its implementation has considerable flexibility. Therapists are encouraged to use it in session with clients to facilitate dialogue about therapeutic change, between sessions in the process of case conceptualization and treatment planning, as well as in training, supervision, and consultation to better understand why client change is not taking place. In the next chapter, we explore its use as a supervision tool for identifying when therapists are hindering the change process.

12

Rating Therapist Interference in the Change Process

This chapter deals with what is probably the most underestimated aspect of therapy with difficult clients: therapist disposition and reactivity. It is usually referred to as countertransference and is often given lip service but is seldom given the attention it deserves. The idea of countertransference is one of the most valuable contributions made by psychodynamic schools of therapy. Unfortunately, the intricate phenomenon itself has been obscured by terminology that is not readily translatable into popular cognitive and behavioral languages (Holmes, 2017; Mills, 2004).

Transference is when a patient treats the therapist as they would a significant other, such as a parent. *Countertransference* is defined as a therapist's reactions to a client's transference. Freud (1910) originally described countertransference as the therapist's unconscious emotional response to the patient. Freud recognized the potential adverse effects that a therapist's emotional reactions can have on a client. Psychodynamic scholars eventually broadened the concept to include conscious and unconscious reactions to a client based on a therapist's own past relationships (e.g., Kernberg, 1967; Reich, 1951; Segal, 1977).

Modern psychodynamic therapists and scholars tend to agree that therapists' reactions to clients' provocative and evocative behaviors and statements must remain under conscious control (Bager-Charleson, 2010). It is further agreed that the therapist must develop sufficient maturity to avoid seeking to meet their own needs with clients in therapy sessions. When therapy has stalled, countertransference

---

Case examples have been disguised to protect client confidentiality.

https://doi.org/10.1037/0000451-013
Therapeutic Change With Difficult Clients: Precursors and Techniques in the CHANGES Model, Second Edition, by B. D. Wilkinson and F. J. Hanna

is often the cause (Holmes, 2017; Weiner, 1982). Blaming treatment failure on the client's difficulty or resistance is often a rationalization—and a poor one.

Unfortunately, this aspect of therapy is discussed almost exclusively by the psychodynamic schools and is too often ignored or mentioned only in passing by other approaches. When it comes to working with a large portion of difficult clients, a therapist of any theoretical persuasion can get frustrated, irritated, sad, anxious, angry, or bored and can have their own issues, biases, or sensitivities inflamed. Fromm-Reichmann (1950) gave the example of a therapist who, as a child, was forced to listen to his elderly grandmother drone on in a seemingly endless chatter. As a result, he automatically detached from any long-winded communication with anyone, including clients.

Countertransference reactions are not limited to particular diagnoses. A depressed person can provoke anger in a therapist, and so can an antisocial client (Giovacchini, 1989). As a consequence, the relationship degrades; the therapist is no longer an empathic helper and the effectiveness of therapy declines. Whenever a therapist experiences frustration, anger, resentment, hurt, or loss of confidence with a client, the potential is there for these feelings to interfere with client change. When the therapist acts on those feelings, therapy deteriorates into a power struggle or inquiry into "who wronged whom." Therapeutic change, as a goal of therapy, is then disregarded.

DIFFICULT CLIENTS OR DIFFICULT THERAPISTS?

For over 100 years, case studies and research have shown how countertransference can interfere with the change process in even the most well-intentioned therapists (Stefana, 2017). The client influences the therapist far more than is generally acknowledged in the psychotherapy literature (Holmes, 2017; Singer & Luborsky, 1977; Valerio, 2017). Outside of psychodynamic programs, countertransference is rarely prioritized in therapist training. It is also seldom controlled for in research since the phenomenon is difficult to study due to its subjective nature, and the methodological question persists as to how to reliably identify its effects. Countertransference could be confounding a wide range of therapeutic outcome and process studies without our knowledge (Persons, 1991).

In the CHANGES model, the key is understanding that there is nothing pathological or disordered about a therapist experiencing countertransference feelings and attitudes. Quite the contrary, it is a completely natural and routine aspect of doing therapy. What is vitally important to understand is that there is a difference between merely experiencing countertransference and acting on those feelings and attitudes. The feelings evoked and provoked can be used as tools to further understand a client, as psychodynamic therapists know so well (Stefana, 2017). The lesson highlighted across a long history of psychotherapy outcome and process research is that the difference between average therapists and excellent therapists seems to be how well they can manage their countertransference reactions (Hayes et al., 2018; Van Wagoner et al., 1991).

Many difficult clients are experts at thwarting well-intended attempts to establish a therapeutic relationship. They perceive help as a threat and can undermine it with great finesse, which is often one of the reasons they are seen as difficult. Some therapists react with frustration, such as one who said in supervision, "Here I am trying to help this woman, and all she does is block my work at every turn! Frankly, I'm sick of it." This chapter helps therapists make sense of countertransference reactions and uses the CHANGES assessment to show how change processes degrade in the therapist.

THERAPIST INTERFERENCE: A NEW TERM FOR A VENERABLE CONCEPT

The term countertransference represents a vitally important concept with a considerable amount of historical and theoretical baggage that needs repackaging. As an alternative, the term *therapist interference* directly conveys the idea of a therapist's hindrance of the change process, in or out of the context of countertransference. Therapist interference has the advantage of describing the detrimental effects of a therapist's reactions toward a client purely in terms of interpersonal interaction. It can include countertransference issues as well as other factors, ranging from lack of skill to being overwhelmed by a client's complexity, difficulty, or degree of suffering and misfortune. The benefit of this perspective lies in the fact that interference can be viewed in the context of each of the precursors. A therapist's set of precursors toward a defiant, insulting, and arrogant client can be far lower than toward a cooperative, willing, and respectful client. This difference within and between therapists can profoundly affect the change process.

When the therapist acts on negative feelings by criticizing the client under the guise of helping, making covertly hostile comments, or prematurely terminating therapy, a valuable opportunity to better know the client is lost. This is often the hidden benefit of understanding therapist interference. Although many therapists know of it, few develop this essential skill.

ASSESSING THERAPIST INTERFERENCE VIA THE CHANGES ASSESSMENT

The CHANGES assessment can be used to rate the potential of a therapist to inhibit the therapeutic change process. In this section, we list each precursor and show how a therapist with a deficit in that category can interfere with client progress in therapy. This tool can be helpful in supervision, and therapists working with difficult clients can use it to draw a more complete picture of their own possible contribution to an impasse in therapy.

Deficit in Confronting the Client's Problems

The primary clue to the lack of this precursor lies in the disposition of the therapist toward the client's issues. Just as a client can be aware of issues and not confront them, a therapist can also be daunted by a client's problems and choose to avoid them. A therapist must be able to directly identify, address, and work toward the resolution of the client's issues and persevere in a sustained, steadfast manner. If not, the client may not be inclined to confront those issues either, and change will be mysteriously elusive.

For example, Colleen worked in a university counseling center for 7 years before returning to school to earn a doctorate. Colleen was always well dressed, energetic, and likable. George, her client, was a graduate student in history who was in his late 20s and working on his master's thesis. He was low-key, unexpressive, and interpersonally awkward, paying little attention to his dress or appearance. He sought therapy at the university because his wife was threatening to leave him, and he was deeply troubled by the possibility. After 4 months, no change had occurred.

Supervision eventually revealed that Colleen had focused primarily on developing George's social skills but, for some reason, was not addressing the marital relationship itself. Colleen told her supervisor that she thought if George were more "appealing," his wife might not want to leave him. Meanwhile, it was apparent that George had become romantically attracted to Colleen. It was a good way to forget about his troubles with his wife. He interpreted her interventions as a means for him to become more appealing to her instead of his wife. This entanglement became clear when Colleen revealed that, in a way, George reminded her of her husband, whom she wanted to change to become more "sensitive." Not surprisingly, she also had avoided dealing with the relationship issues in her marriage. Colleen eventually confronted this issue in her own therapy.

Sometimes, therapists avoid confronting a client's problem when it seems foreign or bizarre. In one case, a married woman disclosed that her job was in danger and that she needed help processing how to manage interpersonal issues at the office. After a few weeks, she revealed that she was involved in encounters involving sexual dominance with random men she had met online. She met these men first in chat rooms and then in person, where she was having them tie her up in ropes and chains for sexual interludes. Although her therapist admitted concern in consultation, she had not discussed the issue in any depth with her client. Despite the potential danger, the therapist avoided the topic because it was unfamiliar and, per her own admission, frightening. For some therapists with a deficit in confronting, staying in familiar territory feels more comfortable.

Other potentially important issues that can be ignored are unethical business practices, thievery, cheating on exams, and insensitivity to others. If a therapist is uncomfortable with and thus avoids a client's problem, that problem is unlikely to be resolved.

Deficit in Hope for Client Change

If a therapist has little hope that a client will change, it is likely to be contagious through their nonverbal signals and cues to the client. It can show up in vocal intonations and inflections as well as physical gestures and postures. The expectations of a therapist for a client's success indicate how much hope the therapist has for a client. Just as a longstanding body of research substantiates the power of expectancy effects for clients (Constantino et al., 2023; Weinberger & Eig, 1999), a growing body of contemporary research shows that a therapist's positive expectations for client change are profoundly impactful in terms of client outcomes (Bartholomew et al., 2020). The degree to which a therapist maintains hope for client change may even explain 7.3% of the variance in positive change outcomes, as determined by the client (Connor & Callahan, 2015).

Unreasonably positive expectations for a client, however, can amount to fantasy and are not helpful at all. Just as the precursor of hope must be realistic in a client, it helps for a therapist to be able to envision the realistic possibility of a client making changes. Hope is also encouraged by the knowledge that in work with difficult clients, a therapeutic window can open at almost any time, and change, although not evident at the moment, can nevertheless happen as a result. This is a realistic expectation born of actual experience for many therapists. This contagion of hope communicates to and affects a client in various ways, one of which is showing a client that improvement and a better future is possible.

Deficit in Awareness of Client Issues or Own Corresponding Issues

The lack of awareness in a therapist primarily manifests as a lack of empathy and a preoccupation with one's own issues, agenda, or needs. For example, some therapists resent difficult clients who do not change. They may not readily admit to this, of course, but it often results from a lack of self-esteem in the therapist. Being unaware of their own self-esteem needs, a therapist might be using therapy to meet these needs. Such a person needs the belief and assurance that they are competent and successful at doing therapy, as a source of self-esteem. A difficult client can cast doubt on that belief, making a therapist feel awkward, inept, or incompetent. The client becomes a threat to the therapist's self-esteem, and the therapist then detests and resents the client precisely because the therapist detests and resents their own lack of self-esteem. In supervision, this usually comes as a great insight to therapists, who quickly see the new awareness as beneficial.

Another manifestation of the lack of awareness is when a therapist does not know that a client is difficult. In some cases, this is because the level of dysfunction is not apparent. For example, a supervisee worked with a client who was likely to be misusing alcohol but had not disclosed this to the therapist. Since the client did not mention it, the therapist overlooked warning signs and failed to address the issue. When asked if he had suspected alcohol use, it came as a surprise, and he responded, "I wondered what was going on, but I wasn't sure and didn't know how to ask." While the symptoms would have been clear to any advanced practitioner who has studied addictive behaviors, it constituted a fundamental blind spot to this early career therapist.

Other therapist issues can be evoked when doing therapy, and odd consequences can occur if they are not managed appropriately. A male and female therapist co-led a group of substance-abusing teens aged 14–18. During one group session, a female client disclosed that cocaine made her feel sexy and that she would flirt with men of all ages when she was high. At this point, the female cotherapist disclosed that while using cocaine she had had sex with many men and never found fulfillment. She ended by saying that she still had not found fulfillment. The entire group was intensely interested and focused on her startling self-disclosure.

A few weeks later, one of the boys from the group, Timmy, spread the rumor that he had had sex with the female cotherapist over the weekend. It was not true, of course, but the female cotherapist was obviously horrified. In consultation, it was determined that nearly a third of the client population in that agency believed the story. Tina could not get Timmy to confess his deception and asked the male cotherapist to intervene. After considerable effort, Timmy finally admitted his ruse. However, the damage had already been done, as the group dynamic was negatively impacted and the female cotherapist had to deal with the ongoing embarrassment of the issue within the agency setting.

The change process becomes derailed when therapists have so little awareness of their issues that they have difficulty identifying when client issues resonate with their own. A therapist will be inclined to treat such an issue in a client the same way they treat it in themselves or may treat the client in the exact opposite way, perhaps out of guilt. For example, if a therapist has a problem communicating with a partner, they might ignore the same issue in a client. Or they might overemphasize it and coerce a client to deal with it above and before all else. When seen through the filter of the therapist's own issues, a client's problems can be obscured. Empathy becomes impaired. In short, a lack of awareness of one's issues can ruin clinical perception and empathy.

Deficit in Necessity to Help the Client

A therapist can lack a sense of necessity to help a client, which can manifest as indifference or lack of interest. It can result from "giving up" on a client and "giving in" to the unconscious conclusion that change is probably never going to happen. In such instances, a therapist is merely going through the motions of therapy, engaging in conversation without a true intent to help.

The most important characteristic for identifying a lack of this precursor is a distinct absence of the therapist's felt sense of a client's need for change. In other words, the helping instinct that may have been strong at one time in that therapist has diminished or is no longer present. The therapist may feel defeated, apathetic, or bored; they may daydream during sessions with this client or shift the conversation into areas more of interest to the therapist and not of any particular therapeutic value.

Another possibility contributing to a lack of a sense of necessity is if the therapist has the same or similar issue as a client that also has not been addressed, such as drinking or a failing relationship. Self-awareness is required on the part of a therapist to recognize and admit that one's apathy about, or lack of attention to, an issue may be stirred up by a client.

Deficit in Grit, or the Willingness to Experience Anxiety or Difficulty With a Client

Sometimes, a therapist can be overwhelmed by the disrespectful treatment from clients. Such treatment can be discouraging and daunting, especially if the client is overtly or covertly critical of the therapist. For example, some narcissistic clients find it necessary to criticize the therapist to keep their own envy and jealousy under control (Adler, 1992). The thought of wading through this kind of treatment can be disconcerting to a therapist who is not aware that this behavior is to be expected. The end result is that the therapist becomes unwilling to experience the anxiety or difficulty of being with the client. The same is also true of work with antisocial or borderline clients, who can be a source of considerable discomfort to a therapist.

On a different front, some therapists can become overwhelmed by the vast amount of raw, painful emotion of a client. Similarly, when therapists are continuously exposed to the pain of client after client, they might begin to avoid any further exposure to this type of painful experience due to vicarious traumatization (Aafjes-van Doorn et al., 2020; McNeillie & Rose, 2021). As a result, a therapist will avoid any inroads into a client's case that lead to more or similar painful emotions. The therapist may have also reached their threshold of tolerance for the pain of others. If this occurs, the therapist and client may end up with an unconscious collusion that is designed to spare the client any more painful experience, even when appropriate. That willingness or readiness to undergo the anxiety of helping a client with this process is the chief aspect of this precursor.

In other cases, a therapist can be discouraged by the sheer amount of work a client has to do to change, especially when the therapist's assessment of the amount of change needed is vastly greater than what the client believes. Normally, an experienced therapist patiently prepares for the long haul, but less experienced or less patient therapists can become discouraged. In supervision, a supervisee once said, "There is so much work to do here, and the client is so difficult to deal with. She has so little awareness and insight. I don't know if I have the energy to go through it all." When the therapist no longer wants to "go through it all," this precursor is nearly gone.

Deficit in Effort and Will to Work Through Issues With a Client

There is a myth that a therapist should kick back and let the therapeutic process take care of itself. Some therapists believe they can just reflect the feelings and statements of the client without getting involved, which is justified as "maintaining professional distance." Although important, the concept of distance is often misunderstood. Some therapists believe that to roll up one's sleeves and get involved with a client's problem is to risk becoming enmeshed. This is also a mistake.

Lazarus (1989a) noted that success in therapy requires effort on the part of the therapist as well as the client. Simply stated, a therapist has to work hard not only at confronting the problem with the client but also at persuading the client to work hard. Being persuasive is part of working with difficult clients, and so is modeling for a client how to exert energy toward change.

However, when a therapist is doing all the work and the therapy itself is going nowhere, it may be time for a slight withdrawal. If all that effort is not leading to change, it may be time for confrontation or even limited provocation (see Chapter 7, this volume) to activate precursors. A therapist may be helped by the Zen state of being fully engaged in actions while remaining unattached to the rewards, as recommended by Horney (1952/1987). Exerting effort toward helping a client is not the same as becoming enmeshed. It is the therapist's responsibility to model effortful action.

Deficit in Social Support for Facilitating Change

Some therapists are in desperate need of social support. If social support is lacking in the therapist's personal life, therapist and client can become so friendly and close that the therapist may inadvertently seek to keep that fuzzy feeling. Consequently, the therapist may find confronting the client on sensitive issues threatening to the delicate security of the relationship. This most often occurs when a therapist is lonely and wants to be friends with the client or desperately needs empathic supervision or collegial support. To avoid this scenario, therapists must ensure that their social support systems are adequate and fulfilling.

Another social support problem arises when the therapist lacks a professional support system. Although isolation is obviously a unique challenge for therapists in private practice, professional burnout due to a lack of social support is most often observed in community agency settings despite ready access to supervision support (Yang & Hayes, 2020). A therapist should feel, as much as possible, part of a therapeutic team. This can be accomplished by attending conferences and workshops, but it is much more fruitful to engage in positive and productive group, individual, or peer supervision. These latter sources of social support can alleviate feelings of isolation and bolster the presence of a therapist's other precursors. The unique benefits of clinical and reflective supervision to prevent burnout and bolster the precursors will be discussed further in Chapter 16 in this volume.

CASE EXAMPLES

The CHANGES assessment form can be helpful to therapists not only in rating clients but in rating themselves. It can also be effectively applied in supervision or consultation. In Chapter 2 in this volume, we review examples of therapists who had "trained" their clients to be difficult. Such unnecessary difficulties arise when therapist interference goes unrestrained and uncorrected, thereby diluting the change process. We now examine two of those examples in further detail and provide an additional example involving a severe ethical violation. Following each example, the case study therapist is rated according to their own precursors.

Rating therapists is similar to rating clients. The therapist's potential is not the focus of the rating; what is rated is their current attitude and actions with a particular client. Just as client precursors can vary on different issues, therapist precursors can vary widely from client to client. The focus is on the therapist's actions with a particular client in a particular moment or with a particular client over several sessions. The score serves as a general indicator of a therapist's potency as a change agent for that particular client at that particular time.

Rating Kurt's Precursors

Kurt was a 39-year-old therapist working with Janey, a female university senior in her mid-20s. Janey's major complaint was that the men in her life verbally mistreated her. Although she was an engaging person in therapy, there was a certain naivete about her and a tendency to smile even while in pain and to laugh with a shrill, almost tinny tone. After 20 therapy sessions, her current male partner continued to verbally abuse her, and she stopped showing up for sessions and then terminated by telephone.

In reflective supervision, Kurt discovered that he harbored a hidden belief formed in high school that "girls with fake laughter" and who "smiled for no reason" were "stupid" and not likely to ever achieve any significance in their lives. At a deeper level, he never took Janey seriously as a person. When confronted further, he also realized that he was attracted to women like Janey in high school but that he also "resented the popular girls" because they wouldn't go out with him. He expressed genuine surprise that these "old attitudes can creep into a counseling session."

Kurt's CHANGES assessment could be rated as follows:

1. Confronting (rating: 1): Kurt only superficially attempted to get Janey to confront her problem with verbally abusive men. Although he did get her to try to escape from them, part of his approach was to subtly, almost imperceptibly blame her for causing her problems.

2. Hope (rating: 2): Due to his maladaptive beliefs about women like Janey, he had little hope for her improvement and did not envision her empowerment. He did, however, believe in the therapy process and spoke with her as though she could improve.

3. Awareness (rating: 1): Kurt was unaware of gender issues affecting his performance as a therapist. He was also unaware of the gender issues affecting Janey's problems with her current and past partners.

4. Necessity (rating: 1): Never taking her seriously, Kurt did not see her problems as worthy of concern and solution, other than just doing his job.

5. Grit (rating: 1): As a part of considering her at some level "stupid" and insignificant, Kurt was not willing to experience her pain as part of an empathic process beyond a superficial devotion to duty.

6. Effort or will (rating: 1): Kurt's exertion of effort amounted to going through the motions with no real dedication or focus.

7. Social support (rating: 3): Kurt did not provide a therapeutic relationship of warmth and support for Janey, but he did have the support of a supervisor and other therapists in the counseling center.

With this small presence of precursors and the corresponding sum score of 10, it is not surprising that Kurt did not act as an agent of change for Janey nor that she terminated therapy prematurely. To his credit, he readily admitted that he understood why his effort was unsuccessful and sought his own therapy to work through some of the underlying issues that arose in reflective supervision.

Rating Nancy's Precursors

Nancy was a 38-year-old therapist working toward her doctoral degree. Her client was Jerry, a pleasant 30-year-old man who reported feeling "lost" in his life. Although intelligent, he had no career plans, and nothing seemed to inspire him to want to do anything with his life. However, he was aware enough to worry about it and sought counseling for help. Jerry was courteous and friendly and genuinely tried to cooperate with Nancy's probes and questions. He would even sometimes apologize for being so noncommittal about any goals or future direction. After 16 sessions, little progress was made, and Jerry was still worried about "wasting" his life.

In supervision, Nancy reported that Jerry was so "totally passive" and so "resistant" that she could not get him to do anything about his problem. She also named a variety of personality disorder traits that Jerry was exhibiting, such as those of avoidant and obsessive–compulsive personality disorders. When asked to report her feelings when in the presence of Jerry, she said she found him "irritating" and "maddening" to work with. She felt bad about feeling this way about him but also said she was not able to help and requested that he be transferred to another therapist. Before doing so, she agreed to have the supervisor explore the dynamics between the two of them.

Nancy's CHANGES assessment could be rated as follows:

1. Confronting (rating: 0): Nancy was unsuccessful in getting Jerry to confront anything of magnitude or substance, and she did not do so with herself in relation to him.

2. Hope (rating: 1): Nancy had not envisioned a future for Jerry that had a realistically positive outcome. Such was her frustration that the future she did

envision for Jerry was referring him to another therapist, although she did believe another therapist might be able to help.

3. Awareness (rating: 0): Nancy spoke of Jerry's issues superficially, occasionally speaking of him as though he were lazy and docile, which was inaccurate. She was not aware of her own issues being stirred up by his behaviors.

4. Necessity (rating: 2): Nancy did recognize Jerry's predicament, in spite of her feeling irritated.

5. Grit (rating: 0): Nancy found it difficult to empathize with Jerry and was hesitant to form a close relationship with him. She never really engaged him in a warm and genuine manner as she did her other clients. It was clear that rather than being ready for the difficulty of working with him, she was waiting to terminate.

6. Effort or will (rating: 2): Although Jerry seemed cooperative and willing to work, Nancy was hesitant to apply herself to the task of working with him. Most of her session time was spent getting him to talk about various aspects of his life while she reflected and summarized. Her effort was in "doing her job."

7. Social support (rating: 3): Nancy did enjoy a fairly strong social support system. She also had several supportive friendships with other therapists and an empathic supervisor.

With a sum score of 8, the lack of change was unsurprising. As noted in Chapter 2 in this volume, the supervisor asked Nancy to write down all the people in her life whom Jerry reminded her of. She later reported that Jerry's mannerisms were similar to her sexually abusive brother, whom she had not spoken to in 20 years. With continued reflective supervision support, Nancy actively worked through the countertransference issue with Jerry, and therapy proceeded in a much more effective way. Nancy also sought personal therapy to work through the issue further on her own terms. If the CHANGES assessment had been done again following Nancy's insight and subsequent change of behavior toward Jerry, her precursors rating would surely have been much higher.

Rating James's Precursors

Any therapist who would engage in a sexual relationship with a client would, of course, be severely lacking in precursors of change. James was a 35-year-old man who took great pride in his ability as a therapist. Psychodynamic by theoretical orientation, he had 10 years of experience working as a counselor in a small East Coast business college. He had been married for 17 years and had three children, all under age 15. He arranged to see a fellow therapist one day for peer consultation and, almost as an aside, told the therapist that he had just met "the woman of his dreams."

Her name was Rachel. He said she was 24 years old, recently divorced, and "incredibly understanding and loving." He made it a point to tell the peer consultant several times how attractive she was, how "perfect" they were for each other, and that he was going to leave his wife and children to be with his new love.

"Unfortunately," he added hesitantly, "she was my client." He immediately emphasized with great sincerity, "But that doesn't matter." He explained that they had, just a week earlier, mutually decided to end therapy because they "knew" that their relationship was "meant to happen," and it would have happened after termination anyway. Fate had just so arranged it, he claimed, that they were to meet in the therapeutic encounter. He explained that their mutual decision was made during their eighth session together, and he asked the peer consultant for his view of the situation.

The consultant decided to be as direct as possible. "James, she doesn't know you." James looked incredulous and, with great frustration in his voice, said, "She knows me better than anyone I've ever met!" When the consultant reminded James that such behavior was unethical and harmful, James pleaded for understanding. The consultant paused, leaned forward, and said, "James, please listen. She only knows the idealizations she projected onto you. You know this. You've thoroughly studied this aspect of therapy. She was your client, James. The sessions were all about her, right?" James nodded. The consultant continued. "She doesn't know you, James. She has obviously filled in all the mysteries about you with her fantasies and desires. You were her understanding, caring therapist. It's natural she would feel this way. You're deceiving yourself and her." The consultant then reminded James of the American Psychological Association ethical codes and implored him to consider the potential harm.

Unfortunately, James responded that "rules don't apply 100% of the time" and that anyone who saw him and Rachel together would understand. James was entrenched, so the consultant acknowledged the impasse and said, "Please do one thing regardless of what you think about me and the rules. Answer this question for your sake and hers: What unmet need is this client fulfilling for you?" As might have been predicted, James ignored the peer consultant as well as numerous other psychotherapists whom he had told about the affair. He promptly left his family for Rachel.

James's CHANGES assessment could be rated as follows:

1. Confronting (rating: 0): James carefully avoided direct examination of Rachel's or his own issues.

2. Hope (rating: 1): James envisioned a bright future for the two of them. Was it realistic? It seemed so to him, but it seemed like fantasy to outside observers.

3. Awareness (rating: 0): It is clear that James had little or no idea of what actual issues Rachel faced. In addition, he had no apparent awareness of his own unmet needs or unresolved marital problems.

4. Necessity (rating: 4): James had an apparently sincere, heartfelt sense of necessity to help Rachel with her emotional issues and problems.

5. Grit (rating: 0): James, being in love, was probably more interested in helping Rachel escape from her anxiety rather than experience it. He was obviously unwilling to experience his own anxiety in terms of issues brought up in his interactions with her as a client.

6. Effort or will (rating: 0): Curiously, James was going to great effort to help Rachel gain what he thought was happiness and growth. But the effort was not toward therapeutic change so much as it was toward the gratification of needs.

7. Social support (rating: 3): James had many friends and a good deal of social support, although no one that I knew of approved of his actions. He ignored his professional and personal social support systems.

This scenario involves the harmful exploitation of a client, ethical violations, and a lack of concern for a client's therapeutic change. With a sum score of 8, James was unlikely to ever be an effective agent of change. There were ongoing ramifications for his actions, as well. His social support system collapsed when he was reported and disciplined for unethical behavior. His wife divorced him, and he lost his job. After a year and a half, his relationship with Rachel came to an end, leaving James severely depressed and alone.

After seeking out therapy, James told the peer consultant that if he had been aware of his issues and needs, "it never would have happened." In spite of his training and intellectual understanding of this cardinal rule of therapy, James did not have sufficient self-awareness to recognize the harm he was doing to his client, as well as himself, until it was too late. The lesson learned from this tragic incident is that a helper can exert great effort, feel tremendous urgency for change, possess great affection for a client, and still utterly fail in helping that client to change. This case demonstrates that change does not arise out of only two precursors on the part of the therapist. A dynamic interplay of precursors seems to be necessary for therapists as well as clients.

A FINAL NOTE ON RATING THERAPIST INTERFERENCE

Just as the CHANGES assessment can be used to measure the precursor activation of clients, it is also an effective measure of the same among therapists. Therapist interference is akin to countertransference but casts a wider net insofar as it includes any behavior that impedes the therapeutic relationship and/or client change efforts. It is important for therapists who use the CHANGES model to consider how their own issues and histories impact client outcomes.

A therapist who turns the light of awareness on themselves to examine deficits in precursors with a client or issue can dramatically alter the course of treatment. With this in mind, we suggest that therapists consider the value of supervision, consultation, and personal therapy at any career stage. Therapists have an ethical duty to examine and work through barriers to empathy, not only at the prelicensure training levels but throughout their many years of practice. Additionally, it is important for therapists to honestly assess their limits. We cannot work with every client, and each of us has limits. Owning such limits requires self-honesty and, at times, the candid feedback of supervisors or consultants to help a therapist overcome blind spots or even a lack of humility.

IV

SPECIALIZED APPLICATIONS

13

Guidance for Advanced Training and Supervision

A unique aspect of the CHANGES model is that therapists can be rated according to their own precursors. The previous chapter looks at rating therapists according to their precursors, which can enhance an understanding of how therapists contribute, or not, to the change process in that client (see Chapter 12, this volume). Since the configuration of precursors can vary from problem to problem or even from day to day, a therapist can be more oriented toward change with one client and less so with another. It is crucial for therapists to self-monitor the precursors in practice.

However, supervision during clinical training is an equally important avenue by which to monitor the precursors. The CHANGES model has clear value in supervision and training, not just in helping supervisees learn ways to foster client change in therapy, but because it highlights the central and deeply relational role played by therapists in the change process. The obvious way to incorporate precursors into supervision involves using the CHANGES assessment to identify whether client progress is hindered or facilitated by unidentified therapist effects.

It is important for supervisors, consultants, and trainers to be able to identify the observable source points of therapist interference, as well as strategies to help therapists monitor and deal with their own interference in the change process with difficult clients. Rating therapist interference can lead to thoughtful dialogues in supervision as to what is happening for the trainee or supervisee while working with a difficult client. Yet there are also notable markers of therapist interference that should be actively identified and targeted for reduction or elimination in training to improve therapist skill and increase the probability of therapeutic change outcomes for clients.

---

https://doi.org/10.1037/0000451-014

Therapeutic Change With Difficult Clients: Precursors and Techniques in the CHANGES Model, Second Edition, by B. D. Wilkinson and F. J. Hanna

In kind, supervisors and trainers who recognize the signs of wisdom in therapy can highlight the path toward greater efficacy in facilitating therapeutic change for difficult clients. As such, another consequence of understanding the CHANGES model is that the knowledge gained sheds indirect light on the central characteristics of the most effective "master" therapists. A complete model of therapeutic change must define the kind of therapist most adept at facilitating it. As seen later in this chapter, the CHANGES model makes the characteristics of effective therapists stand out in bold relief and helps us better understand exactly what they do.

MARKERS OF THERAPIST INTERFERENCE

It is important for therapists to recognize when they play a role in preventing therapeutic change. We have identified 13 ways in which therapists inadvertently undermine client outcomes.

Wanting to Be Liked

Many therapists believe that difficult clients will be more likely to work in therapy if they like their therapists. While there is evidence to support this assertion (Fletcher & Delgadillo, 2022; Orlinsky et al., 1994; Russell et al., 2022), placing too much emphasis on it can be a mistake. If a therapist has a neurotic craving to be liked by clients, the client may only validate and reinforce certain therapist actions that lead to being liked but do not lead to client change. It is more important to be respected than liked. If a client respects a therapist, this is a tacit permission for the therapist to operate as an active change agent rather than a passive supporter of the client.

Engaging in Long-Winded Explanations

Packing a lot of meaning into a single sentence is an art form that is seldom appreciated. It gets easier with practice. If a therapist fumbles for words in an explanation, the verbiage can hinder the therapeutic process. For example, instead of a long-winded explanation about drug use to an addicted client, one could say instead, "So you figure you are your own physician, and you are prescribing illegal medicine to heal your pain. Am I getting it?" The client will usually correct the therapist with a better description or approximation, leading the conversation in the direction of further awareness and confronting.

Prioritizing Care Over Empathy

Caring and empathy are not the same. In fact, a therapist can show caring toward a client and still cause the client to deteriorate (Hardy, 2019; Lambert et al., 1977). For example, when a therapist genuinely cares for the client but lacks empathy and is authoritarian and intrusive, not only is change unlikely, but such attitudes disempower a client. Empathy can also degrade when a therapist is deeply affected by a client's stories of abuse and tragedy. Therapists can get caught up in feelings of protest, sympathy, protectiveness, and righteous anger toward those who hurt the client, which can interfere with the therapist's ability to empathically see the world from the client's perspective. The therapeutic process can stop at this point if one is not aware.

Losing Focus in Session

When the therapist's thoughts are swirling and feelings and emotions are in turmoil in the presence of a client, the therapist has likely lost the sense of being centered and should seek consultation. In some cases, the depersonalization and emotional exhaustion associated with therapist burnout serve as a means to cope when working with many difficult clients during the same day or week. In a closely related vein, difficulty focusing on a client may also be a sign that one has taken on the emotional baggage of clients' unresolved issues, as with compassion fatigue (Figley, 2013).

   When one loses focus, it is time to get centered and proactive. Therapists are encouraged to identify client behaviors and attitudes that are stressful or curry one's attention and try to consciously let them go, one by one (Teater & Ludgate, 2014). There can also be value in reflecting upon the rewarding aspects of work as a therapist to help maintain perspective and sense of purpose. Kottler (2022) developed a helpful, six-step self-reflection exercise for identifying and confronting points of therapist interference that stymie client progress and lead to compassion fatigue and burnout:

1. List what one is doing to exacerbate the situation.
2. List the therapist's "buttons" that are being pushed by the client.
3. List the people from the therapist's past with behaviors similar to the client.
4. List the ways the therapist acts out their impatience.
5. List the therapist's expectations of the client and if they are being met.
6. List the therapist's needs that are not being met by the client.

Challenging Clients Too Soon

When working with difficult clients, the temptation to confront and challenge can come too soon and can actually contribute to uncooperativeness. Before engaging in confrontation, the therapist must thoroughly convince the client that they are understood through empathic reflections of meaning and feelings to the point where the client has little choice but to believe the therapist genuinely understands. Only then can challenges and confrontations be made that will be respected and not dismissed out of hand. Kiesler (1988) called this approach "hooking and unhooking," and it is quite effective with difficult clients.

Asserting One's Credentials or Degrees

When a client is particularly difficult, it is easy for therapists to "pull rank" and try to assert one's college degrees, license, credentials, or years of experience as proof of value and competency. This is seldom effective and typically serves as a symptom of the therapist's frustration and a sign of burnout. It is also a possible indicator of a power struggle the therapist is losing. Any attempt to one-up clients will create barriers that prevent genuine interaction and hinder the therapeutic process. It is often a last-ditch attempt by the therapist to gain respect, but unfortunately, respect usually has to be earned in other ways.

Many difficult clients will take an adolescent "whatever" attitude toward this display and become resentful and rebellious. As part of their metalogue, some privately ridicule people with degrees and see the assertion of one's degrees or education as similar to boasting about one's wealth or property. The therapist should be aware of any inclinations to do so and note carefully when the urge arises, which often signals the arrival of an impasse.

Engaging in Power Struggles

Many difficult clients expect a power struggle with a therapist, just as they would with anyone who has a potential influence on their lives. One way to avoid power struggles is to call out or identify any agenda or "game" the client is playing, whether it involves sex, intimidation, or simple evasiveness. To win the struggle, the client must keep their game a secret. For the change process to occur, the therapist must bring the game into the open and call it faster than the client can reset it. Empathy is key and is indispensable in identifying the client's power agenda. Calling the game is superior to winning the struggle, especially when the client admits to the game itself.

Take, for instance, the 16-year-old girl who had steadfastly refused to disclose anything for more than 90 days in a unit for adolescent criminal offenders. The therapy team described her as a "classic borderline," and the agency director decided to call in a consultant. Upon meeting the girl, the consultant told her that she must be remarkably intelligent and powerful to be able to frustrate and resist all the highly educated people in that agency. It was about time someone gave her credit for being so savvy. "You've won," the consultant said. "You've proved that you can stop these people from ever affecting your life." The consultant then told her she was so smart that she might be outsmarting herself by not letting these people help her. That acknowledgment was all she needed, and her change process began with the knowing smile she radiated in spite of herself.

Some therapists feel a need to be in continuous control of a session and feel threatened by a client who rebels against that control (Shamoon et al., 2017). In many cases, if the therapist was not enforcing the control, the client would not be so likely to rebel against it, creating a power struggle. It is sometimes helpful to reverse the interaction by getting a rebellious client to admit that they hate being told what to do, even by a therapist. Role reversals can be used with defiant teenagers to great effect, whereby a therapist asks a client to "boss me around for a while," within reason, of course. If done in a group setting, the process can be entertaining.

Confronting With Impatience or Rancor

Some therapists, counselors, and social workers in community-based treatment programs confront clients in a hostile way. Such confrontation, replete with accusations of denial and dishonesty, are still seen in the addictions field. Defenders of this approach have described it to us as "tear 'em down and build 'em up." Unfortunately, these people are ignoring the basic tenets of motivational interviewing (W. R. Miller & Moyers, 2021; W. R. Miller & Rollnick, 2012). Heavy confrontation tactics are a mistake of considerable magnitude made by people who have neglected to resolve their own hostilities and frustrations or who are tormented by their own unresolved issues. Being so tormented, they also torment clients.

Confrontation can be an extremely effective tool when it is done with curiosity, empathy, compassion, serenity, and the intention to help. When done in anger, it simply activates a power struggle with the client, who may become defiant or hostile or, conversely, submissive and docile, or it may only produce premature termination. Either way, change is unlikely. Therapy with difficult clients is not the same as training soldiers or disciplining inmates. It requires finesse.

Avoiding Confrontation

Some therapists eschew confrontation altogether, instead prioritizing unconditional positive regard to such an extent that confrontation becomes a dirty word. From this perspective, the warm feeling that accompanies a therapeutic relationship must be preserved at any cost, and confrontation is framed as a dire threat to the relationship. This threat can cause a therapist to retreat from sharing even basic observations that might upset the client or otherwise "rock the boat." Many clients happily engage in such warm, supportive therapy for years without making therapeutic progress.

Becoming Either Too Rigid or Too Flexible

A therapist who has been adversely affected by working with difficult clients is at risk of becoming rigid, which serves as a last-ditch effort to gain a sense of control. When one notices this tendency in oneself, it is important to take a step back to determine when it began and what was said or done that led to the rigidity. On the other hand, most therapists are nice people rather than taskmasters and do not want to be controlling or dominating. Some difficult clients are adept at persuading such exceedingly flexible therapists to take a break from all the "hard work," saying something like, "Do we have to do this now? I'm not really in the mood." Once again, when one becomes lackadaisical in terms of sustaining efforts toward client change, the tendency should be explored with attention to when and how it started. Chances are there is a lesson to be learned in reflection upon that moment. Either extreme is a potential move away from therapeutic change.

Defending Oneself Against Clients

There are times when an overworked therapist is so weary from seeing difficult clients that they might create artificial distance, unconsciously perceiving clients as a threat to their sanity or peace of mind. Again, this can be a sign of burnout, but it can also result from the fear of becoming somehow "polluted" by the negative attitudes and problems of unsavory clients. An indicator that this may be happening is a reluctance to form a relationship, perhaps coupled with bitterness, sadness, or helplessness. Numerous therapists have shared with us how they erect mental walls to maintain a personal space that difficult clients cannot touch or violate. The problem with walls is that they also incarcerate therapists, keeping them from making empathic contact with clients. When this kind of distancing occurs, it is time to seek help.

Accusing Clients of Defensiveness

Some therapists will directly say to a client, "You're being defensive" or "You're in denial." This might work on some occasions but more often makes clients resentful and recalcitrant. To many difficult clients, such a statement appears to be an accusation. Such "in-your-face" confrontation tactics are outmoded and have been shown to be ineffective (W. R. Miller & Rollnick, 2012). Rather than accuse the client of being defensive, ask whether the client dislikes someone trying to get inside their head. Also, using the term "protective" can be helpful. Saying, "Are you trying to protect yourself by not answering my question?" may be far more to the point. One might also say, "Did you notice how you did not answer my question just then? Do you think it is too much of a hassle to deal with?" This latter question addresses grit as being willing to experience difficulty.

Disliking a Client Because They Do Not Change

In consulting and supervision, many therapists will reveal that they dislike certain clients. To be clear, we do not maintain that a therapist has to like their client to facilitate change. However, further exploration of this issue with some therapists reveals that the dislike arises when a client is not responding to therapist interventions and strategies or attempts to form a relationship. In other words, dislike can arise when a client threatens a therapist's self-esteem. The same can occur when a client does not change, as the therapist begins to question their own competence, and self-esteem is diminished. From that point forward, the client becomes a symbol of the therapist's low self-esteem, and the therapist is likely to respond in ways that further interfere with client progress.

GUIDEPOSTS TO WISDOM IN THERAPY

Standardized and formulaic approaches to therapy tend to be of limited value when working with difficult clients. When a client has refined the skills of averting and avoiding positive change, standard treatment methods tend to fall short. Many difficult clients are more adept at undermining the therapeutic process than therapists are at facilitating therapeutic engagement toward change. Remarkably, it is in work with difficult clients that a therapist's skills become honed and refined, and a therapist's knowledge of human beings becomes deepened and seasoned. Mere theories, techniques, and even empathy are often not enough. Influencing difficult clients to change often calls for therapeutic wisdom, a set of abilities that transcend formal therapy training (Karasu, 1992).

Wisdom is not the same as intelligence (Grossmann et al., 2013; Sternberg & Glück, 2021). It involves abilities and kinds of understanding that are not assessed by an IQ test. Such abilities include dialectical thinking, self-awareness, self-transcendence, impeccable timing, and the ability to formulate reframes and metaphors that can easily transfer into and out of a client's worldview (Hanna & Ottens, 1995). Therefore, the wise therapist is centered, genuine, engaged, empathic, and committed to helping clients activate the precursors so as to facilitate therapeutic change. The therapist is intellectually and intuitively present in awareness to all verbal and nonverbal client offerings and remains open to facing any difficulties that arise in the therapeutic relationship.

Difficulty for the therapist surfaces when a client engages in behaviors that compromise or undermine these foundational conditions of therapeutic wisdom. A client may do or say something that introverts and collapses the therapist into their own issues, knocking them off center, breaking contact between client and therapist, and compromising the therapist's empathy. Wisdom helps a therapist to maintain empathy and poise despite inclinations to the contrary. Therapists should remain alert to the breakdown of this essential state and learn to recognize certain behaviors and states of mind that tend to indicate one is operating from a place of wisdom. In what follows, we explore a subset of such healthy behaviors and states of mind.

Seeing Empathy as an Act of Will

Empathy does not always occur naturally and automatically. If it did, the entire human race and the living of life would be qualitatively and radically different. A rule of thumb: Empathy will tend to break down to the degree that one's unresolved issues begin to emerge. Another rule is that empathy breaks down to the degree that the other person presents with viewpoints or perspectives that seem strange or foreign. Thus, when these conditions manifest, empathy requires other-directed intentionality as an act of will to be maintained (Margulies, 1989; Zahavi, 2014). In addition, some clients are uncomfortable with empathy and prove adept at discouraging it in a therapist. Mindfulness of this phenomenon in the moment that the client is making the attempt is extraordinarily helpful in recognizing how and why one's empathy begins to dissipate. At that point, empathy must be intentionally recalled, reestablished, and maintained as an act of will.

Cultivating Nonattachment to the Fruits of One's Actions

A personal state of equanimity is invaluable when working with difficult clients. To learn how to develop it, we highly recommend *Everyday Zen: Love and Work* by C. J. Beck (1989), which provides invaluable mindfulness guidance with remarkable implications for therapists. Horney (1952/1987) noted that Zen can teach therapists to be wholeheartedly and fully present, paying full attention to the client without any involvement in self. Of course, this is not a matter of being a cold observer, and the therapist should not have any "personal axe to grind and no neurotic craving" (p. 31) attached to therapeutic outcomes. This means having, as Horney put it, both "the highest presence and the highest absence" (p. 34). She also recommended being so totally absorbed in the practice of therapy that one is putting "all of yourself in what you do" (p. 31).

Some difficult clients are extremely alert to a therapist's desire that they improve and will react to that desire by attempting to frustrate the therapist and sabotage therapy in a variety of ways. Such clients learned these skills long before meeting the therapist, perhaps as a result of their interactions with those who oppressed them or denied them in their families, schools, neighborhoods, and other environments. If a therapist is open and not egotistically craving a particular outcome, or if they are not defending their ego or sense of competence, a difficult client has no "hook" or "tug" that undermines the change process. Remaining unattached to our ego-driven need for control and admiration helps therapists maintain a calmness that fosters creativity and tolerance for ambiguity.

Maintaining Self-Compassion

Working with difficult clients can make one feel foolish and inept. The benefits of maintaining a positive and empathic attitude toward oneself are wide reaching, with extensive research supporting the value of self-compassion as a means of coping with stress and hardship (Ewert et al., 2021; Muris & Otgaar, 2020; Neff, 2023). If one is understanding toward oneself, it is easier to recover from the inevitable mistakes one makes with difficult clients. This has the added benefit of indirectly modeling self-compassion for clients. No therapist needs a critical, invalidating stream of negative self-talk sabotaging awareness and spontaneity in therapy; this can be handled through standard cognitive and mindfulness-based methods (see Hayes, 2005; Leahy, 2017).

Attending to One's Own Metalogue

Both clients and therapists alike have a metalogue, or unspoken streams of thoughts, whether we attend to them or not. Well-trained therapists naturally attend to the metalogue of clients. It can be extremely revealing when therapists listen attentively to their own thought streams during sessions, especially when listening to a difficult client tell a story or describe a problem. One thought stream might think the client is being deceptive, while another wants to believe the client. Simultaneously, another reaction could be disgust, yet another sympathy, and still another a desire to console the client. Accompanying all this may be the thought that it may take years for this client to change, while a concurrent stream is weighing the value of various approaches and strategies that may help. Still another stream may wonder if therapy is having any beneficial effect.

These reactions can be extremely revealing to a therapist who is unsure where to go with a client or what to believe about what a client says. The more these parallel processes are present in one's mind at a given time, the more concerned the therapist should be about the success of the therapy. Noting all these thought streams may be helpful in the case of difficult clients who are confusing, misleading, or extraordinarily complex. Of course, one must be able to do this while still maintaining active contact in the relationship. It takes practice, but attending to one's metalogue can be extraordinarily helpful as a barometer or centeredness, as well as insight, in session.

Monitoring One's Own Visceral Reactions

That queasy feeling in the pit of one's stomach may be communicating something of inestimable value. One may be going along listening and reflecting a client's statements, not suspecting anything amiss at the intellectual level, yet one's "gut" may be churning in a way that says something is wrong. The gut feeling may be a nearly imperceptible tightness in the stomach, an empty feeling, or some other indication of anxiety. It is all too easy to ignore.

Gut feelings are often a sign that something is going on at the level of one's own metalogue that needs to be examined. Therapists who recognize these feelings can then suspend them and explore how and why they arose. Often, there is much more to such a client than meets the intellectual eye. Perhaps this client is intimidating or threatening in a way that is easy to ignore, and the therapist wants to give them the benefit of the doubt. On the other hand, perhaps the therapist is feeling nervous, self-conscious, or worried and wants to escape. Or it could be a projective identification on the part of the client. Whatever the case, monitoring and attending to gut reactions reap rewards in terms of greater learning and insight.

Confronting With Compassion and Empathy

It can be very difficult to care about some difficult clients, such as those who are cruel, demeaning, or insulting or who make sexist, racist, or other prejudicial and harmful comments. Some difficult clients blatantly lie, cajole, and deny responsibility regardless of the evidence at hand. It can be challenging to meet such clients with compassion and empathy, much less confront the client with an open heart. Then, when it would be most useful to confront such a client, the agitated therapist may feel so much hostility or disgust that they become afraid it will be revealed and therefore avoid confronting altogether, or otherwise does so ineffectively, as a sort of half measure.

Confrontation can be an effective tool if done with care and respect. If a therapist does not honestly like a client and a confrontation is necessary, the therapist should be respectful and courteous to that individual despite their own feelings. Ideally, a therapist would work through any negative feelings in therapy or peer supervision. If this is not possible, a therapist can suspend or bracket those feelings, leaving the mind clear to go ahead with the confrontation, knowing that their negative reactions to a client are natural and, to some degree, expected. Suspending or bracketing negative feelings is a skill that one is well advised to develop. It allows one's natural helping instincts to come to the fore and take over the process. One should never ignore such feelings but rather suspend them with full awareness of what one is doing.

Meeting Hostility With Equanimity and Humor

If a client knows that a therapist shrinks away from open hostility, the client may use it as a control tactic. Clients tend to respect therapists who genuinely show no negative or fearful reaction in the face of hostility. Equanimity serves a dual purpose. It shows the client that the therapist will not act out, and it models how to respond to hostility. If the hostility continues, it needs to be discussed empathically with the client. If it continues, termination may be necessary, but this is rare.

Defiance and hostility may also present an opportunity to use humor. Therapists can occasionally use self-deprecating humor to place themselves on an even status with the client. This is especially helpful with aggressive adolescents who use obscene language. If a therapist can insult themselves more severely than the client can, the act not only diminishes their momentum but can paradoxically garner respect. Of course, the use of humor must be natural and not strained.

For instance, if a client calls the therapist an "ass," one reply might be "Have you been talking to my friends?" If a client calls the therapist stupid, one response might be, "I wish I was smart enough to see that." These cannot be canned lines, however. They must be spontaneously delivered in the moment to be fully effective. The purpose is to lessen the client's impression of the therapist as a symbol of authority or a bundle of predictable responses. Role-playing such situations with a supervisor or with another therapist can be extremely helpful along these lines.

The value of humor in therapy cannot be overestimated. If a difficult client can be helped to see the humor in a situation or a behavior, the aura of seriousness and tragedy can diminish and make it easier to confront. It is vital, of course, to remain sensitive to the needs and condition of the client in the moment. Empathy rules. The therapist should avoid any humor that has traces of residual anger or resentment toward a client. For some therapists, healthy humor tends toward tongue-in-cheek situational quips or observations laden with existential irony, whereas sarcasm or dark cynicism tends to indicate unresolved issues being stirred up by a client. The therapist's duty is to resolve personal issues that a client evokes, and healthy humor tends to be a good barometer of effective boundaries and a lack of countertransference in the room.

Recognizing Projective Identification in Action

Projective identification involves feelings produced in a therapist by a client that do not originate with the therapist (Ogden, 2018). It is the responsibility of therapists to thoughtfully assess whether such feelings originated within oneself or are a projection of the client. For example, if a therapist feels intimidated by a client, it could be the client's projection of power. If a therapist experiences sexual feelings for no apparent reason, it could be the client's projection of sexuality. If a therapist feels indebted to a client, or as though they owe something to a client, it could be a projection of ingratiation. If a therapist is disgusted by a client, it could be a projection of repugnance. All of these reactions can be used in therapy to deepen empathy with and insight into the client through the recognition that this may be how people in the client's environment feel in their presence.

Projective identifications can be approached passively or actively. For example, in the case of an intimidating client, one may feel afraid, powerless, or weak. Although it is not a good idea to admit when one is afraid of a client, one can ask, "Do you find that people in your life are scared of you?" A client will often respond to this in the affirmative in some manner. The therapist can then ask how the client came to be that way. One can also ask if it works for the client's life in terms of advantages and disadvantages. In addition, one can find out who the client's intimidating models have been. If the client can identify and describe the models, the therapist can work with the client to reconsider the value of those models. Each of these approaches can be fruitful.

Knowing When Discouragement or Disgust Is Not Your Own

When working with difficult clients, it is common to feel discouraged, disgusted, or hopeless. Such feelings may actually be an empathic "borrowing" of how that client habitually feels toward themselves. To test this, it is sometimes possible to describe to the client the feeling of disgust, discouragement, or hopelessness that one is experiencing as a therapist and to inquire whether this is, in fact, what the client is experiencing. It is often accurate to some degree. Clients can sometimes be so surprised by this revelation that trust is deepened. This is also true of anger and resentment. Phrasing is important; one would never tell a client that they are disgusting or hopeless.

Drawing Clear Boundaries Around What Is Tolerable and Acceptable

Some clients have a way of making a therapist feel silly about not being willing to discuss their personal lives or fantasies, not being willing to meet outside the office, or not being able to "take a joke." Too many of these clients on one's caseload can eventually cause a therapist to doubt their sanity. The only course of action is to be sensitive to one's sense of propriety, personal space, privacy, and limits. These must be communicated to the client clearly and unhesitatingly for the sake of the therapeutic change process. It is also important to stay in contact with colleagues or a supervisor to maintain one's social support system.

Asking "Therapy Veterans" How They Managed to Defeat Previous Therapists

Occasionally, a therapist will run into a client with a long history of confounding and defeating therapists. Some even seem to have made it a hobby. Many enjoy being so complex and mysterious that no one can understand or reach them. In a convoluted twist, many clients believe that to be understood is to be humiliated. It is advisable to ask such "therapy veterans" how they managed to foil the attempts of so many intelligent people, as well as to praise their intelligence and credit them for the accomplishment. It can be helpful to reframe their "failure" as a client as a "success" in defeating a therapist, which can be noted as a skill born of intelligence, craftiness, or shrewdness.

Therapists can also say that the client will, no doubt, defeat them well. Therapists should make no pretense about being better than other therapists or more capable of handling the client's difficulties. Instead, the therapist can convey curiosity and a desire to learn from the client about how to defeat therapists. One might even suggest the client could probably give lectures on therapy if they were so inclined. Eventually, it is important to point out that the client has not really tried therapy yet, and that maybe they could try it for the first time. If the client can be persuaded to teach their skills, a therapeutic window may open. Many such clients are secretly convinced that they are empty inside, devoid of soul or self. If a therapist, or anyone, were to discover their true nature, it would result in a kind of mortal disintegration.

Understanding That Difficult Clients Function as Teachers

Here is a simple rule: Treat a client who does not change as an opportunity for learning rather than a professional failure. There are times when it is helpful to tell a client that they are functioning as a teacher. This approach can produce a shift in how the client regards the therapist in a way that reduces power struggles and promotes the genuineness of the relationship. For instance, a power-seeking client will sometimes be responsive to admiration. Thus, the therapist might say, "From what you've told me, I'm willing to bet you've learned some pretty remarkable lessons about life and people. Do you ever share any of that knowledge? I'll bet there's a lot I could learn from you."

A FINAL NOTE ON GUIDANCE FOR ADVANCED TRAINING AND SUPERVISION

Jung (1934/1969) suggested that we may better understand ourselves by examining what we dislike about others. The client who evokes graded reactions of irritation, annoyance, frustration, or even utter disgust provides a wonderful opportunity for therapists to learn more about their own values and biases. Recognizing the various markers of therapist interference can lead to personal and professional growth, but such recognition may require the observation or input of supervisors, consultants, or other therapists. The path to wisdom is seldom an isolated affair. We learn from our interactions with, and the supportive insight provided by, others. There are few careers in which one's professional talents may grow in close tandem with one's evolutions in personal wisdom. It would surely be wise for all of us to take this unique opportunity seriously.

14

Oppression, Perspicacity, and Liberation

The prioritization of multicultural awareness has become a pillar of knowledge and practice in the fields of counseling and psychotherapy during the 21st century. After years of neglect, it has finally been widely acknowledged that clients from cultures different from those of a therapist need to be understood from within their own unique sociocultural perspectives. Significant emphasis has been placed on studying various customs and beliefs to develop cultural competency in tandem with better communication of empathic understanding in therapy (Fuertes et al., 2006; Sue et al., 2022).

At the same time, there is a fundamental and profound limit to a therapist's capacity to understand the lived experience of clients from different cultural backgrounds. White therapists are unable to fully grasp the trauma of racism due to cultural privilege, for example, and the same can be applied beyond race or ethnicity to areas such as gender, sexuality, age, disability, religion, and so forth. It is vital to acknowledge such limits while still seeking to build sociocultural knowledge and understanding that grows empathy. Effective multicultural practice therefore requires cultural humility, by which "therapists are able to have an accurate perception of their own cultural values as well as maintain an other-oriented perspective that involves respect, lack of superiority and attunement regarding their own cultural beliefs and values" (Hook et al., 2017, p. 29).

Another dimension of multiculturalism that must be acknowledged in practice is the phenomenon of oppression, which clarifies the context or situatedness of many difficult clients. If one examines the wide range of problems

---

Case examples have been disguised to protect client confidentiality.

https://doi.org/10.1037/0000451-015
Therapeutic Change With Difficult Clients: Precursors and Techniques in the CHANGES Model, Second Edition, by B. D. Wilkinson and F. J. Hanna

encountered in psychotherapy from this perspective, it is readily apparent that oppression is an active ingredient in the formation of psychological and emotional problems. Yet there is also a curious and widely overlooked perceptual skill that arises from oppression that has implications for empowerment with difficult clients: *perspicacity*, a characteristic of wisdom that enables one to see beyond appearances (Sternberg, 1990) and "intuitively understand, read, and accurately interpret the environment" (Hanna et al., 2000; p. 433). In this chapter, we examine the nature and trauma of oppression, the power of perception, and how an integrative existential-cognitive therapy can support psychological liberation for oppressed clients.

THE NATURE OF OPPRESSION

Oppression may be defined as an abuse of power at the expense of the well-being of others. As a phenomenon, oppression is the central concern guiding both professional and broader sociocultural discourses on multiculturalism and social justice. It manifests in our relationships as well as through institutional and systemic influences that, while pervasive, are sometimes more difficult to identify, diagnose, and modify than interpersonal abuses of power. However, in both interpersonal and systemic cases, oppression involves two modalities: force and deprivation.

Oppression by force, coercion, or *duress* is the act of imposing an object, label, role, experience, or set of living conditions on another or others that is unwanted, brings needless pain, or detracts from physical or psychological well-being (David & Derthick, 2018; Hanna et al., 2000). An imposed object, in the context of oppression, can be a bullet, a bomb, shackles, a bludgeon, a fist, a penis, unhealthy food, or abusive messages designed to degrade or reduce the self-determination of the person in question. Other examples of oppression by force can be coerced labor, enforced religion, degrading jobs, and negative media images and messages that foster distorted, negative beliefs. Oppression by force is directly tied to physical harm in interpersonal relationships, as seen in cases of intimate partner violence or child abuse.

Oppression by deprivation is the act of denying to another an object, role, experience, or set of living conditions that is desirable and conducive to physical or psychological well-being (Hanna et al., 2000; Sue, 2010). Neglect is a central form of oppression by deprivation, whether in terms of neglecting to provide basic needs such as food, shelter, or clothing or withholding relational needs such as respect, dignity, or love. Objects deprived can be a house, a plot of land in a desirable neighborhood, various forms of wealth, or gainful employment. Oppression can deprive one of one's children, parents, friends, freedom, or even one's childhood. Religious practice can also be deprived, as was the case from 1890 to 1940 when the United States banned certain practices of the Sioux tribes (D. Brown, 1970).

Implicit Oppression

There has been a steady, multigenerational transition in American culture from explicit and thus wholly undeniable acts of oppression to implicit, easily deniable acts of oppression grounded in phenomena such as color blindness and microaggressions. By no means are we suggesting that oppression by force is not a major contemporary cultural issue. The Black Lives Matter movement is a clear example of protests designed to address explicit and ongoing oppression by force in American culture. However, the blatant nature of daily prejudicial acts that buoyed the civil rights movement has largely been replaced with subtler, more easily deniable acts of discrimination.

As proposed by the cultural philosopher Harvey (2015), the transition from explicit acts of oppression that are sanctioned and normalized by a dominant cultural group to the outright denial of oppression as a phenomenon of sociocultural interest or concern by many individuals and organizations within the same dominant group marks the sociocultural onset of

> *Civilized oppression* ... [which] refer[s] to oppression that involves neither violence, nor the use of law. It is systematic and disadvantages and demeans members of certain groups and in Western society it is pervasive. The phenomena involved are routinely trivialized, given their subtle nature, yet both their effects and their nonconsequentialist implications are highly significant. (p. 1; italics added)

The visceral nature of abuse and violence in oppression by force tends to take center stage in our collective consciousness. When one thinks of oppression, it is quite natural to first think of harms that are obviously imposing or abusive. At a systemic level of analysis, we reference examples of enslavement, genocide, or other violent acts in which a group of people are disproportionally and deleteriously impacted. At an interpersonal level, we may identify specific instances of physical or verbal violence in the home, such as an alcoholic parent belittling their child or a physically abusive partner striking their spouse. In systemic and interpersonal conditions, oppression by force is often the default reference when wrangling with the complexities of harmful acts.

In contrast, the notion of implicit oppression by deprivation, or civilized oppression, can be more difficult to grasp while simultaneously being central to contemporary discussions on the role of social justice and multicultural awareness in therapy. At the interpersonal level, we can easily cite issues of child neglect or a partner unwilling to apologize for abusive actions as oppression by deprivation. Yet deprivation also includes interpersonal acts that are not so obviously identifiable, such as microinvalidations that arise from implicit biases, or denials of difference that arise from "color blindness," or a disavowal of oppression as a concern for some group of people altogether.

For instance, the White therapist who decides not to broach the topic of race with a client of color is engaging, inadvertently or not, in oppression by deprivation because avoiding the discussion amounts to a denial of difference. Such a choice also runs counter to research that has established the value of broaching, particularly since therapists occupy a position of privilege (Day-Vines et al., 2020; Lee et al., 2022). It has also been shown that unresolved countertransference issues and self-ascribed color blindness increase the likelihood that a therapist will either microinvalidate or overpathologize racial and sexual minority clients (Dictado & Torres-Harding, 2023).

Epistemic Injustices

Invaluable scholarly work has been done on epistemic injustice in therapy. It has been argued that therapists should avoid epistemic injustice in two forms: testimonial injustice and hermeneutical injustice (Lee et al., 2022). Testimonial injustice clearly serves as a form of interpersonal oppression by deprivation. For instance, a therapist might explicitly (and without malintent) deny the validity of an experience by casually reframing a client's report of racial profiling at work as "a misunderstanding." Such a denial of lived experience amounts to "an ontological violation" that perpetuates an erroneous yet oft-perceived "credibility deficit" among marginalized clients in therapeutic settings (Fricker, 2007, p. 137).

While hermeneutical injustice is also enacted interpersonally, it more directly speaks to systemic oppression by deprivation. For instance, even if the therapist validates a testimonial provided by a client who reports racial profiling at work, the therapist may have little to no grasp of the deep significance of this event for the client due to the therapist's own privilege. In such an event, the therapist actively reflects the perspective of the client, yet the client feels viscerally unheard anyway. Such instances speak to structural inequities in larger social systems, whereby a client experiences systemic oppression by deprivation in an encounter with a therapist who, despite good intentions, has not done the self-work necessary to empathize with that client.

In either case, therapists should obviously avoid perpetuating such epistemic injustices. There is strong evidence that therapy can be traumatizing for minoritized clients when therapists, however well-intended, perpetuate oppression (Bennett-Leighton, 2018). Therapists are ethically bound to communicate with deep empathy to avoid testimonial injustices, as well as to engage in the self-work required to avoid hermeneutical injustices. The self-reflection and personal work required is perpetual, in the sense that one must always work to deepen empathy and awareness; it is an ongoing journey without a final destination or state of being.

THE TRAUMA OF OPPRESSION

Our discussion thus far primarily focuses on the duty of therapists to avoid oppressive acts. From the client perspective, oppression can be a stalwart barrier to therapeutic change, whether it is interpersonal or systemic in nature. It can feel impossible for many clients to imagine positive change when one has experienced a lifetime of relational and systemic disempowerment. Most difficult clients encountered in therapy have had tough lives, often filled with pain and suffering inflicted upon them by others. Many difficult clients cause similar pain and suffering for others, perpetuating a traumatic cycle of anguish and misfortune. Arguably, various forms of oppression are at the root of all traumatic coping (Bennett-Leighton, 2018; Jacobs, 1994; Watson et al., 2016).

The therapist's duty is to validate feelings and perceptions and not discourage anger. Anger management strategies, in our estimation, risk failure with oppressed groups when they do not acknowledge that oppression causes justifiable anger (Archer & Mills, 2019). Anger often derives from hurt and serves as a coping response to protect against further hurt. Anger is also a much safer emotion to display than hurt, which demands some vulnerability and, thus, perceived risk. At the same time, we maintain that hurt is more of a sensation than an emotion, making it easier for clients to identify than contextual feelings that can be difficult to grasp. The following story is an actual occurrence showing how this approach can be used with traumatized clients.

The Story of Carlos

A consultant was providing training to staff in an adolescent runaway shelter at the time of this case example. The shelter was for kids living on the streets with no place to sleep. There was no court involvement here, and kids could stay to get possible placement in a foster home or stay one night and move on. There was no leverage to get kids to engage in therapy, but all adolescents who stayed there were encouraged to seek on-site counseling services. The staff ranged from licensed therapists to social workers with bachelor's degrees to volunteers without degrees. The consultant provided training days once every 2 weeks and also worked with some of the teens on-site.

Carlos was a 17-year-old who had been at the shelter for only 24 hours. The consultant entered the building that morning to find Carlos yelling and cussing at staff and other kids. Apparently, he had been throwing furniture. The consultant walked directly up to Carlos in a nonthreatening manner and spoke to him loudly. People do not listen well when angry, so the standard therapy statements can be made, but the volume often needs to be turned up without any hint of hostility or disrespect:

THERAPIST: (loudly, but respectful and unimposing) Wow! Man, are you angry! Wow! Look at all of that anger!

CARLOS: (turning around, breathing hard) You're goddam right! I'm pissed off!

THERAPIST: (loudly) I can see that! What's got you so pissed off?

CARLOS: I'm sick and tired of this shit!

THERAPIST: (more softly now) I hear you, Carlos. I am sorry you are taking a lot of shit. Come on, man. Let's get away from all this and go talk somewhere. (shakes hands with Carlos and leads him to a group room followed by three trainees from the program designated to sit in to observe that day)

THERAPIST:	Can we talk, Carlos? If I make you angry, you just tell me to back off.
CARLOS:	(sits down with arms crossed) Whatever.
THERAPIST:	What's got you so angry?
CARLOS:	I'm sick and tired of people all the time telling me what to do.
THERAPIST:	Yeah. I get it. That shit gets old fast.
CARLOS:	(a bit calmer) Yep.
THERAPIST:	Do you get angry a lot, Carlos?
CARLOS:	Yeah. Like, all the time, almost.
THERAPIST:	Can I ask you a tough question, Carlos? You don't have to answer.
CARLOS:	Yeah.
THERAPIST:	Have you been through a lot of shit in your life? Don't tell me what it was.
CARLOS:	(calmly) Hell yeah.
THERAPIST:	Have you ever been hurt?
CARLOS:	(stiffens up a bit) Hell no. (pausing) What do you mean?
THERAPIST:	Like somebody cut you deep, but in your feelings where no knife or bullet could ever go.
CARLOS:	(hesitantly, turning away slightly) Yeah.
THERAPIST:	Thank you for telling me. Do you think about it much?
CARLOS:	I think about it a lot. Yeah, and f*** him.
THERAPIST:	Don't tell me who it was, but is there a place in your body where you feel the hurt?
CARLOS:	(points at his chest area) Here.
THERAPIST:	That's where you feel the hurt?
CARLOS:	(nodding)
THERAPIST:	Thank you, Carlos. Can I ask you another question? If all that hurt inside of you went away, what would happen to your anger?
CARLOS:	(thinks about it, then laughs) If it went away? Man, I wouldn't be angry.
THERAPIST:	Okay. Have you ever been told you have an anger problem?

CARLOS:	(still laughing) All my life.
THERAPIST:	Maybe you don't have an anger problem. Maybe what you really have is a hurt problem. Do you like having all that hurt inside you?
CARLOS:	(quietly, looking down) No.
THERAPIST:	What do you do to get rid of the hurt?
CARLOS:	I don't know. I get high. If people mess with me, I mess with them back.
THERAPIST:	Does any of that actually make the hurt go away?
CARLOS:	(smiling) Yep, sure does.
THERAPIST:	Okay, but does the hurt go away for good, or does it come back?
CARLOS:	(looking down, not smiling) Nah, it comes back.
THERAPIST:	So, hurting others doesn't *really* make the hurt go away.
CARLOS:	Not really. No.
THERAPIST:	Would you like to try something that actually works?
CARLOS:	Yeah, what's that?
THERAPIST:	It's called counseling. (smile) It can make the hurt go away, Carlos. Not like getting high or fighting people, but it works, and it makes you feel a lot better. You want to try it? You can get it right here. You don't have to do it forever. But maybe you can give it a try and see if it helps.
CARLOS:	(hesitating)
THERAPIST:	You've already given drugs and (smiling) throwing furniture around your best shot, and I give you credit for trying to feel better. But maybe getting high and breaking stuff and yelling at people isn't really the answer.
CARLOS:	Yeah, okay. But I'll only talk to you.

This session was done with a client who was never introduced to the therapist and the two had never seen each other previously. The therapist identified the underlying issue behind the anger that seemed to disturb Carlos the most, which was hurt. By offering Carlos the option of reducing the hurt, Carlos became motivated to engage in therapy, and he did, although with limited success.

Activating Anger Related to Systemic Oppression

Effective multicultural therapists recognize the depth of traumatic tension, anger, and resentment felt by marginalized groups toward dominant groups (L. S. Brown, 2017). In regard to systemic forms of oppression, anger can be an effective catalyst of action. The key to validating anger is to help clients express, manage, and redirect it toward worthwhile goals such as community engagement and activism. While it may be helpful in some cases to suggest that clients make anger a "friend" so as to become acquainted with it, in many other cases, the anger is so destructive that only acknowledging it, validating it, and reflecting its intensity and meaningfulness can take oppressed clients beyond it. On the other side of destructive anger lies the potential for healing, personal transformation, and constructive sociopolitical action (Comas-Díaz, 2016).

In most cases, detailed discussions should move into the relationship between anger and cultural positioning. The following questions can foster discussion on the impact of oppression in the lives of minoritized clients. Such questions, even if pursued briefly, can be helpful in relationship building:

- What beliefs does the dominant culture have about the client's cultural group?
- How does the dominant culture hold control over the client's cultural group?
- How does the dominant culture want marginalized persons to be, think, and behave?
- What messages about the client's cultural group are seen in movies and television?
- What behaviors by the client's cultural group are rewarded in this society?
- What attitudes by the client's cultural group are rewarded in this society?

The purpose of this approach is not to build resentment or fan the flames of anger but to produce a sense of liberation from negative beliefs about oneself and one's cultural group (David et al., 2019; Vickery et al., 2023). The minority stress model (Meyer, 2003) highlights the mental health strain that arises for clients who identify with historically marginalized groups. While originally developed to address the challenges faced by gender and sexual minorities, it has been expanded to examine the intersectional identities among racial and ethnic minoritized groups (Cyrus, 2017) and people with disabilities (Botha & Frost, 2020). It emphasizes the complex relationship between external, sociocultural experiences of discrimination and the internalization of oppressive ideals.

When clients from historically marginalized communities internalize stigmatizing ideas and beliefs held by dominant cultural groups, there is an increased likelihood of negative physical and mental health outcomes (Boykin et al., 2016; Hendricks & Testa, 2012). Ever since Crenshaw's (1989) examination of the sociopolitical ramifications of ignoring how overlapping axes of gender and race "reveal how Black women are theoretically erased" (p. 139), research has made it increasingly clear that such outcomes are even more deleterious for minoritized clients with intersectional identities (Vargas et al., 2020).

Of course, there is also considerable variation in the attitudes of members of oppressed groups toward oppressors. Some may not have experienced the intensity of oppression that other members of their groups have. Assuming that all

Latino Americans, for example, have had the same experiences or attitudes is a mistake and could be called "benign stereotyping." As a presenting issue, discrimination may not be of the same magnitude for all clients from oppressed groups.

LIBERATION AND THE POWER OF PERCEPTION

As that which arises by means of dismantling oppression, *liberation* may be defined as the sociopolitical freedom to live under self-determined conditions, unconstrained or unaffected by oppressive forces (Martín-Baró, 1996; Watkins, 2002). According to the CHANGES model, psychological liberation may occur when a person engages in practices that facilitate therapeutic change via the activation of precursors, the bulk of which are inhibited by harmful messages imparted by means of racism and discrimination. Psychotherapists are in a particularly good position to support clients in the process of confronting the impact of internalized racism, misogyny, homophobia, ableism, and other forms of discrimination (David & Derthick, 2018).

The path to psychological liberation partly involves identifying, challenging, and altering one's relation to negative internalized beliefs imposed by individuals, institutions, and systems. Asking an individual from an underrepresented group to adjust or adapt to an oppressive society that does not work toward the best interests of some of its members clearly reduces the integrity of that client. However, working with minoritized clients to identify the traumatic impact of dominant narratives on self-concept can be a path to psychological liberation, particularly if we view trauma as "any experience that is subjectively unbearable" (Greenberg, 2019, p. 1144) and which subsequently results in some form of psychological and behavioral adaptation to environmental conditions.

Since oppression arises from power imbalances, those who are denied power must cope somehow to survive under threat. As noted by J. B. Miller (1986), a primary mechanism for coping with the threat of harm arises through an enhanced perception of the oppressor, be it an individual or a group. In this context, perception has to do with cognizance, recognition, or noticing and is thus related to the awareness precursor. It also relates to what Sternberg (1990) called *perspicacity*, an aspect of wisdom that involves the ability to see beyond appearances, to "see through" situations, or to "read between the lines."

For example, when a battered spouse becomes increasingly aware of how her abusive partner reacts to certain situations, she learns to deftly maneuver around sensitive topics. Her enhanced empathic attunement to the oppressor allows her to read into subtle verbal and nonverbal cues so as to better predict danger and ensure self-preservation. As her awareness becomes more acute, she may also come to see through and understand the mechanisms used by her partner to entrap her and how her life has become limited by abusive actions. Eventually, as awareness increases in therapy, she may learn how to maneuver herself safely out of the relationship. Perspicacity, born to ensure safety in the face of suffering, may yet serve as the catalyst for freedom and well-being.

Deprivation of power can awaken perception (J. B. Miller, 1986). Being rejected from a group or excluded from its benefits can inspire one to notice and study the oppressive group. Whether within or between cultures or among individuals of the same or differing cultures, this phenomenon of heightened perception has the paradoxical yet remarkable advantage of keeping the oppressed person or group alive and aware. Although an oppressed client's life may be ruled by harsh realities, their therapeutic ticket is often the raw and penetrating perception that develops out of those painful experiences. In this light, their accurate perception can be reframed in therapy as a strength, not only in perceiving their current situation but as a way out of it.

Leveraging Perspicacity

Although oppressed people are largely unaware of any hidden benefit, it is within this dynamic that we find a critical mechanism of empowerment that can stimulate the precursor of hope. This mechanism operates in members of systemically oppressed groups and among oppressed persons who have been relationally abused. It can be useful to empower certain clients by pointing out, or helping them realize, that they possess the hard-won, valuable perceptual skill of perspicacity. The therapeutic aim is to get a client to describe the oppressor in as much detail as possible.

Victims of intimate partner violence and domestic abuse, for example, can typically provide very descriptive accounts of the batterer's triggers, behaviors, attitudes, and emotions, complete with predictions of when and under what circumstances the abuse will occur. They seldom see evidence of this being a skill, however. When told that this same perceptive ability can be used to read people in a variety of settings, from the workplace to romantic relationships, they are often surprised to learn that they possess a valuable ability. For instance, group work with heterosexual women and teenager girls can be guided by questions to refine, clarify, and heighten perception:

- How does this society expect women to be, think, or behave?
- What kinds of behavior by women are rewarded in this society?
- How does society treat women who are considered overweight?
- How are women's bodies typically portrayed in popular culture?
- What does a man gain from having a woman with low self-esteem?
- What kind of partner is a man with little or no empathy?
- What kind of man is likely to physically abuse women or girls?
- How do women benefit, or suffer from, being dependent on men?
- Why are women more often depressed than men?

The phenomenon of perspicacity is also transcultural. It is observable among members of many culturally oppressed groups, such as the Tamils of Sri Lanka, the Uighurs of Northwest China, the untouchables of India, and the Bataks of Sumatra in Indonesia (see Hanna, 1998). In nearly all cases, members of the oppressed groups make accurate, detailed observations about the behavior and attitudes of their oppressors. Even a cursory examination of descriptions of oppressors by members of oppressed groups reveals remarkable insights. For example, the writings of Douglass (1855) are far more detailed and accurate than any of the bankrupt descriptions by enslavers. Northup (1853/1968) was a free African American who was kidnapped from New York State and forced into enslavement in Louisiana. He had no education and no status but was intelligent and wise, as seen in the following systemic clinical analysis of enslavers:

> It is not the fault of the slaveholder that he is cruel, so much as it is the fault of the system under which he lives. He cannot withstand the influence of habit and associations that surround him. Taught from earliest childhood, by all that he sees and hears, that the rod is for the slave's back, he will not be apt to change his opinions in maturer years. (pp. 157–158)

During the years of Northup's bondage, he observed how being an oppressor hardens a person, turning men and women alike into callous and cold beings:

> The existence of Slavery in its most cruel form ... has a tendency to brutalize the humane and finer feelings of their [the slaveholders'] nature. Daily witnesses of human suffering—listening to the agonizing screeches of the slave—beholding him writhing beneath the merciless lash—bitten and torn by dogs—dying without attention, and buried without shroud or coffin—it cannot otherwise be expected, than that they should become brutified and reckless of human life. (p. 157)

Acton (1887) offered an oft-quoted observation: "Power tends to corrupt, and absolute power corrupts absolutely" (p. 3). Members of dominant groups tend to describe members of subordinate groups in ways that justify their own possession and superiority (Gevisser, 2020). In both remote and well-traveled parts of the world, one may hear standard, stereotypical accusations against members of subordinate groups as "lazy," "dirty," and "stupid" and accused of not caring about or being harmful for or toward children. In this same way, boys come to believe that women are sex objects, heterosexuals frame sexual orientation as a moral quandary, and whole societies become convinced that underrepresented groups are somehow "less than." To be immersed in a culture is to be immersed in its context, and context, at its core, is made up of beliefs (David & Derthick, 2018).

Power corrupts, whether it is abused in the context of a country, culture, workplace, family, or marriage. The road to healing for oppressors is through recovering empathy and awareness lost due to the effects of excessive power on accurate perception. The goal is to bring them out of a state of obliviousness that prevents empathy for the oppressed and to increase awareness of their own psychological states. There are also mixed cases in which a client is oppressed in one context but an oppressor in another. For example, a woman may be oppressed at the workplace but be abusing her children at home. In these not-uncommon cases, the client needs to be helped to restore empathy for anyone they oppress and be liberated from their own oppressors in kind.

INTEGRATIVE EXISTENTIAL-COGNITIVE THERAPY FOR OPPRESSED CLIENTS

Liberation is, at the most fundamental level, a process of being freed from limiting beliefs. Many difficult clients have trouble isolating and identifying distorted cognitions or beliefs. However, there is an alternative approach that may make it easier for some clients who have been oppressed. The freedom-from-oppression model (FOM) promotes the use of clients' advanced perception to identify the beliefs of those who have hurt and forced dysfunctional beliefs upon them (Vickery et al., 2023). Many oppressed clients with heightened perceptive capabilities can identify the irrational beliefs and messages of oppressors, which they consequently absorb.

An oppressed person's negative beliefs are heavily influenced by oppressors, whether a group or an individual. Part of this oppression is a series of beliefs that the oppressor "inflicts" on the victim. As noted by Vickery et al. (2023), "Repeated exposure to oppressive messages or actions is coercive, resulting in the internalization of an oppressive and undermining self-structure" (p. 175). For example, a belief that one is stupid, worthless, incompetent, or unlovable can be seen as inflicted rather than self-determined. The standard cognitive approach would be to help a client identify irrational or dysfunctional beliefs as though they generated them. Yet a client is often not the origin of such beliefs; the oppressor is. The client's mistake is in agreeing with the beliefs inflicted or forced upon them, creating a negative array of feelings and behaviors.

The therapeutic goal is to end the agreement and replace the dysfunctional beliefs with those that are accurate and self-determined. To this end, the FOM includes three existential stages and 12 cognitive steps that support clients in relinquishing internalized, oppressive belief structures. Moving across stages that emphasize awareness, empowerment, and liberation, clients are supported in discovering their perspicacity and applying it with resoluteness to discover liberation from internalized oppression (Vickery et al., 2023). In every stage of the FOM process, it is incumbent upon the therapist to maintain empathy and compassion for the client. The approach is based on Heidegger's (1927/1962) descriptions of how a person may lose authenticity.

Stage 1: Awareness

In the first stage, the therapist must help the client gain awareness by identifying the oppressive persons or groups that impact their life. Following identification and description of the oppressor and oppressive beliefs, the therapist asks the client, "What did [the oppressive group or person] want you to believe about yourself?" For example, if a man was oppressed by his father, his father may have given him beliefs that he was a mistake or that he was worthless or ugly. African Americans may identify the dominant group as White society that conveys messages that Black people are lazy or incompetent. Specific people, such as teachers, neighbors, or employers, can be cited as oppressors as well.

Women have long been inundated with messages of inferiority (Saini, 2017). A therapeutic focus therein might be on listing dysfunctional beliefs imparted by messaging from popular culture, as well as men or boys in the client's life. It is important to cite actual sources when possible, such as movies, musicians, social media influencers, or family members. For example, when asked, a severely battered woman once listed the following beliefs forced upon her by her abusive husband:

- I'm stupid.
- I'm immoral.
- I'm a terrible mother.
- I'm fat and ugly.
- I can't make it without him.
- I'm a chronic liar.

She could easily recognize how much she had agreed with these beliefs and how he not only wanted but needed her to believe all these things so that she would not leave him. Once again, client perception needs to be validated to highlight that the belief was not created by the client but rather imposed by the oppressive source. Such perception is not perfectly accurate, of course, and like any skill, it often needs to be honed. In this instance, the approach may be framed in terms of the idea that women should not be blamed for having negative self-beliefs when those beliefs are so often a direct consequence of patriarchal culture.

It can be relatively easy for perceptive clients to spot the beliefs and tactics of oppressive individuals, but it is more difficult when those beliefs come from institutions or systems. In such cases, the therapist should help clients identify those oppressive beliefs. For example, if a lesbian were asked to list beliefs forced upon her by a rigidly heterosexual society, it is possible that she might omit certain oppressive beliefs, such as "All gays are immoral." The therapist could help by submitting that belief for the client's verification and then determine if she agrees with it and, if so, to what extent.

Alternatively, if a teenage girl reports a negative self-belief but has difficulty grappling with the possibility that her family plays some role in imparting that belief, she can be asked if there is any group in the world that might like a young woman such as herself to believe it. Helping the client address that larger group may provide the distance needed to directly challenge the belief and identify that the client's only mistake was in agreeing with something false. Sometimes, broader sources of oppression can be easier to discredit than more specific and proximal ones, and it is important to remember that challenging the internalized belief remains the therapeutic goal.

After isolating beliefs that were inflicted or otherwise fed to the client, the therapist must ask how much the client agreed with the message. A little? A lot? It might be rated on a scale from 1 to 10, with 10 being the most that one could ever believe anything and 1 being just a tiny bit. The belief will have its most damaging effect, of course, if the client still heavily agrees with it.

Stage 2: Empowerment

In the second stage, a therapist helps the client examine the consequences of agreeing with the negative internalized belief and any reasons the oppressor wanted or demanded agreement. For example, a client's agreement with the negative belief, "I'm not attractive because I'm not skinny enough," serves the purpose of always having the client doubt themself and never feeling worthy enough to challenge their partner on possible sexual manipulations or power schemes. The therapist must then work with the client to confront the pain associated with the belief in an effort to build tolerance as grit, or the willingness to experience anxiety and difficulty. After closely examining how one feels and acts as a result of agreeing with the belief, the client is then supported to dispute the belief to reclaim power and self-determination from the oppressor.

This process involves identifying evidence against an imposed belief and identifying evidence that discredits the standing of the oppressor. Sometimes, these processes merge in a broader effort of grasping intergenerational transmission patterns. For example, a young bisexual Latina woman named Maria once shared how her family's enactment of marianismo culture derived primarily from her grandfather's values. She came to believe that her mother and grandmother had long been depressed because they had submitted to familial expectations that ran counter to their nature. Her grandmother was raised in Guadalajara by an artistic, willful mother and progressive father, both of whom died in a tragic accident when her grandmother was just a teenager. Her paternal aunt soon pressed her to marry into a wealthy family with rigid views on traditional gender roles.

At the intersection of race, gender, sexual orientation, and first-generation immigrant status, Maria was confronting a highly complex, multigenerational family pattern. In observing how her grandmother and her mother would quietly shift from expressiveness to submissiveness around the men in her family, she had come to see her depression as a result of internalizing the belief that "women only have value as quiet homemakers, wives, and mothers." Determined to break the pattern, she not only identified and disputed the belief but discredited the oppressive message not by attacking her grandfather (although this was her initial path, she found it difficult to maintain focus on the issue due to deep, cultural guilt) but confronting embedded cultural patriarchy.

Finally, clients consciously and actively terminate agreement with the belief. If the client does not readily see the benefit of terminating agreement, the therapist can ask that they try it just as an experiment to see how the act of disagreeing with the belief feels. The Jamesian device technique (see Chapter 5, this volume) can also be used here to determine the truth or falsehood of an enforced belief. This approach is not about clients cutting themselves off from or ending all ties with the oppressor; that is another decision entirely, and the therapist should explicitly discuss the distinction.

Stage 3: Liberation

In the third stage, clients work toward liberation. Once harmful or dysfunctional aspects of a belief are revealed through disputation, the client can proceed to disagree with it and then replace it with more accurate, self-determined beliefs. This approach can be easily adapted to group therapy. Finding hope and social support for clients in this stage is also important. Therapists can tell stories of, and help clients connect with, people who have escaped difficult conditions, such as gang involvement or abusive relationships. Such exemplars demonstrate a path to establishing self-determined and empowering beliefs and show that achieving a degree of happiness or fulfillment is possible. Therapists can also link clients directly with community resources or organizations that offer help to people in need.

A FINAL NOTE ON OPPRESSION, PERSPICACITY, AND LIBERATION

For people who have faced a lifetime of disempowerment by others and by society, it can be hard to imagine life getting better. The various traumas of interpersonal and systemic oppression often underlie the suffering and ineffective coping mechanisms of difficult clients. At the same time, a significant increase in perspicacity can arise among oppressed persons and groups, as the trauma of oppression tends to enhance perceptive awareness and empathic attunement. A therapeutic path to liberation for oppressed clients involves recognizing how oppressors maintain coercive power by introjecting destructive beliefs at both individual and sociocultural narrative levels. Helping clients see how dominant narratives have shaped their self-image can be a powerful way to heal.

15

Addiction and Substance Use

Therapy with addicted clients is one of the most challenging and difficult kinds of therapy, especially if considered in the context of achieving successful outcomes. This kind of therapy can be plodding, stressful, disappointing, and discouraging to therapists. Burnout is a common side effect of doing therapy with these clients, especially if the agency or setting does not provide support, encouragement, and high-quality additional training (J. J. Kim et al., 2018; Yang & Hayes, 2020). Such additional training should not only be on the nature of drugs, alcohol, and addictions but also on how to work with difficult clients. Burnout is often due to empathy degradation and other countertransference phenomena, such as resisting resistance, as well as inadequate training.

This chapter demonstrates how the activation of precursors helps clients enter the change mindset needed for successful treatment. A combination of practical strategies and techniques are provided to illustrate the ideas behind the CHANGES model approach to drug and alcohol treatment. There is no single strategy or technique that will lead to sobriety, so a competent addictions therapist needs a well-assembled toolbox of techniques. We will begin with a reframe of addiction itself.

DRUG USE VERSUS THERAPY: THE GRAND REFRAME

Some therapeutic approaches to addictions therapy suggest that clients are wrong in their use of drugs or alcohol, gambling, or whatever the addiction happens to be. It is common in psychoeducation-focused addictions groups for clients to

---

Case examples have been disguised to protect client confidentiality.

https://doi.org/10.1037/0000451-016
Therapeutic Change With Difficult Clients: Precursors and Techniques in the CHANGES Model, Second Edition, by B. D. Wilkinson and F. J. Hanna

learn that their beliefs, attitudes, and behaviors are simply wrong. The moral implication is clear: They would not be in active treatment for drug and alcohol use if such uses were the "right" thing to do.

The grand reframe takes a different tack by establishing why the client is using in the first place and how addictive drug use in general is often pursued as a solution to the client's problems in life. Eschewing the impulse to repudiate addiction as immoral, therapists can demonstrate how drug or alcohol use can be understood as an attempt, at least initially, to improve one's life experience.

Many reasons explain why a person uses substances, becomes addicted, or becomes chemically dependent, including genetic makeup, family dynamics, social pressure, reducing stress, self-medication, thrill seeking, or sheer boredom. This technique works best, in our experience, with the self-medicating user. Clients have reported self-medicating to address a wide variety of symptoms, including physical pain, emotional pain, anxiety, depression, emptiness, loneliness, relationship problems, low self-esteem, self-loathing, bitterness, and apathy.

The grand reframe is that drug use and psychotherapy have the same purpose: to produce positive changes in thinking, feeling, behaving, and relating. Thus, the grand reframe presents drug use as purposeful in a manner similar to psychotherapy and counseling. When clients are presented with this reframe, they tend to be surprised, if not shocked, to hear a mental health professional say such a thing. It can also increase interest in therapy and bolster the motivation to do the work. In essence, clients can learn that their behavior has been purposeful, even if the use of drugs is not the optimal solution to attain their goal. Rather, psychotherapy is.

Step 1: The Backdoor Question—Finding Out Why the Client Is Using

This technique aims to discover why a client is using and reframe the entire endeavor. Of course, one cannot ask a client, "Why do you use?" We have tried variations of this many, many times, but the typical responses are "to feel good" or "to get high." However, a strategy that we refer to as "the backdoor" approach often renders clinically useful responses.

The reframe can be initiated in the first session after intake. It is important to mention that the technique may need to be repeated several times, depending on the client's awareness level or cognitive condition, before it takes hold, or "bites." Once the client has disclosed their drug of choice, it is appropriate to inquire as to why the client uses at all. This is done in a context that reveals their purpose through inference, as a direct answer is unlikely. The backdoor question is presented next with a typical dialogue with an opiate user that includes follow-up questions:

THERAPIST: (backdoor question) What do you get out of being high?

CLIENT: It makes me feel relaxed.

THERAPIST: Does that mean that when you're not high, you're not relaxed?

CLIENT:	Yep. Getting high relaxes me.
THERAPIST:	What are you trying to get relaxed about?
CLIENT:	I just feel uptight a lot, like everything is all messed up.

At this point, a dialogue may ensue that invites self-disclosure from the client. The therapist can ask questions that do not demand specific information but rather emphasize what burdens the client is experiencing and the purpose that using a substance serves in that context.

THERAPIST:	Don't tell me what it is, but are there some things in life that are keeping you from feeling relaxed?
CLIENT:	Yeah. (looking down) I don't want to talk about it.
THERAPIST:	Fair enough. Don't tell me what it is, but can I ask how it's stopping you? And listen, if I start to bother you, just tell me to back off and I will.
CLIENT:	Okay.
THERAPIST:	I'm going to guess that you've been through a lot in life. Is that fair to say?
CLIENT:	Yeah. I've been through more shit than anybody knows.
THERAPIST:	You mean you've never told anyone about it?
CLIENT:	Nope. (shifting in seat) Nah ... what's the point? Nobody cares anyway.
THERAPIST:	What's it like to be carrying around all of that bad stuff inside of you 24/7?
CLIENT:	That's why I use. It helps me forget.

Step 2: The Grand Reframe: Admiring the Intention

THERAPIST:	You know, I've gotta give you credit for finding a way to forget and relax.
CLIENT:	(surprised) Really?
THERAPIST:	Yeah. You're trying to fix the problem. Are the painkillers working for you?
CLIENT:	Yeah, a little.
THERAPIST:	How much?
CLIENT:	What do you mean, how much? Like, enough, I guess.
THERAPIST:	As a percentage, how much is the codeine working to fix your problem and help you relax?

CLIENT:	Maybe, like, half the time it works, so 50%. Used to be a lot more.
THERAPIST:	Pardon me, but 50% isn't much. It sounds like you've noticed the drug is less and less effective in helping you relax and forget.
CLIENT:	Yeah, my tolerance is up, so I take more, but it's never enough.
THERAPIST:	You know, counseling and drug use are very similar. Both aim to help you find some relief. The big difference is that counseling works over the long haul. Codeine is not a method that works forever, you know?
CLIENT:	Yeah, I get that, but it works right now, and that feels like enough sometimes.
THERAPIST:	Right, but now you're addicted to a pain pill that controls your life through addiction, and you're stuck in this treatment center. Here you are, having to talk to someone like me for something that only helps half the time, at best?
CLIENT:	Well, it's better than nothing.

Step 3: The Redirect

THERAPIST:	Fair enough, it is better than nothing. Nothing would be no help at all. Can I say something else, and you tell me what you think?
CLIENT:	Sure.
THERAPIST:	The goals of counseling and drug use are the same, but the methods are way different. Counseling has the same goal to help you relax, but unlike drugs, it actually works. You've given oxy and other drugs a shot, and you deserve credit for trying to fix problems. But it hasn't helped, 'cause here you are.
CLIENT:	Yeah, okay. So what?
THERAPIST:	So, you gave drugs your best shot. Are you willing to try something that really works? The good thing about counseling is that you can easily quit if you don't like it (laughing). You're in treatment now, so it might be a good time to give it a try. And if you want to get out of this program, working in counseling is the best way to do it.
CLIENT:	Well, I'm here, so why not. I'll give it a shot.

We have found that this reframe can be remarkably motivating, activating the precursors of grit, awareness, confronting, and necessity. Although the use of affirmations in motivational interviewing involves praising positive behavior (W. R. Miller & Rollnick, 2012), few addiction therapists would naturally consider affirming or admiring drug use itself as an attempt to fix a problem. As such, admiring clients for their intention to feel better is a big part of the effectiveness of the grand reframe. When used early in treatment, it can lay the groundwork for treatment success and eventual sobriety. If it doesn't work for a client early in treatment, it can always be attempted later in the therapy process.

CLIENTS UNDERGOING PHARMACOTHERAPY

It is widely acknowledged that medication is best combined with psychotherapy to facilitate change. For most people, medication alone is an insufficient condition for change. In terms of the CHANGES model, medications may make it easier for some clients to activate the precursors and achieve lasting changes. Many clients who report even minor improvements in daily functioning due to medication use are better able to work toward change in therapy. A good metaphor might be weightlifting: Accomplishing therapeutic change is the equivalent of lifting a 500-pound weight. An appropriately prescribed medication can reduce that weight to something more manageable. The effects of the medications vary from person to person, of course; a medication might reduce that 500-pound burden for some people to 100 pounds but for others, only to 400 pounds.

FIRST HIGH, BEST HIGH

This strategy is best done in group therapy but can be done individually as well. After years of work with drug-using clients, we found that there is a large percentage of clients who had their most euphoric and impacting experience the very first time they became intoxicated on their drug of choice. This can be a powerful topic to pursue, demonstrating that drug use is so insidious that it holds out a promise for happiness on the first high and then yanks it away by never again delivering a high as good as the first one or, in some few cases, a second. Meanwhile, the user tries over and over to achieve the intensity and wonder of that first high. It usually doesn't happen again.

The drug experience can be reframed to show that

> Drugs are like con artists or swindlers. They suck us in, getting us to buy some line of crap about how great it all is, making us think that we just discovered the secret of happiness. But it's seldom, if ever, that good again. And we are left holding an addiction as a reward for our efforts, along with a life in ruins.

This type of phrasing gets to the essence of the issue but can be varied to fit the situation at hand.

This technique can be done in groups, where each group member recounts their first high and talks about how great it was. After recounting the experience, the therapist or the other group members ask, "Was it ever that good again?" The therapist or group members then go further by comparing drug use to "buying a line of crap" or something to that effect.

Clients typically report that it was never that good again, and indeed, drug users begin to see that it is even harder to get high with continued use as tolerance of the drug builds. Presenting therapy as an alternative has the advantage of providing hope for the client rather than their compulsively pursuing drugs to squeeze every last bit of joy out of them, as often happens. This technique can increase a sense of necessity, grit, awareness, confronting, and hope.

SUBPERSONALITY TECHNIQUE FOR ADDICTION

The subpersonality technique was explored in relation to the sense of necessity precursor (see Chapter 7, this volume). The term itself refers to different parts of the personality (Assagioli, 1965, 1973; Rowan, 1990), and it has an important role in addictions counseling as a way of using the person's inner resources to work toward change. It can be done relatively quickly when a client expresses apathy or defiance about stopping their drug or alcohol use. Listen for statements about their drug use or regarding quitting drug use, such as "I don't care" or "I'm never going to quit using."

Therapists must first acknowledge, fully accept, and show empathy for the defiance, apathy, and resentment. Defiance can often be reframed as the love of freedom. Make sure that the client feels understood. In our experience, ignoring this first step will lead to technique failure. Then, ask the client, "I know you said you really don't care, but is there a small, perhaps 'little teeny' part of you that worries about what's going to happen to you—a little part of you that does care?" Often, the addicted client will nod or give a simple "yeah." Other possible sub-personality questions are provided next, but do not utilize more than one, as it will disperse the focus of the technique:

- Is there a part of you that thinks you use too much?
- Is there a part of you that wants to quit using?
- Is there a part of you that is tired of living like this?
- Is there a part of you that knows you can't go on like this for much longer?
- Is there a part of you that knows you need to make a change?

If the answer is positive, the therapist can then ask what percentage of their mind is that part, from 0% to 100%. Answers tend to range from 3% to 40%, and any client-identified percentage can be addressed. It is important to note that this percentage step can also be done later in the process if the therapist thinks it better to wait. However, getting a percentage estimate will give the therapist an indication of how much of the client wants to improve. The next step is crucial and involves directly addressing the newly discovered subpersonality. The following question should be asked:

• Can I talk to that part of you?

If the client can identify that there is a part of them that runs contrary to what they have been saying, and if they feel understood by the therapist, the client will almost always let the therapist talk to that positive part of them. However, if the client does not experience the empathy of the therapist, the technique is unlikely to work. This approach can change the entire tone of the conversation and the counseling process itself. It is common to see a completely new part of the client that had not previously been present. The goal is to strengthen the positive part and make it bigger and stronger. In theory, at least, this could be the real client. Other questions to identify the positive subpersonality, according to the issue at hand, could be

• Is there a part of you that wants to change?
• Is there a part of you that wants to quit using drugs?
• Is there a part of you that wants to stay alive? (in the case of suicidal ideation)
• Is there a part of you that is tired of living this way?
• Is there a part of you that thinks you use too much?

When the client acknowledges that there is indeed a part of them that wants to change, and the therapist is given permission to talk directly to that part of them that is interested in positive change, the clinical adventure begins. This technique can be done in the first session, and we have demonstrated this in live consulting practice with actual clients in treatment programs before a small audience, without ever meeting the client previously.

The next step involves speaking directly to the positive part. The therapist can say to the positive part of the client, "What is it like to watch yourself using and taking risks with drug use?" Or, the client could be asked, "What are you thinking when you watch yourself using and getting wasted day after day?" This can sometimes lead to some very positive and encouraging conversations.

Finally, the procedure calls for an assessment on that part of the client. The client subpersonality is asked something on the order of, "You said that you're 5% of the total you, but I wonder how big you'd like to be?" At this point, the client may answer with a much larger percentage. The response from the therapist might then be, "How about we work on making you bigger and stronger so that you are no longer controlled by your using self?" If they get this far, the client is usually interested in pursuing this line of therapy. Validate the client for their good intentions and ask to make this a goal of future sessions. If the client moves back into defiance or apathy in the following sessions, the therapist can ask politely to again speak to the subpersonality that wants to change.

EMPTY CHAIR WORK FOR ADDICTION

It should be mentioned at the outset that in order to use the empty chair technique from gestalt therapy (Mann, 2010; Perls, 1969, 1973; Polster & Polster, 1973), it is helpful to have studied the technique itself, as it is commonly misapplied. Done correctly, this technique can be remarkably powerful as evidenced by our own experience both as therapists and as clients in therapy. It is not within the purview of this book to teach the use of the empty chair technique, as this can be obtained elsewhere easily enough. However, we feel it important to mention that maintaining the dialogue between the entities in the chairs is what brings about resolution and closure. A common mistake, seen even in online training videos, is that the dialogue is compromised by too much conversation between therapist and client and there is not enough focus on continuing the interchange carried by the dialogue itself. It is in that dialogue that the personality integration takes place.

Empty Chair With Subpersonalities

Once the subpersonality is identified, the empty chair technique can help resolve the split between personality parts by bringing about a personality integration. In one chair is placed the part that wants to quit using and in the other chair is placed the subpersonality that wants to continue using. The empty chair procedure is conducted, continuing the interaction until the aforementioned personality integration takes place. Addressing subpersonalities, or disowned parts of the personality, as they are called in gestalt therapy (Mann, 2010; Perls, 1969, 1973; Polster & Polster, 1973), is a standard utilization of the empty chair. The results can be remarkable. We have seen this technique occasionally turn the tide of drug use in some clients.

Other Applications of the Empty Chair Technique in Substance Use Therapy

In addition to use with subpersonalities, there are other applications of the empty chair technique that can be effective in addictions work. The following list includes various applications of the empty chair in substance use that we have found helpful. However, do not attempt the technique unless the client can actively visualize something or someone in the empty chair. If they cannot visualize it, the technique will likely fail, or the client will be unwilling to enact it.

- Place a supportive deceased person in the empty chair.
- Place an oppressive deceased person in the empty chair.
- Place the addiction itself in the empty chair.
- Place the drug of choice or the craving in the empty chair.
- Place an influential drug-using person in the empty chair.

That said, some clients find this technique unappealing and will not attempt it at all, although they might do so later in the therapy process. Unfortunately, we have seen several occasions where a client declares, "I'm not talking to an empty chair," and that's that. Confronting the problem, grit, and the awareness precursor are most operative herein.

THE DRUG HERO TECHNIQUE

Clients occasionally disclose that they have a friend who can consume any amount of alcohol or any quantity of a particular drug with no ill effects at all. When asked, clients in such a situation will typically say that they think about this "drug hero" during psychoeducation sessions or videos illustrating the dangers and destructiveness of drugs. The memory or image of the drug hero will invalidate any therapeutic message or information about the problems that come with drug use.

Clients have reported that they often see these videos in treatment programs. However, many of them listen to and then dismiss the messages because they think, "Yeah, but that doesn't apply to Joey." In this instance, the client will keep their drug hero, Joey, alive in their mind as a means to hold onto the defiant or desperate wish that drug use really is not all that bad.

Although this technique can be done individually, it is perhaps best in group therapy by having each client tell a story about how their drug hero (if they have one) was virtually immune to the negative effects of alcohol and/or drugs. The group therapist can also share an example of a drug hero from their life, if applicable. The next step consists of having clients talk about what the hero is like in the present, presumably after years and years of drug use. Clients will often report that their hero is now in jail, on the street, lost their job, rejected by their family, selling drugs, or committing other crimes to support their addiction. If not, the hero is the exception, not the rule.

Either way, it is better to bring the hero out of the client's mind and into therapy than allow them to take up space in the mind playing an oppositional role that is illusory if not delusional. Clients tend to enjoy this technique when done in groups and can tell interesting stories. The point of this technique is to show that some people indeed have higher resistance to drug effects than others, but eventually, the drug wins, and it destroys the hero's life just like it does for everyone else.

Finally, it is a good idea to ask clients in group if they were ever considered a drug hero, capable of consuming huge doses with minimal negative effects. This is particularly helpful when clients hear that a fellow group member has been so badly affected that they are here, in the same treatment program as the rest of the group. When the heroes can self-disclose in group, it can be beneficial to the group as a whole to see how drugs can take down the hardiest among us. The awareness, necessity, and hope precursors are primary here, but when used in a group dynamic, this technique can obviously influence social support, as well.

VALUE DISSONANCE AND REALIGNMENT

This is another technique that can be done individually and in group therapy. It is a cognitive approach that is combined with an existential component. It is a way of restoring value systems among users who have had their values devastated by drug and alcohol addiction. Like most of the techniques presented in this chapter, this technique is not powerful enough to get the user to quit using altogether, but it may be powerful enough to put a dent in the user's drug mindset.

The technique begins with asking group members, in a round, to name the three most important things in their lives. They can briefly describe each and explain why each is important. Typical values can include family, friends, love, jobs, money, romantic partners, and freedom. The second step is to have each group member discuss how drug use has impacted each of these values. For example, using can destroy families, lead to loss of freedom, break up marriages, and so on.

The third step consists of asking, still using rounds, how much the drug is valued compared with the three major values. In the fourth step, the therapist asks the client to insert the drug into the list of values. This begins to reveal cognitive dissonance in the client's mindset in terms of how the pursuit of the drug has degraded the precious things in life that the client has held dear. Finally, the group is asked, one client at a time and still in the rounds format, how they would or could realign their values without the drug taking precedence and what this might look like.

This technique can help a client build a clearer picture of what they want their life to look like. It makes goal setting easier due to removing a good portion of the conflicting value that arises between drug use and the living of life itself. It is also valuable because it presents a very stark image of how drug use is destroying the important things in their lives and yet how there remains hope in recovery. Awareness, confronting, necessity, and hope are the operative precursors in this technique.

EXISTENTIAL-COGNITIVE THERAPY OF OPPRESSION FOR DRUG USE

This technique has been described elsewhere (Hanna & Cardona, 2013; Hanna et al., 2000; Vickery et al., 2023) and can be used in the drug and alcohol context simply by identifying the specific people in the client's life who have been harmful to them. Make a list of these people and ask who among them seems to be related to their drug or alcohol use. With each of these people, list the beliefs that the oppressive person forced or imposed upon the client and how much the client agreed with each of the beliefs on a scale from 1 to 10.

By getting the client to disagree with and let go of the enforced harmful beliefs, the client may be able to free themselves of the psychological attachment to these oppressors and become empowered to stop drug use and aim for sobriety. Another way of addressing this is by asking the client if they are hard on themselves, hate themselves, or "give themselves a lot of shit." All that is necessary for therapeutic benefit is for the client to disagree with the imposed messages.

If this is insufficient to get a client to disagree, the therapist can ask what they say to themselves in classic cognitive behavior style (Meichenbaum & Cameron, 1974; Meichenbaum, 1977) and then restructure the self-talk. Sometimes, discrediting the source of the messages can help dismiss the harmful belief. This technique involves confronting the problem and liberating the client from the oppressive influence rather than merely adjusting to the situation.

ROLE-PLAY: THE DEVELOPMENT OF REFUSAL SKILLS

Refusal skills are an important strategy in the establishment and maintenance of sobriety. Role-playing situations in which the client has been, or is likely to be, offered drugs and/or alcohol can be empowering. This role-play is best done in group therapy, with each group member getting a turn to play the client. The technique is carried out in stages. The emphasis is on situations where the offer is strong and a simple "no" is an insufficient response due to active social pressure.

The first stage consists of the therapist and client sitting in the middle of the group. A marijuana blunt, for instance, can be easily simulated by rolling up a piece of paper. The therapist mimics smoking from the blunt before offering it to the client, saying with insistence, "Hit it." as if the therapist's lungs are filled with smoke. The therapist, as in real life, pushes the blunt toward the face of the client, insisting they take it. Meanwhile, the client is informed only that they should mindfully observe the process, watching for thoughts or feelings that arise in role-play. The client is then asked if any memories are triggered. Thoughts and feelings that arise during the role-play are actively processed in the group setting.

The second stage of the role-play involves having a group member sit in for the therapist and offer the blunt to add an element of reality to the scene. The group member foists the blunt on the client, using condescending or ridiculing statements to get them to use the drug. Once again, the client does not answer but mindfully observes any feelings and thoughts that arise as well as any memories that might be triggered. These are also processed in the group.

The third stage of the role-play involves an element of psychodrama called doubling (Goldman & Morrison, 1984). The client is again offered the blunt by a group member while being mindful, as in the earlier stages. However, in this stage, two group members are asked to provide verbal, audible "self-talk" by standing alongside the seated client and speaking into the client's ear. When the client is offered the blunt, the two standing "doubles" actively participate. The double on the client's right side speaks positive statements into the client's right ear, saying, "You know you shouldn't hit it," or "You've been clean; don't wreck it now." Meanwhile, the double on the left side says in the client's left ear, "You know you want to hit it," or "Go ahead, get high." Clients consistently report that this method is close to their lived experience and reproduces their mindset in the real world. They also tend to report how helpful it is to role-play such situations.

The fourth stage is called refusal dialogue, and this is the stage in which the refusal itself is role-played. With the continued engagement of mindfulness, the third stage scenario is duplicated with an additional step of speaking actual refusal lines that convince the person foisting the drug or alcohol to back off or give up. Done properly, this stage can be remarkably empowering and encouraging for clients, if not a bit humorous as well.

In the midst of being offered the drug, and with the doubles continuing their messages in the ears of the client, a list of refusal lines is provided. Refusal lines go beyond the simple "no" for an answer in a way that discourages the person from continuing to offer the drug. Some of these responses are intentionally sarcastic or absurd so as to activate cognitive dissonance. Please note that refusals should be spoken respectfully, as rude as they may appear in writing. There is no point in antagonizing others, and it is preferable for the lines to be spoken with a sense of irony, sarcasm, or humor. Here are some refusal lines we have found to be effective in group therapy:

- I appreciate your wanting to get me high, but sorry, I'm into depression!
- I don't do that anymore. Drugs make me too happy. I hate being happy.
- Nah, I like feeling like shit. Can't be getting high and messing that up.
- Thanks, but I got better things to do than to feel good.

Of course, group members can work to come up with their own refusal lines. Clients in outpatient programs often come back to the treatment program laughing at the effects these kinds of lines have on sellers or people who try to get them high. The confronting precursor as well as grit and awareness precursors are clearly at work here.

ALCOHOL AND DRUG USE IN THE SERVICE OF THE FAMILY

There is an aspect of family systems that is often overlooked by therapists, which may be because the *Diagnostic and Statistical Manual of Mental Disorders*, in its various iterations, does not take systems theory into account (Bonino & Hanna, 2018). There are some instances we have found where the only way to reach the client was by treating the client as the family healer (Whitaker, 1989). As is well known, in systems theory, the problematic person in a family is often referred to as the scapegoat or symptom bearer (Bowen, 1976). Whitaker (1989) added the concept that the symptom bearer or scapegoat can also serve as the family healer.

A drug or alcohol user may be engaged in addictive behavior not only because of addiction but to actually serve the family. Hanna (2004) told the story of how even a 2-year-old boy with serious symptoms could function as the family healer. Whitaker (1989) informed us that we should not be too quick to label maladaptive behavior as psychopathology. What follows is the story of Jimmy, an 18-year-old boy with a serious alcohol problem. It illustrates how negative behavior can be well-intended and purposive. But as the saying goes, "The road to hell is paved with good intentions."

The Story of Marco

At 18 years old, Marco had been in an inpatient facility for 2 months. He was reported to the consultant by the clinical supervisor of the agency as being unmotivated to quit drinking and disinterested in sobriety. The consultant was informed that he had made no progress at all. Marco openly admitted that he was going to drink as soon as he was released from the facility, and he was highly defiant toward therapists and staff members, as well as showing a certain amount of contempt for therapy itself. The consultant was also informed that Marco's father was a severe alcoholic who had been hospitalized several times because of it and had developed a serious liver disease.

The consultant was asked if he would see Marco with the goal of getting him motivated to participate in counseling and make positive changes. The consultant met with the treatment team to learn what had been previously done with Marco to help with his excessive alcohol use. They reported that no discernible progress had been made during Marco's time in treatment. The treatment team reported using cognitive behavioral therapy and motivational interviewing to talk with Marco about his father, with particular emphasis on building some dissonance around ending up sick like his father had been.

The consultant sat down with Marco, who had been informed of this session. Initial probing and precursors techniques such as admiration of his defiance as an expression of freedom were just effective enough to establish some small amount of rapport. After the consultant asked Marco if he was worried that he might end up like his father, Marco, as predicted, replied that he was not worried at all. He also said that he did not care if he became addicted and was not concerned that alcohol could ruin his life. He said that he did not know why he loved to drink and did not care to find out.

The consultant attempted the subpersonalities technique, addressing the hurt, freedom challenge, admiring negatives, and others, but none were effective. The only reason Marco was talking to the consultant was due to a few effective expressions of empathy. Seeing no pathway into his mindset, it dawned on the consultant that Marco might be an alcoholic in service of the family when the following sequence occurred in the conversation:

CONSULTANT: Do you like your father?

MARCO: Nope.

CONSULTANT: How well do you know your father?

MARCO: I mean, I don't really know him. Nobody does.

CONSULTANT: Did you ever try to get close to him, talk with him, anything like that?

MARCO: Yeah, he didn't want to know me.

CONSULTANT: I see. So, you somehow became much like the guy you don't like or know?

MARCO: (hesitantly) I guess.

At this point, the consultant sensed an inroad. Through a series of questions and reflections, the consultant highlighted how Marco's father chose alcohol as his only meaningful relationship, over and above that of Marco and his siblings. The consultant validated the difficulty of knowing an alcoholic and suggested that Marco was trying to not only understand his father but to save him:

CONSULTANT: Is it possible that you're drinking to learn all that you can about alcohol ... as a way to better understand your father?

MARCO: Uh, I don't know. Maybe? Never thought about it like that ...

CONSULTANT: Think about it ... take your time ...

MARCO: Maybe, yeah. I just assumed we were both addicts.

CONSULTANT: Maybe. But maybe it's different for you. Maybe you started drinking because you wanted to learn about it so that you might be able to save him. You started drinking to feel close to your father, to save your father.

MARCO: (staring at the ground) Yeah, I mean, I was just curious, when I started, about why he loved it so much. I just wanted to know what it was like ...

CONSULTANT: Jimmy, you're a hero.

MARCO: (looking up with a scowl) Yeah, right. What are you talking about?

CONSULTANT: (reframes) You could have had a very different life, but you're such a good person—such a good son—that you decided to help your father with his drinking regardless of what it does to you. That's what heroes do; they help others despite the risk to themselves. And that's what you're doing.

MARCO: (with tears in his eyes but shrugging his shoulders) If you say so.

CONSULTANT: Well, to your credit, you've become very familiar with drinking. Maybe it's time to learn about sobriety and how to stop drinking. What do you think?

MARCO: (wiping tears) Yeah, maybe it's time to do that.

From that session forward, Marco responded to most therapy techniques and, after a few weeks, had become active as a leader in group therapy and strongly involved in individual therapy as well. The consultant informed the treatment team, the clinical supervisor, and the director of the agency that Marco was not a typical kid with an alcohol problem. He was a family healer attempting to acquire knowledge of alcohol use through experiential learning and that he was now ready to work toward sobriety. It was a classic example of how systems can play a major role in addictions.

TECHNIQUES FOR REDUCING CRAVINGS

According to research, cravings are among the most important phenomena to address in drug and alcohol treatment due to evidence showing that once the cravings are greatly reduced, the urge or need to use is also greatly reduced (Tapper, 2018). In addition, the presence of cravings is related to the urge to relapse, and conversely, without cravings, the user will be much more likely to achieve stable sobriety (Vallejo & Amara, 2009). Mindfulness practice has been shown to be consistently effective in reducing cravings (Tapper, 2018). What follows in this section are various techniques and approaches to reducing cravings through the application of mindfulness.

Craving Management

Ask the client to locate in the body where exactly they feel the craving. This is done so that the client can "anchor" the craving and reduce its vagueness so they can identify some specific details about how they experience it. Typical responses are that the craving is in the area of the chest, solar plexus, or throat. Teach the client how to be mindful of the craving and whether the intensity varies, as well as when and in what situations the craving becomes most and least intense. Ask the client to set their phone to sound an alarm every 30 minutes (or whatever is most appropriate) so they can then enter a craving intensity rating into a tracking app. This will give the client and therapist a good indication of what kind of state the client is in relative to the nature of the cravings on a daily basis. Part of craving management also involves tracking the craving itself, noting if it grows or shrinks in the body at various times and across various situations.

Mindfully "Riding" the Craving

Also known as "urge surfing" (Shonin & Van Gordon, 2016), this technique involves deliberately confronting a craving but not reacting to it. This technique is best done in the beginning with the therapist present. Inform the client that cravings do not have to be the most controlling phenomenon in their life. The therapist then asks the client to establish a mindful state, enter the craving itself, and describe the sensations, feelings, and temptations associated with it.

The key is to fully concentrate on the craving and stay with it until the client achieves some stability in the sense that they can accept its presence and not feel overpowered by it. If a client can immerse oneself in the craving without reacting, the craving has been observed to reduce in some cases. But at first, the riding of the craving should be done with the therapist present and guiding. The "riding" is essentially the capacity to experience the craving itself and watch how one is "drawn into" or "sucked into" the craving, and noticing where and how one loses control to it. Once again, mindfulness is the key practice in this technique, which requires deliberate client practice.

Influencing the Craving

Once the client has shown some skill in riding the craving, they can begin to influence it. The key here is to consciously increase the intensity of the craving while continuing to ride it. Once the craving has increased, it can be somewhat controlled by intentionally reducing its intensity. Mindfulness reveals that some of the intensity of a craving is due to resisting it, whereas accepting it (as is done by riding the craving) removes some of the power of the craving.

Working with the therapist in session, some clients start to show self-determined degrees of direct influence by taking a measure of control of cravings.. The effect of this technique for some clients is significant in that the client is no longer helpless before the craving and not controlled by it to the degree they were previously. The result, when successful, gives a client a sense of hope for the possibility of achieving sobriety. But as we said, one cannot become overconfident here.

A FINAL NOTE ON ADDICTION AND SUBSTANCE USE

In important ways, this technique-focused chapter serves as an appropriate endcap to the book due to its fully pragmatic bent. Since the purpose of the CHANGES model is to help therapists facilitate change with difficult clients, it is reasonable to conclude with the immense challenge faced in the battle against addiction and substance use. In the last chapter, we review the advantages of the CHANGES model, highlight potential applications of the CHANGES model in the business sector, and discuss how the CHANGES model informs the development of a metatheoretical framework on teleological freedom that uniquely contributes to the psychotherapy integration movement.

V

CONCLUSION

CONCLUSION

16

At the Horizon of Change

The CHANGES model may be a valuable step in isolating change principles that are not bound by jargon, techniques, theory, stages, or personality traits. The model moves in a direction that cuts to the essence of therapy in attempting to isolate the necessary conditions or common factors of therapeutic change itself. Such an approach has several practical advantages.

The first advantage arises when a difficult, perplexing client seems unlikely to change. Rating difficult clients using the CHANGES assessment may help formulate new approaches to change, and using the techniques provided in this book could assist in implementing the missing precursors. There are, of course, many techniques and strategies that can be developed for each precursor beyond what is listed herein. We leave it to therapists and researchers to add new approaches and techniques. When one understands the nature of the precursors, suitable techniques for each tend to spontaneously develop. Indeed, many therapists do this already.

A second advantage is gained through rating the precursors of a therapist. Possibly for the first time, a gauge is provided that supervisors and trainers can use to take some measure of a therapist's potential as a change agent with specific clients. Similarly, when having difficulty with a client, the CHANGES assessment can help practitioners rate themselves and pinpoint missing precursors. The aim in this context is to bolster missing precursors to help therapists maximize helping efforts. It can also be of assistance in rehabilitating impaired therapists or those suffering from burnout.

A third advantage is that the CHANGES model can help a therapist better understand therapist interference. When therapists recognize that their actions or attitudes are diminishing the presence of specific precursors in clients, corrections can be made to increase, rather than reduce, those precursors. For example,

https://doi.org/10.1037/0000451-017

Therapeutic Change With Difficult Clients: Precursors and Techniques in the CHANGES Model, Second Edition, by B. D. Wilkinson and F. J. Hanna

sometimes therapists make the mistake of thinking that certain actions or attitudes that were helpful with one client will be helpful with others. Unfortunately, this can impede the emergence of precursors in some clients. Awareness of therapist interference is important for developing self-awareness, facilitating self-correction, and growing wisdom. It also helps therapists avoid automatizing their approach with difficult clients.

A fourth advantage is that focusing on precursors may help train therapists and counselors in client-specific change processes and variables. When trainees are taught to think in terms of therapeutic change, including what causes it and what discourages it, the psychotherapy enterprise is seen as a process of removing the obstacles to change and implementing elements that expedite its progress. Manuals and treatment procedures should be a secondary priority after change itself.

When trained in the CHANGES model, students can recognize that resistance and difficulty are spontaneously removed by increasing the precursors. A resistant or difficult client, then, is not to be thought of in rigidly stereotypical or diagnostic terms. A person who is difficult to work with may simply be a person who is missing precursors at that time. Because the precursors wax and wane from day to day or week to week, almost everyone is bound to be difficult now and then.

Finally, research seems to indicate that the production and enhancement of client change in psychotherapy lies in four areas: (a) intensifying the client's motivation to change, (b) augmenting involvement in the change process, (c) enhancing the feasibility of change, and (d) removing obstacles to change. If each of these four areas of change is addressed, the rate and magnitude of client change in psychotherapy will likely increase. If the field had a variety of procedures designed to increase each of these areas for clients, the efficiency of therapy might be enhanced, and psychotherapy may become far more reliable in terms of expected outcomes.

Figure 16.1 outlines precursors that play a role in enhancing each of these four areas. Of course, the therapeutic relationship is assumed to be operational in each area. The CHANGES model lends itself to these tasks by pinpointing specific avenues of approach with difficult clients.

POTENTIAL FUTURE APPLICATIONS OF THE CHANGES MODEL

The CHANGES model can support new frameworks for enhancing clinical outcomes by fully centralizing the potency of client-specific change factors. We explore two such prospective frameworks in the following two sections. First, we briefly demonstrate how the CHANGES model might be applied as a client-specific change factor framework in organizational leadership, emphasizing identifying barriers to business and corporate reorganizational change efforts.

Second, and more importantly, we examine how the concept of freedom may serve as a teleological approach to psychotherapy integration. Our proposed

FIGURE 16.1. Increasing the Rate and Magnitude of Change

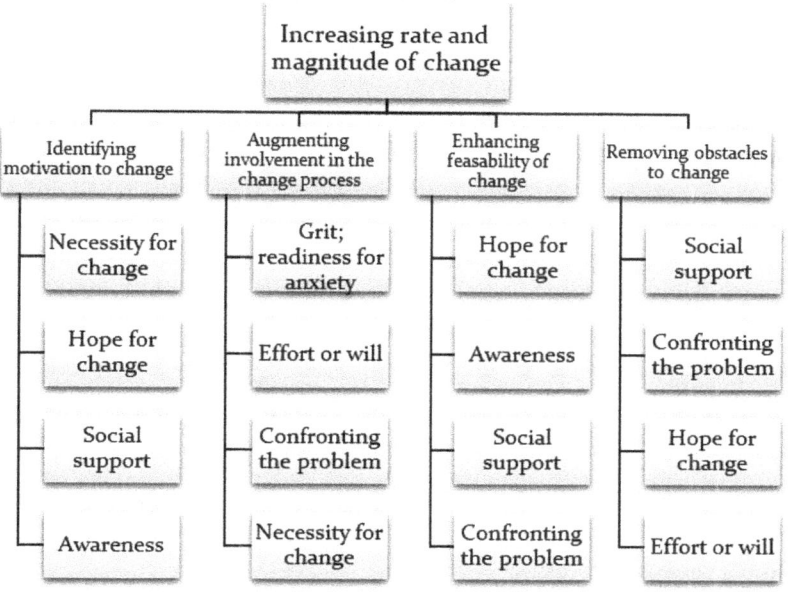

metatheoretical framework suggests that the purpose of psychotherapy is to facilitate psychological freedom, which occurs via activation of the precursors as client-specific factors in the CHANGES model. Such a teleological integration preserves the value of different theories, techniques, and even the common factors but uniquely positions psychotherapy as an integrative endeavor with an overarching purpose. By acknowledging that freedom is the guiding purpose of therapeutic change efforts, we can begin to collectively focus on the pivotal nature of client-specific factors in counseling and psychotherapy.

ASSESSING INDIVIDUAL, TEAM, AND ORGANIZATIONAL CHANGE

Just as the CHANGES model is used to determine the change potential of groups and families, it might also be used for the same with employees, departments, or entire businesses. A particularly rigid, compulsive, or driven executive, for example, may be lacking in certain precursors and thus negatively impact the precursors of employees during a corporate transition. A modified version of the CHANGES assessment form has the potential to help business leaders and employees think in terms of generating, tolerating, and working toward constructive organizational change.

The CHANGES Assessment for Businesses and Corporations (CHANGES-ABC) is a prospective tool for understanding and supporting employees, management teams, and other units during organizational transitions. The proposed assessment form is not yet empirically validated, but it is empirically informed and may serve as a guide for change agents in the business sector to identify the presence or absence of the seven change factors from the

CHANGES model. CHANGES-ABC can identify where a team is in the change process, which deficits may be preventing development along the change process continuum, and whether specified change factors need to be activated in order to better facilitate the leadership or organizational transition.

Scoring the CHANGES-ABC allows assessors to determine the likelihood that change will occur based on individual scores, whether for project coordinators, midlevel managers, or executives. The assessment could be taken at a number of points throughout the change initiative process, letting assessors track the probability of project success based on normed metrics and within-group comparisons across project teams, units, departments, or full organizations. The CHANGES-ABC would support business leaders across various sectors to ensure the efficient facilitation of change initiatives and transitions by

- Assessing a business's overall readiness for change when preparing for a transition of any kind.

- Supporting new team leaders and/or managers who want to understand their teams' readiness for change and to identify gaps that need to be filled in order for the change process to be realized.

- Onboarding executives placed directly in leadership roles who must join with and adapt to a new organizational culture. Research indicates that a significant percentage of business executives derail in the first 18 months due to an inability to join with company culture.

- Training leaders and executives responsible for organizational change, providing a framework for understanding how to increase change-related opportunities and reduce barriers to change.

- Monitoring executives perceived to be in "derailment" who need to make immediate and sustainable positive changes in their role to get on track and maintain their current position.

- Helping leaders determine the probability of success during major business transitions by measuring how responsive employees/teams are to specific change initiatives.

- Being integrated into company culture as part of a 360° feedback assessment. Human resources departments can use it as an educational/training tool on adaptability to change and what is required to facilitate new initiatives. Managers can be trained to understand and grow change readiness—a problem that can be fixed via training—and to support new talent acquisitions.

To support CHANGES-ABC, each of the precursors in the CHANGES model can be updated to capture their applicability to the business sector, as seen in the following expanded definitions:

1. *Confronting the problem:* This is the culmination of awareness but is not the same. This is the steady and deliberate attending to and observing of anything intimidating, painful, or confusing in the change process. It is looking at the

problem dead in the face and continuing to look in spite of the tendency to avoid it. *Expanded definition:* This precursor involves the individual's, team's, or organization's willingness and perceived ability to constructively confront the problem(s) the organization is presently seeking/struggling to overcome through initiating the change process. The ability to constructively confront the problem also involves the willingness of the individual, team, or organization to learn new skill sets that they may not possess but are necessary to learn in order to confront the problem areas and develop a sustainable solution. At the organizational level, this precursor is indicated through one's willingness to accept and offer constructive feedback to or from fellow employees regarding their role in creating and sustaining the problem and/or the change process. This precursor is most closely interrelated to the grit precursor in that the individual, team, or organization must be willing to experience discomfort/anxiety so they can effectively and constructively confront the problem they are facing. Often, fear or anxiety are the underlying psychological mechanisms that prevent obstacles from being overcome and goals achieved.

2. *Hope for change:* This is the realistic expectation that change can and will occur. It is not wishing, longing, desiring, or yearning. Hope sees the possibility of change and motivates a person, knowing that change can be accomplished. *Expanded definition:* When an employee has hope, they can envision a positive outcome and how it can be achieved. This precursor is intimately linked to the effort precursor, as hope, more often than not, precedes will, and effort and is needed to stimulate their development. If one has a low hope score, it is likely that effort will also be low. This is important because motivation has no force in and of itself without a strong and emerging foundation of hope guiding it forward.

3. *Awareness of the problem:* This is knowing that a problem exists and having a good sense of what the problem or issue is. Awareness is the opposite of denial. Without it, a person has no idea where to direct their resources toward change. Awareness has to do with the ability to identify thoughts, feelings, and perceptions that may be obstructing change processes and those needed to embrace it. *Expanded definition:* Awareness can also be defined as the employee, team, or organization understanding of their role in creating, developing, and maintaining the present issue and/or problem that needs to be changed; the role they play in obstructing change processes; and the role they can play in affecting positive change to procure a future solution. Once an awareness precursor score has been determined, the change agent can determine the individual's underlying assumptions and limiting and mistaken beliefs that hinder them from developing the insight necessary to effectively participate in and influence the change process. This precursor helps to measure the level of leadership interference that may be present in the organization.

4. *Necessity for change:* This is the recognized urgency or need that change take place. It considers that change is important and that current conditions are

not satisfactory and must give way to a different set of circumstances. *Expanded definition:* This precursor indicates the employee's, team's, or organization's level of understanding that change is essential for problems to be resolved and a solution developed. It indicates that current dispositional, environmental, and situational conditions are not satisfactory and must give way to a different set of circumstances if the change process is to be initiated and change outcomes are to be achieved.

5. *Grit, or the willingness to experience anxiety/difficulty:* This is the simple surrender to the change process. It is the recognition that one is willing to feel the discomfort that comes with change. Defensiveness is usually defined as an attempt to avoid anxiety. This precursor is the diametric opposite. The person is open to and allows for the presence of any anxiety or difficulty in order to bring about change. The willingness to take risks and be open to experience is also an important aspect of this precursor. *Expanded definition:* This precursor indicates the employee's, team's, or organization's willingness to experience the anxiety, discomfort, uncertainty, and fear that originate from not understanding what to do and how to effectively initiate and/or engage in the transitional process. This precursor involves employee, team, or organizational acceptance of their own limitations and creates a platform for learning new skillsets needed to initiate and participate in the change process. A fundamental part of this is being willing to confront the very things one has been actively avoiding.

6. *Effort toward change:* This is the precursor that indicates action engaged and taken to solve the problem. It is the actual expending of energy as well as movement taken. It also involves the will, in the sense of commitment and a decision to change. Effort takes place in changing the mind, behavior, feelings, or environment. *Expanded definition:* This precursor measures the will to action that is essential to effectively achieve the change being targeted through an initiative. It equally measures the level of anabolic and/or catabolic energy the individual puts forth to resolve the issue. From the score, the change manager can then process with the employee the factors influencing their levels and/or type of energy and how those influential factors are preventing them from overcoming the obstacles to participating in and fulfilling change initiatives. Such obstacles may be motivational factors that can be questioned and addressed once the individual's level of energy and effort has been determined. The level and type of energy indicate the obstacle the client is not willing to confront.

7. *Social support for change:* This consists of confiding, supportive relationships that are dedicated to the well-being of the person. Such relationships make the change process more tolerable and can inspire each of the other precursors. Conversely, relationships not dedicated to the well-being of the person negatively impact a person's ability to change. *Expanded definition:* Supportive relationships in an organization make overall change processes far more tolerable and achievable and can motivate the formation and

development of each of the other precursors. Without high scores in social support, all other precursors can be extremely difficult to inspire or motivate. This precursor has a secondary gain in that it helps to identify relational problem areas in departments, teams, and between individuals within the organization. Conversely, professional relationships that are not dedicated to the well-being and future growth of employees, teams, or the organization as a whole negatively impact change initiatives. Once the score of this precursor has been determined, change agents can explore the depth of the problem and how to establish and/or reestablish relationships that have been damaged or severed between departments or among employees. The purpose of this is to affect substantive change for team building processes and motivate team members and departments to work more constructively toward the realization of an initiative.

FROM MODEL TO METATHEORETICAL FRAMEWORK: THE FREEDOM PARADIGM

The driving ideological force behind the psychotherapy integration movement has been the pursuit of consensus, without which we are ostensibly left stranded within the much-frowned-upon realm of preparadigmatic scientific status. The CHANGES model finds its footing in the ground between the common factors model and longstanding calls from integrative researchers (see Goldfried, 1980, 2019) to closely examine principles of change that arise "at an intermediate level of abstraction between theoretical frameworks … and specific techniques or clinical procedures" (Gaines & Goldfried, 2021, p. 268). Based on such relative positioning of the CHANGES model, there is the possibility that it can support conceptual extrapolations into metatheoretical territory.

We believe that all effective psychotherapists have a distinct capacity for phenomenological engagement; that is to say, being predisposed to examine the structures of consciousness both as a general form of experiential-psychological inquiry (i.e., psychological mindedness) and an ability to attune to the inner universe of others by means of deep relational contact (i.e., presence). When such therapists engage clients in a second-order change process, they are not just trying to reduce symptoms. There is a deeper, more meaningful transformation taking place to which the savvy therapist is distinctly attuned. This transformative process transcends the language of particular theories and thus may only be conceptualized in terms of a metatheory or paradigm.

The metatheoretical framework we propose as an extension of the CHANGES model is rooted in the concept of freedom. Simply put, the purpose of nearly all psychotherapy endeavors, at some level and to some degree, is to set people free (Hanna, 2011). This deceivingly simple statement, hidden in plain sight, reflects what might be considered the preeminent goal of therapy for individuals, families, groups, and communities. We propose that coordinating therapeutic practices under the metatheoretical framework of freedom provides a common teleology, or purpose, to the act of therapeutic engagement that fosters a client-specific change emphasis (Hanna & Black, 2007).

Controversy and suspicion have long surrounded the notion of freedom, particularly among traditional behavioral scientists inclined to doubt its existence. Whereas James (1981/1890) held the subject of freedom in high regard, Skinner (1971) regarded it as an illusion (see Korn et al., 1991). The free will–determinism debate continues today, as seen between various philosophical heavyweights such as Daniel Dennett and Robert Sapolosky (D. Miller, 2024). Clarifying the concept of freedom in its present use is thus necessary to skirt controversy.

To begin, freedom as discussed herein is not the same as free will, which is a metaphysical perspective on freedom that denotes that the human condition is one of rational, freely chosen actions, behaviors, and decisions. Freedom in its use here does not relate to free will. The debate between determinism and free will cannot be empirically validated because it is an antinomy (see Kant, 1787/1929), and the freedom paradigm is not designed to address, much less resolve, that philosophical dispute.

Furthermore, freedom in its present use is related to political freedom only indirectly and should not be considered in a political or liberty-related context. Within our purview, freedom is considered through a psychological rather than a physical lens. As such, the 27-year imprisonment of Nelson Mandela by the South African Apartheid government signifies the difference between political freedom or liberty and psychological freedom. Reflecting on his experience, Mandela (1995) said, "I learned that courage was not the absence of fear, but the triumph over it. The brave man is not he who does not feel afraid, but he who conquers that fear" (p. 622). A similar perspective is expressed by Frankl (1992), who wrote, "Everything can be taken from a man but one thing: the last of the human freedoms—to choose one's attitude in any given set of circumstances" (p. 86). Such statements appropriately convey the disparity between physical and psychological freedom.

With these parameters in mind, freedom may be defined in terms of a psychological state absent those psychological restrictions and inhibitions that result in symptoms of depression, anxiety, compulsions, obsessive thoughts, or emotional pain. This definition of freedom includes the active capacity to ameliorate or alter undesired thoughts, emotions, and behaviors so as to enhance positive conditions and increase the range of available options for consideration. This also corresponds with a mastery of or the ability to navigate conflictual conditions by acquiring whatever skills necessary to handle mental, interpersonal, systemic, or societal challenges. Responsibility is another key component of such freedom (Sartre, 1943/2003) insofar as the individual is willing to proactively manage, influence, or otherwise respond to such conditions without succumbing to a sense of burden, duty, or blame. In this manner, empathy, understanding, and tolerance supersede forms of prejudice, bias, and obliviousness when the individual chooses responsibility and freedom.

Maintaining a permanent state of freedom is clearly not possible. However, it is assumed that greater degrees of freedom can be attained through intentional and constructive change processes. Influenced by myriad internal/psychological and external/environmental factors, freedom involves a capacity to alter or amend our response to influences. As such, the metatheoretical freedom framework highlights the importance of understanding the process of becoming free such that one may adaptively respond to a variety of influences with empathy, compassion, and common sense.

This conception of freedom is closely related to previous discussions in this book on active agency, although it represents a more fluid take on the concept. In many ways, the metatheoretical freedom framework is more closely akin to liberation as conceptualized in certain ancient Indian philosophies (Pereira, 1976), particularly regarding the attainment of *mukti* or *moksha* as rendered in Sanskrit. The ancient Yoga concept of *kaivalya* is also similar (Aranya, 1983; Srinivasan, 2021), by which freedom is an attainable state of being. The foundational concept of *nirvana* in Buddhism also relates to freedom as an attained state corresponding to the cessation of suffering (Rahula, 1978).

The similarity between these ancient philosophical paradigms and the proposed metatheoretical freedom framework rests in the shared idea that freedom can be attained only by degrees, is never complete, and is neither intrinsic to human action nor divinely given. To be absolutely clear, we are not recommending *moksha*, *kaivalya*, or *nirvana* as a psychotherapeutic goal or practice. It cannot be disputed, however, that ideas originating from such Asian philosophies have begun to deeply influence psychotherapy research and practice in the Western world (see Moodley et al., 2017). Mindfulness and meditation practices taken from the ancient Buddhist and Hindu traditions have been adopted and adapted, rapidly becoming a central tenet in many psychotherapy practices.

All this aside, the idea is that clients benefit when therapists trade a restrictive mindset imposed by singular theories for a metatheoretical framework that emphasizes the value of increasing a client's degree of freedom. Such teleological integration signifies an attempt to align classical psychotherapy theories and subspecialties under a common conceptual heading that may result in greater cohesion, collaboration, and innovation across helping professions. In an effort to support and unify the field, the teleological approach aims to enhance distinct subspecialty areas through the integration process rather than attenuate them. Freedom-based teleological integration purposefully aligns theories and subspecialties so that they may retain their tradition, authority, and power (Hanna & Black, 2007).

Defining Four Modes of Freedoms

According to Weiss (1958), we can conceptualize freedom via four different modes: freedom-from, freedom-to, freedom-with, and freedom-for. These modes are interdependent and interactive, and they align with majortheories and practices in psychotherapy. For each freedom mode, corresponding knowledge and practices must be applied to increase them in accordance with the other modes.

Freedom-From

This mode of freedom relates to the alleviation of symptoms such as depression, anxiety, obsessions, compulsions, and emotional pain, including freedom from addictions. *Freedom-from* is a psychological state absent those psychological restrictions and inhibitions resulting in symptomatology. Freedom-from relates to internally oppressive conditions seen in psychotherapy, such as negative self-talk, distorted beliefs, disturbing images, and otherwise harmful, violent, and self-defeating impulses and behaviors. It also refers to a reprieve or escape from oppressive external conditions that may include abuse, bullying, racism, sexism, and homophobia. Metacognitive skills are a key component of freedom-from insofar as the process of increasing freedom necessitates an ability to disidentify with issues, choose how to conceptualize particular problems or psychological phenomena, and cultivate an understanding of both one's awareness and the limits of that awareness.

Freedom-To

This mode of freedom involves personal growth and development toward self-determined goals that enhance well-being and self-efficacy. *Freedom-to* includes the active capacity to ameliorate undesired thoughts, emotions, and behaviors so as to enhance adaptiveness, improve decision-making and self-regulation, and expand behavioral options. It thus includes the ability to actively change aspects of psychological experience, such as fluidly replacing maladaptive beliefs or directly altering, controlling, or dissolving mental phenomena such as memories, images, thoughts, and emotions (see Puhakka & Hanna, 1988). Freedom-to also suggests an enhanced ability to navigate conflictual conditions by acquiring the skills to handle mental, interpersonal, systemic, or societal challenges. Perspicacity and wisdom are relevant considerations here such that adaptability in any given situation reflects a heightened capacity to perceive reasonable courses of action from a broad range of possibilities. Furthermore, freedom-to involves a sense of autonomy and personal responsibility whereby thoughts and behaviors remain independent from internal and external pressures that can result in abandoning one's integrity or rationality.

Freedom-With

This mode of freedom involves respecting the agency of others and recognizing the interpersonal or systemic nature of the human condition (Hanna et al., 1999). *Freedom-with* highlights both that personal development is inextricably linked to social relationships and denials of others' freedom diminishes our own freedom in kind (Sartre, 1943/2003). Individuals typically do not live in isolation but rather in a complex web of social relationships that thrive when imbued with empathy, compassion, tolerance, and a desire for the freedom of others. The bifurcation of competitive societies and the accompanying issues of privilege, status, and exclusivity result from a lack of freedom-with. Enhancing receptivity and respect toward others makes communicating differences in opinion or perspective possible without harboring ill will. At the same time, freedom-with demands a capacity to maintain boundaries such that the individual self-protects against verbal, emotional, or physical harm. Balancing autonomy and interdependence is, at its foundation, an attempt to establish freedom-with while sustaining one's freedom-to.

Freedom-For

This mode of freedom involves proactively responding to, assessing, managing, or otherwise influencing sociocultural conditions without succumbing to a sense of burden, duty, or blame. *Freedom-for* is the grounds for advocacy, a central goal in the fields of psychotherapy and counseling that both includes and transcends the provision of services that lead to the other three freedoms. Those who are actively denied freedom due to oppressive conditions or circumstances need liberation, as is so often seen among clients (Hanna et al., 2000; Ivey, 1995). As such, the therapists actively seek to combat social oppressions such as sexism, racism, and homophobia by supporting the development of freedom-with. However, it is not restricted to therapists or other health and human service providers. Insofar as clients can serve as advocates for others, freedom-for can be an active client goal in psychotherapy. Positively transforming the world necessitates all people providing freedom for others. By seeking freedom-for, counseling and psychotherapy become instruments of transformation across interpersonal, institutional, and systemic levels.

Freedom as a Teleological Approach to Integration

According to teleological integration, *freedom* is a state that includes the absence of restrictive or inhibitive psychological symptoms, the ability to enhance positive psychological conditions, the experience of respect for the agency of others, and the sense of responsibility for supporting or otherwise enhancing the agency of others. Such a broad conception of freedom is notably related to the concept of human agency outlined in social-cognitive theory, insofar as "freedom is conceived not just passively as the absence of constraints, but also proactively as the exercise of self-influence in the service of selected goals and desired outcomes" (Bandura, 2006, p. 165). Furthermore, freedom is not an isolated activity, as "in thus willing freedom, we discover that it depends entirely upon the freedom of others and that the freedom of others depends upon our own" (Sartre, 1943/2003, p. 48). Freedom is an expression of agency at both personal and communal levels (Bandura, 2006).

Rather than alter, combine, or otherwise integrate psychotherapy theories and practices, the proposed approach is meant to focus and coordinate them within the framework of freedom as a common teleology, or purpose (Hanna & Black, 2007). The traditionally espoused purpose of theory has been to provide a framework for conceptualization, a coherent explanation for presenting concerns, and a general guide for clinical interventions (Fall et al., 2017). A freedom-based teleological approach to integration supports each of these goals, whereas selectivity is paramount across the four standard approaches to integration. Technical eclecticism focuses on techniques, common factors identifies nonspecific change principles, assimilative integration selects a single theoretical basis, and theoretical integration seeks a unified theory (Zvi-Beiman & Shahar, 2015).

The teleological approach serves as a lens through which to view theories as unique approaches to enabling client freedom. Such a perspective circumvents the competitive nature of divergent theoretical perspectives and replaces it with the remedial view that each theory or approach provides insight into different facets of lived experience. The purposes of the four freedoms align with four major models in counseling and psychotherapy: the medical model, the wellness model, the systems model, and social justice and advocacy models (see Table 16.1). This conceptual alignment indicates that each model lends a unique perspective to the therapeutic process as it relates to freedom. If the purpose of counseling is freedom, then all theories, subspecialties, and therapeutic change factors serve a role for clients in attaining freedom. The proposed teleological approach to integration suggests that each model centralizes and restores a particular form of freedom.

Freedom-From: Symptoms, as a Medical Model Perspective

The medical model arises from "a scientific process involving observation, description and differentiation which moves from recognizing and treating symptoms to identifying disease etiologies and developing specific treatments" (Shah & Mountain, 2007, p. 375). From the perspective of the medical model, psychotherapy denotes a process of alleviating symptoms of psychological distress, which, in turn, may enhance mental health. Teleological integration in freedom-from aligns with efforts to reduce maladaptive symptomatology, highlighting an inverse relationship between negative symptoms and client freedom. In effect, the medical model approach to psychotherapy aims to promote freedom-from symptoms within a disease-oriented framework of mental health.

Freedom-To: Grow, as a Wellness Perspective

The wellness model emphasizes holistic and strength-based mental health along with practices that increase "a positive state of well-being, through developmental, preventive, and wellness-enhancing interventions" (Myers & Sweeney,

TABLE 16.1. Johari's Window of the Four Freedoms

	Being stance	Becoming stance
Individual lens	Freedom-from: symptoms *Medical model*	Freedom-to: grow *Wellness model*
Relational lens	Freedom-with: relationships *Systems model*	Freedom-for: engagement *Social justice/advocacy model*

2008, p. 482). The wellness model prioritizes developmental, humanistic, and other growth-oriented perspectives on mental health. Teleological integration in freedom-toward aligns with efforts to grow adaptive psychological functioning, asserting that client freedom is enhanced when capacities for personal growth are promoted and enhanced. In effect, the wellness model approach to psychotherapy promotes freedom-toward growth by encouraging personal development within a holistic-oriented framework of mental health.

Freedom-With: Relationships, as a Systems Perspective

The systems model emphasizes the influence of interpersonal relationships within and across interconnected social structures (McDowell et al., 2022). The systems model examines relationships through the lens of nonlinear dynamics, with an eye toward disentangling how various intersecting points of complex interaction influence individual development and system functioning. Teleological integration in freedom-with aligns with efforts to support effective interpersonal dynamics, maintaining that client freedom is enhanced by forming meaningful, congruent, and authentic relationships with others. In effect, the systems model approach to psychotherapy promotes freedom-with by improving the quality of interpersonal relationships within and across various ecological systems.

Freedom-For: Engagement, as a Social Justice/Advocacy Perspective

Social justice advocacy has been defined as "intentional and sustained action intended to influence public policy outcomes, with and/or on behalf of a vulnerable individual, group, community, or the public at large" (Marshall-Lee et al., 2020, p. 12). Taken together, social justice and advocacy models in psychotherapy encourage political, economic, and sociocultural engagement as a professional practice to address metasystemic issues of oppression, discrimination, and inequality. Teleological integration in freedom-for upholds the idea that denying others freedom diminishes our own freedom in kind, such that no one can truly be free until everyone is free. In effect, social justice and advocacy models promote freedom-for by motivating psychotherapists to acknowledge and confront oppressive sociocultural forces that impede mental health and wellness.

Teleological Freedom and the CHANGES Model

The CHANGES model identifies the necessary preconditions for any effective implementation of theory-based therapeutic interventions. As such, precursors are the conditions upon which freedom manifests, particularly in relation to freedom-from and freedom-to. Freedom-with is incorporated into the CHANGES model vis-à-vis the development of client empathy through the awareness and social support precursors. The metatheoretical freedom framework suggests that change precursors are the necessary prerequisites of freedom. By means of activating and maintaining precursors, the path is cleared to enable the exploration of the individual's four freedoms. In sum, we maintain that the CHANGES model is the fundamental catalyst of an individual's freedom. Therapeutic change involves distinctive processes, stages, and precursors which have the capacity to set people free.

FINAL THOUGHTS

As coined by the sociologist Merton (1968), the Matthew effect serves as a foundational principle of inequality in Western capitalist societies, aligning with the old saying that the rich get richer and the poor get poorer. The underlying notion of accumulated advantage indicates that inequality grows over time because those who start with sufficient resources garner compounded resource advantages over time, whereas those who start without resources remain at a perpetual disadvantage (Rigney, 2010). It could be easily argued that such advantages derive not only from wealth, power, prestige, and social status but also from knowledge or education.

As such, a similar phenomenon can be seen in the realm of psychotherapy: Clients who are already in a good state of mental health seem to make the greatest gains in psychotherapy. Alternatively, clients who need change the most tend to be the ones who are least capable of achieving it. So, what are the assets of the rich who get richer in therapy? It may well be that the precursors of change are the mental and emotional equivalent of wealth and resources needed to achieve and maintain mental health. Even a cursory analysis indicates that a person with an ample supply of mental health and wellness would also have an abundance of active precursors. If the rich really do get richer, time invested in establishing precursors among people who find change difficult may pay healthy dividends in terms of the relative degree of productivity per psychotherapy session.

Of course, this line of thought begets still larger questions: Will psychotherapy ever advance to the stage in which every single client, regardless of background or presenting concern, can achieve productive and lasting therapeutic change? What will it take to level the playing field, so to speak, and thereby produce a reliable and reproducible science of psychotherapeutic change? Do we have a professional responsibility to strive for such outcome effectiveness? Is it even possible to establish an efficacious science of change through the efforts of psychotherapy researchers and practitioners alone, or will it require coordinated efforts across multiple fields of study? Is it even ethical to propose such a possibility within our neoliberal, capitalist, sociocultural milieu as we struggle to reconcile mental health with historical economic advantages and social justice?

There are no easy answers to such questions, and we make no claim to the contrary. However, we do wish to acknowledge the value of shifting contemporary dialogues on mental health away from an emphasis on categorical and diagnostic features toward an emphasis on experiential features that may provide greater insight into therapeutic change mechanisms. In other words, we might do well to prioritize the phenomenology of lived experience over and above any intellectual fetish for conceptual abstraction. We are not suggesting that concepts are inherently problematic but rather that a preoccupation with abstract ideas can impede our ability to identify change processes as they unfold, in real time, with clients facing difficult problems while embedded in dynamic situations.

What moves the cynical, callous client from selfishness to relationality, from a sense of disdain to a sense of respect for others? What shifts the hopelessly depressed client from reactivity to proactivity, from a sense of helplessness to a sense of control? What nudges the defiant, mandated client from blaming and withdrawal to responsibility and engagement? There are subtle decision processes involved in replacing closed-mindedness with empathic openness, moving from a reactive to a proactive stance, and replacing blame with responsibility, or disengagement with engagement.

We know far too little about these subtleties. Our knowledge of change processes demarcated by the seven precursors is still remarkably incomplete. An activated precursor denotes a dynamic, contextually embedded psychological act. We may see the dawning of awareness, the shift into a sense of necessity, the onset of grit, or the leaning-into of social supports, but we are limited to observing these psychological acts via behavioral concomitants. What are these psychological acts, and how can they be better addressed in clients to enhance the likelihood of change?

All seven precursors would benefit from rigorous qualitative studies that are thoughtfully informed by advancements in various other academic areas, including the cognitive sciences and philosophy of mind. As noted in the introduction, change process research will also be key to unlocking these mysteries. Studies using neurophenomenology along with functional magnetic resonance imaging may lend insight into the therapeutic change transition as both an experiential and a neurobiological phenomenon. Conceptually driven research informed by works in philosophy of mind may support the phenomenological examination of how meaning is altered at the ontological level. In kind, microphenomenology reports might be conducted into the precise experiential concomitants of, for instance, the therapeutic activation of a sense of necessity for change. Newer methodologies of psychotherapy process analysis (Kiesler, 2017) could help us understand how unique therapist–client communication patterns contribute to the activation of specific precursors.

If the discipline of psychotherapy is to advance to the point of quickly and reliably producing lasting therapeutic change for clients, we must closely examine what it takes to activate each of the precursors. Again, the precursors are not our invention. They have been a part of the mythos of human knowledge and wisdom across the ages. They themselves are indeed broad categories that likely involve an extraordinarily complex array of neurocognitive subprocesses. Yet we are not calling for a complete understanding of the neurobiology of conscious awareness, which is perhaps an insurmountable task, although surely worth the effort (Chalmers, 2020; Gallagher & Zahavi, 2020).

Instead, we are calling for advanced research at the nexus of, for instance, insight, awareness, and change. There is perhaps as much, if not more, to glean from phenomenological investigations into these complex psychological acts than can be found via neuroscientific inquiries. The CHANGES model highlights seven well-established yet subtle change mechanisms that are extraordinarily pervasive and thus taken for granted, often to the point of disappearing from both the conceptual and practical view of therapists. Understanding the nature of within-individual precursors as well as pathways to their activation in the therapeutic encounter should be a top research priority.

REFERENCES

Aafjes-van Doorn, K., Békés, V., Prout, T. A., & Hoffman, L. (2020). Psychotherapists' vicarious traumatization during the COVID-19 pandemic. *Psychological Trauma: Theory, Research, Practice, and Policy, 12*(S1), S148–S150. https://doi.org/10.1037/tra0000868

Acton, L. (1887). *Letter to bishop Mandell Creighton: Historical essays and studies.* Macmillan.

Adler, A. (1927). *Understanding human nature* (W. B. Wolf, Trans.). Greenburg.

Adler, A. (1956). *The individual psychology of Alfred Adler: A systematic presentation in selections from his writings* (H. L. Ansbacher & R. R. Ansbacher, Eds.). Harper & Row.

Adler, A. (1979). *Superiority and social interest* (H. L. Ansbacher & R. R. Ansbacher, Eds.). W. W. Norton.

Adler, G. (1992). Psychotherapy of the narcissistic personality disorder patient: Two contrasting approaches. In N. G. Hamilton (Ed.), *From inner sources: New directions in object relations psychotherapy* (pp. 195–212). Jason Aronson.

Afonseca, M., Sousa, D., Vaz, A., Santos, J. M., & Batista, A. (2023). Psychotherapist's persuasiveness in anxiety: Scale development and relation to the working alliance. *Journal of Psychotherapy Integration, 33*(2), 169–184. https://doi.org/10.1037/int0000288

Ainslie, G. (2021). Willpower with and without effort. *Behavioral and Brain Sciences, 44*, Article e30. https://doi.org/10.1017/s0140525x20000357

Alcoholics Anonymous. (2012). *Alcoholics anonymous—Big book* (4th ed.). AA World Services.

Al-Yagon, M., & Margalit, M. (2017). Hope and coping in individuals with specific learning disorders. In M. W. Gallagher & S. J. Lopez (Eds.), *The Oxford handbook of hope* (pp. 1–21). Oxford University Press.

American Psychiatric Association. (2013). *Diagnostic and statistical manual of mental disorders* (5th ed.). https://doi.org/10.1176/appi.books.9780890425596

American Psychiatric Association. (2022). *Diagnostic and statistical manual of mental disorders* (5th ed., text rev.).

Anderson, T., Finkelstein, J. D., & Horvath, S. A. (2020). The facilitative interpersonal skills method: Difficult psychotherapy moments and appropriate therapist responsiveness. *Counselling & Psychotherapy Research, 20*(3), 463–469. https://doi.org/10.1002/capr.12302

Anderson, T., McClintock, A. S., Himawan, L., Song, X., & Patterson, C. L. (2016). A prospective study of therapist facilitative interpersonal skills as a predictor of treatment outcome. *Journal of Consulting and Clinical Psychology, 84*(1), 57–66. https://doi.org/10.1037/ccp0000060

Arango-Muñoz, S. (2019). Cognitive phenomenology and metacognitive feelings. *Mind & Language, 34*(2), 247–262. https://doi.org/10.1111/mila.12215

Aranya, H. (1983). *Yoga philosophy of Patanjali.* State University of New York Press.

Archer, A., & Mills, G. (2019). Anger, affective injustice, and emotion regulation. *Philosophical Topics, 47*(2), 75–94. https://doi.org/10.5840/philtopics201947216

Ardelt, M., & Ferrari, M. (2014). Wisdom and emotions. In P. Verhaeghen & C. Hertzog (Eds.), *The Oxford handbook of emotion, social cognition, and problem solving in adulthood* (pp. 256–272). Oxford University Press.

Arenson, M., Bernat, E., De Los Reyes, A., Neylan, T. C., & Cohen, B. E. (2021). Social support, social network size, and suicidal ideation: A nine-year longitudinal analysis from the Mind Your Heart Study. *Journal of Psychiatric Research, 135,* 318–324. https://doi.org/10.1016/j.jpsychires.2021.01.017

Arkowitz, H. (1989). From behavior change to insight. *Journal of Eclectic and Integrative Psychotherapy, 8*(3), 222–232.

Arslan, G. (2019). Mediating role of the self-esteem and resilience in the association between social exclusion and life satisfaction among adolescents. *Personality and Individual Differences, 151,* Article 109514. https://doi.org/10.1016/j.paid.2019.109514

Assagioli, R. (1965). *Psychosynthesis: A manual of principles and techniques.* Penguin.

Assagioli, R. (1973). *The act of will.* Penguin.

Aubuchon-Endsley, N. L., Callahan, J. L., González, D. A., Ruggero, C. J., & Abramson, C. I. (2015). The impact of hope in mediating psychotherapy expectations and outcomes: A study of Brazilian clients. *International Journal of Integrative Psychotherapy, 6,* 63–80.

Avdi, E., & Georgaca, E. (2007). Discourse analysis and psychotherapy: A critical review. *European Journal of Psychotherapy and Counselling, 9*(2), 157–176. https://doi.org/10.1080/13642530701363445

Avdi, E., Lerou, V., & Seikkula, J. (2015). Dialogical features, therapist responsiveness, and agency in a therapy for psychosis. *Journal of Constructivist Psychology, 28*(4), 329–341. https://doi.org/10.1080/10720537.2014.994692

Axsom, D. (1989). Cognitive dissonance and behavior change in psychotherapy. *Journal of Experimental Social Psychology, 25*(3), 234–252. https://doi.org/10.1016/0022-1031(89)90021-8

Bager-Charleson, S. (2010). *Reflective practice in counselling and psychotherapy.* Sage Publications.

Bandura, A. (1977). Self-efficacy: Toward a unifying theory of behavioral change. *Psychological Review, 84*(2), 191–215. https://doi.org/10.1037/0033-295X.84.2.191

Bandura, A. (2006). Toward a psychology of human agency. *Perspectives on Psychological Science, 1*(2), 164–180. https://doi.org/10.1111/j.1745-6916.2006.00011.x

Barker, P. (2013). Reframing: The essence of psychotherapy? In J. K. Zeig (Ed.), *Ericksonian methods: The essence of the story* (pp. 211–233). Routledge.

Barlas, Z., Hockley, W. E., & Obhi, S. S. (2017). The effects of freedom of choice in action selection on perceived mental effort and the sense of agency. *Acta Psychologica, 180*, 122–129. https://doi.org/10.1016/j.actpsy.2017.09.004

Barlas, Z., & Obhi, S. S. (2013). Freedom, choice, and the sense of agency. *Frontiers in Human Neuroscience, 7*, Article 514. https://doi.org/10.3389/fnhum.2013.00514

Bartholomew, T. T., Gundel, B. E., Scheel, M. J., Kang, E., Joy, E. E., & Li, H. (2020). Development and initial validation of the Therapist Hope for Clients Scale. *The Counseling Psychologist, 48*(2), 191–222. https://doi.org/10.1177/0011000019886428

Bartlett, R. C. (2019). *Aristotle's art of rhetoric.* University of Chicago Press.

Bateson, G. (1979). *Mind and nature.* Bantam Books.

Bateson, G., & Bateson, C. G. (1987). *Angels fear: Toward an epistemology of the sacred.* Bantam Books.

Bayne, T. (2008). The phenomenology of agency. *Philosophy Compass, 3*(1), 182–202. https://doi.org/10.1111/j.1747-9991.2007.00122.x

Beck, A. T. (1976). *Cognitive therapy and the emotional disorders.* New American Library.

Beck, A. T., Rush, A. J., Shaw, B. F., & Emery, G. (1979). *Cognitive therapy of depression.* Guilford Press.

Beck, A. T., Steer, R. A., Kovacs, M., & Garrison, B. (1985). Hopelessness and eventual suicide: A 10-year prospective study of patients hospitalized with suicidal ideation. *The American Journal of Psychiatry, 142*(5), 559–563. https://doi.org/10.1176/ajp.142.5.559

Beck, A. T., Weissman, A., Lester, D., & Trexler, L. (1974). The measurement of pessimism: The Hopelessness Scale. *Journal of Consulting and Clinical Psychology, 42*(6), 861–865. https://doi.org/10.1037/h0037562

Beck, C. J. (1989). *Everyday Zen: Love and work.* Harper Collins.

Bellaert, L., Van Steenberghe, T., De Maeyer, J., Vander Laenen, F., & Vanderplasschen, W. (2022). Turning points toward drug addiction recovery: Contextualizing underlying dynamics of change. *Addiction Research and Theory, 30*(4), 294–303. https://doi.org/10.1080/16066359.2022.2026934

Bendig, E., Erb, B., Schulze-Thuesing, L., & Baumeister, H. (2022). The next generation: Chatbots in clinical psychology and psychotherapy to foster mental health—A scoping review. *Verhaltenstherapie, 32*(Suppl. 1), 64–76. https://doi.org/10.1159/000501812

Benn, P. (2021). Freedom, resentment and the psychopath. In C. Heginbotham (Ed.), *Philosophy, psychiatry and psychopathy* (pp. 29–46). Routledge.

Bennett-Leighton, L. (2018). The trauma of oppression: A somatic perspective. In C. Caldwell & L. Bennett-Leighton (Eds.), *Oppression and the body: Roots, resistance, and resolutions* (pp. 17–30). North Atlantic Books.

Bernstein, A., Hadash, Y., Lichtash, Y., Tanay, G., Shepherd, K., & Fresco, D. M. (2015). Decentering and related constructs: A critical review and metacognitive processes model. *Perspectives on Psychological Science, 10*(5), 599–617. https://doi.org/10.1177/1745691615594577

Bettelheim, B. (1960). *The informed heart.* Free Press.

Beutler, L. E. (2000). David and Goliath: When empirical and clinical standards of practice meet. *American Psychologist, 55*(9), 997–1007. https://doi.org/10.1037/0003-066X.55.9.997

Beutler, L. E., & Forrester, B. (2014). What needs to change: Moving from "research informed" practice to "empirically effective" practice. *Journal of Psychotherapy Integration, 24*(3), 168–177. https://doi.org/10.1037/a0037587

Birditt, K. S., Polenick, C. A., Luong, G., Charles, S. T., & Fingerman, K. L. (2020). Daily interpersonal tensions and well-being among older adults: The role of emotion regulation strategies. *Psychology and Aging, 35*(4), 578–590. https://doi.org/10.1037/pag0000416

Blais, R. K., Tirone, V., Orlowska, D., Lofgreen, A., Klassen, B., Held, P., Stevens, N., & Zalta, A. K. (2021). Self-reported PTSD symptoms and social support in U.S. military service members and veterans: A meta-analysis. *European Journal of Psychotraumatology, 12*(1), Article 1851078. https://doi.org/10.1080/20008198.2020.1851078

Bohart, A. C. (2000). The client is the most important common factor: Clients' self-healing capacities and psychotherapy. *Journal of Psychotherapy Integration, 10*(2), 127–149. https://doi.org/10.1023/A:1009444132104

Bohart, A. C., & Tallman, K. (1999). *How clients make therapy work: The process of active self-healing.* American Psychological Association.

Bonino, J. L., & Hanna, F. J. (2018). Who owns psychopathology? The *DSM*: Its flaws, its future, and the professional counselor. *The Journal of Humanistic Counseling, 57*(3), 118–137. https://doi.org/10.1002/johc.12071

BonJour, L. (2009). *Epistemology: Classic problems and contemporary responses.* Rowman & Littlefield.

Botha, M., & Frost, D. M. (2020). Extending the minority stress model to understand mental health problems experienced by the autistic population. *Society and Mental Health, 10*(1), 20–34. https://doi.org/10.1177/2156869318804297

Bowen, M. (1976). Theory in the practice of psychotherapy. In P. J. Guerin, Jr. (Ed.), *Family therapy: Theory and practice* (pp. 42–90). Gardner Press.

Boykin, A. W., Dixon, D., Mitchell, D. S. B., Bruce, A. W., Akinola, Y. O., & Holt, N. P. (2016). The intersection of racial and cultural identity for African Americans: Expanding the scope of black self-understanding. In J. M. Sullivan & W. E. Cross, Jr. (Eds.), *Meaning-making, internalized racism, and African American identity* (pp. 159–174). State University of New York Press.

Brodley, B. T. (2002). Client-centered: An expressive therapy. *The Person-Centered Journal, 9*(1), 59–70.

Brooks, H. L., Rushton, K., Lovell, K., Bee, P., Walker, L., Grant, L., & Rogers, A. (2018). The power of support from companion animals for people living with mental health problems: A systematic review and narrative synthesis of the evidence. *BMC Psychiatry, 18*(1), Article 31. https://doi.org/10.1186/s12888-018-1613-2

Brown, D. (1970). *Bury my heart at wounded knee.* Bantam Books.

Brown, L. A., Zandberg, L. J., & Foa, E. B. (2019). Mechanisms of change in prolonged exposure therapy for PTSD: Implications for clinical practice. *Journal of Psychotherapy Integration, 29*(1), 6–14. https://doi.org/10.1037/int0000109

Brown, L. S. (2017). Contributions of feminist and critical psychologies to trauma psychology. In S. N. Gold (Ed.), *APA handbook of trauma psychology: Foundations in knowledge* (pp. 501–526). American Psychological Association. https://doi.org/10.1037/0000019-025

Brown, L. S. (2018). *Feminist therapy* (2nd ed.). American Psychological Association. https://doi.org/10.1037/0000092-000

Browning, S., & Hull, R. (2021). Reframing paradox. *Professional Psychology: Research and Practice, 52*(4), 360–367. https://doi.org/10.1037/pro0000384

Buechner, B. D. (2023). Empathy versus tyranny: Witnessing moral conflict through Adlerian lenses. *Journal of Individual Psychology, 79*(4), 425–442. https://doi.org/10.1353/jip.2023.a915977

Cannon, W. B. (1942). "Voodoo" death. *American Anthropologist, 44*(2), 169–181. https://doi.org/10.1525/aa.1942.44.2.02a00010

Carcione, A., Riccardi, I., Bilotta, E., Leone, L., Pedone, R., Conti, L., Colle, L., Fiore, D., Nicolò, G., Pellecchia, G., Procacci, M., & Semerari, A. (2019). Metacognition as a predictor of improvements in personality disorders. *Frontiers in Psychology, 10,* Article 170. https://doi.org/10.3389/fpsyg.2019.00170

Castonguay, L. G., & Hill, C. E. (Eds.). (2017). *How and why are some therapists better than others? Understanding therapist effects.* American Psychological Association. https://doi.org/10.1037/0000034-000

Cautela, J. R. (1996). Training the client to be empathetic. In J. R. Cautela & W. Ishaq (Eds.), *Contemporary issues in behavior therapy* (pp. 337–353). Plenum.

Chalmers, D. J. (2020). How can we solve the meta-problem of consciousness? *Journal of Consciousness Studies, 27*(5–6), 201–226.

Chemero, A. (2013). Radical embodied cognitive science. *Review of General Psychology, 17*(2), 145–150. https://doi.org/10.1037/a0032923

Christensen, A., & Jacobson, N. S. (1994). Who (or what) can do psychotherapy: The status and challenge of nonprofessional therapies. *Psychological Science, 5*(1), 8–14. https://doi.org/10.1111/j.1467-9280.1994.tb00606.x

Chu, C., Walker, K. L., Stanley, I. H., Hirsch, J. K., Greenberg, J. H., Rudd, M. D., & Joiner, T. E. (2018). Perceived problem-solving deficits and suicidal ideation: Evidence for the explanatory roles of thwarted belongingness and perceived burdensomeness in five samples. *Journal of Personality and Social Psychology, 115*(1), 137–160. https://doi.org/10.1037/pspp0000152

Clark, A. J. (2023). *Empathy and mental health: An integral model for developing therapeutic skills in counseling and psychotherapy.* Routledge.

Cleeremans, A. (2019). The mind is deep. In A. Cleeremans, V. Allakhverdov, & M. Kuvaldina (Eds.), *Implicit learning: 50 years on* (pp. 38–70). Routledge.

Cochran, J. L., & Cochran, N. H. (2015). *The heart of counseling: Counseling skills through therapeutic relationships.* Routledge.

Coffey, K. A., Hartman, M., & Fredrickson, B. L. (2010). Deconstructing mindfulness and constructing mental health: Understanding mindfulness and its mechanisms of action. *Mindfulness, 1*(4), 235–253. https://doi.org/10.1007/s12671-010-0033-2

Comas-Díaz, L. (2016). Racial trauma recovery: A race-informed therapeutic approach to racial wounds. In A. N. Alvarez, C. T. H. Liang, & H. A. Neville (Eds.), *The cost of racism for people of color: Contextualizing experiences of discrimination* (pp. 249–272). American Psychological Association. https://doi.org/10.1037/14852-012

Connor, D. R., & Callahan, J. L. (2015). Impact of psychotherapist expectations on client outcomes. *Psychotherapy, 52*(3), 351–362. https://doi.org/10.1037/a0038890

Constantino, M. J., Goodwin, B. J., Muir, H. J., Coyne, A. E., & Boswell, J. F. (2021). Context-responsive psychotherapy integration applied to cognitive behavioral therapy. In J. C. Watson & H. Wiseman (Eds.), *The responsive psychotherapist: Attuning to clients in the moment* (pp. 151–169). American Psychological Association. https://doi.org/10.1037/0000240-008

Constantino, M. J., Muir, H. J., Gaines, A. N., & Ouimette, K. (2023). Hope and expectancy factors. In S. D. Miller, D. Chow, S. Malins, & M. A. Hubble (Eds.), *The field guide to better results: Evidence-based exercises to improve therapeutic effectiveness* (pp. 131–153). American Psychological Association. https://doi.org/10.1037/0000358-007

Corey, G. (2017). *Theory and practice of counseling and psychotherapy* (10th ed.). Cengage.

Cozolino, L. (2017). *The neuroscience of psychotherapy: Healing the social brain* [Norton Series on Interpersonal Neurobiology]. W. W. Norton.

Crenshaw, K. (1989). Demarginalizing the intersection of race and sex: A Black feminist critique of antidiscrimination doctrine, feminist theory and antiracist politics. *University of Chicago Legal Forum, 1989*(1), 139–167.

Cuijpers, P., Reijnders, M., & Huibers, M. J. H. (2019). The role of common factors in psychotherapy outcomes. *Annual Review of Clinical Psychology, 15*, 207–231. https://doi.org/10.1146/annurev-clinpsy-050718-095424

Cyrus, K. (2017). Multiple minorities as multiply marginalized: Applying the minority stress theory to LGBTQ people of color. *Journal of Gay & Lesbian Mental Health, 21*(3), 194–202. https://doi.org/10.1080/19359705.2017.1320739

Daly, M. (1978). *Gyn/ecology: The metaethics of radical feminism.* Beacon Press.

David, E. R., & Derthick, A. O. (2018). *The psychology of oppression.* Springer.

David, D., Lynn, S. J., & Ellis, A. (2009). *Rational and irrational beliefs: Research, theory, and clinical practice.* Oxford University Press.

David, E. R., Schroeder, T. M., & Fernandez, J. (2019). Internalized racism: A systematic review of the psychological literature on racism's most insidious consequence. *Journal of Social Issues, 75*(4), 1057–1086. https://doi.org/10.1111/josi.12350

Davidson, R. J. (2003). Seven sins in the study of emotion: Correctives from affective neuroscience. *Brain and Cognition, 52*(1), 129–132. https://doi.org/10.1016/s0278-2626(03)00015-0

Davis, D. E., DeBlaere, C., Owen, J., Hook, J. N., Rivera, D. P., Choe, E., Van Tongeren, D. R., Worthington, E. L., & Placeres, V. (2018). The multicultural orientation framework: A narrative review. *Psychotherapy, 55*(1), 89–100. https://doi.org/10.1037/pst0000160

Dawson, G. C. (2018). Years of clinical experience and therapist professional development: A literature review. *Journal of Contemporary Psychotherapy, 48*(2), 89–97. https://doi.org/10.1007/s10879-017-9373-8

Day-Vines, N. L., Cluxton-Keller, F., Agorsor, C., Gubara, S., & Otabil, N. A. A. (2020). The multidimensional model of broaching behavior. *Journal of Counseling and Development, 98*(1), 107–118. https://doi.org/10.1002/jcad.12304

Delgadillo, J., Branson, A., Kellett, S., Myles-Hooton, P., Hardy, G. E., & Shafran, R. (2020). Therapist personality traits as predictors of psychological treatment outcomes. *Psychotherapy Research, 30*(7), 857–870. https://doi.org/10.1080/10503307.2020.1731927

de Shazer, S. (1985). *Keys to solutions in brief therapy.* W. W. Norton.

de Silva, P. (1985). Early Buddhist and modern behavioral strategies for the control of unwanted intrusive cognitions. *The Psychological Record, 35*, 437–443.

De Vos, J., & Pluth, E. (2016). *Neuroscience and critique: Exploring the limits of the neurological turn.* Taylor & Francis.

Decety, J., & Jackson, P. L. (2004). The functional architecture of human empathy. *Behavioral and Cognitive Neuroscience Reviews, 3*(2), 71–100. https://doi.org/10.1177/1534582304267187

Deikman, A. (1982). *The observing self: Mysticism and psychotherapy.* Beacon Press.

DeLisi, M., Tostlebe, J., Burgason, K., Heirigs, M., & Vaughn, M. (2018). Self-control versus psychopathy: A head-to-head test of general theories of antisociality. *Youth Violence and Juvenile Justice, 16*(1), 53–76. https://doi.org/10.1177/1541204016682998

Dictado, J., & Torres-Harding, S. R. (2023). Predictors of therapy trainees' pathologizing and invalidating microaggressions with sexual and racial minority therapy clients. *Training and Education in Professional Psychology, 17*(3), 304–313. https://doi.org/10.1037/tep0000424

Di Giuseppe, M., Perry, J. C., Prout, T. A., & Conversano, C. (2021). Recent empirical research and methodologies in defense mechanisms: Defenses as fundamental contributors to adaptation. *Frontiers in Psychology, 12,* Article 802602. https://doi.org/10.3389/fpsyg.2021.802602

Dinkmeyer, D. C., Dinkmeyer, D. C., Jr., & Sperry, L. (1987). *Adlerian counseling and therapy.* Merrill.

Douglass, F. (1855). *My bondage and my freedom.* Penguin Books.

Drozd, J. F., & Goldfried, M. R. (1996). A critical evaluation of the state-of-the-art in psychotherapy outcome research. *Psychotherapy: Theory, Research, Practice, Training, 33*(2), 171–180. https://doi.org/10.1037/0033-3204.33.2.171

Duckworth, A. L., Milkman, K. L., & Laibson, D. (2018). Beyond willpower: Strategies for reducing failures of self-control. *Psychological Science in the Public Interest, 19*(3), 102–129. https://doi.org/10.1177/1529100618821893

Duckworth, A. L., Peterson, C., Matthews, M. D., & Kelly, D. R. (2007). Grit: Perseverance and passion for long-term goals. *Journal of Personality and Social Psychology, 92*(6), 1087–1101. https://doi.org/10.1037/0022-3514.92.6.1087

Dumont, F. (1991). Expertise in psychotherapy: Inherent liabilities of becoming experienced. *Psychotherapy: Theory, Research, Practice, Training, 28*(3), 422–428. https://doi.org/10.1037/0033-3204.28.3.422

Easwaran, E. (2007). *The upanishads* (Vol. 2). Nilgiri Press.

Eccles, D. W., & Feltovich, P. J. (2008). Implications of domain-general "psychological support skills" for transfer of skill and acquisition of expertise. *Performance Improvement Quarterly, 21*(1), 43–60. https://doi.org/10.1002/piq.20014

Edmondstone, C., Pascual-Leone, A., Soucie, K., & Kramer, U. (2023). Therapist effects on outcome: Meaningful differences exist early in training. *Training and Education in Professional Psychology, 17*(2), 149–157. https://doi.org/10.1037/tep0000402

Elliott, R. (2010). Psychotherapy change process research: Realizing the promise. *Psychotherapy Research, 20*(2), 123–135. https://doi.org/10.1080/10503300903470743

Elliott, R., Bohart, A. C., Watson, J. C., & Murphy, D. (2018). Therapist empathy and client outcome: An updated meta-analysis. *Psychotherapy, 55*(4), 399–410. https://doi.org/10.1037/pst0000175

Epictetus. (1944). *Epictetus: Discourses and enchiridion.* Walter J. Black. (Original work published circa 130)

Esterman, M., & Rothlein, D. (2019). Models of sustained attention. *Current Opinion in Psychology, 29,* 174–180. https://doi.org/10.1016/j.copsyc.2019.03.005

Eubanks, C. F., & Goldfried, M. R. (2019). A principle-based approach to psycho-therapy integration. In J. C. Norcross & M. R. Goldfried (Eds.), *Handbook of psychotherapy integration* (pp. 88–104). Oxford University Press.

Ewert, C., Vater, A., & Schröder-Abé, M. (2021). Self-compassion and coping: A meta-analysis. *Mindfulness, 12*(5), 1063–1077. https://doi.org/10.1007/s12671-020-01563-8

Eysenck, H. J. (1952). The effects of psychotherapy: An evaluation. *Journal of Consulting Psychology, 16*(5), 319–324. https://doi.org/10.1037/h0063633

Fall, K. A., Holden, J. M., & Marquis, A. (2017). *Theoretical models of counseling and psychotherapy*. Routledge.

Farber, M. (1968). *Theory of suicide*. Funk & Wagnalls.

Fear, R. M. (2018). *Systematic desensitization for panic and phobia: An introduction for health professionals*. Routledge.

Feinstein, R. A. (2018). *When rape was legal: The untold history of sexual violence during slavery*. Routledge.

Festinger, L. (1957). *A theory of cognitive dissonance*. Stanford University Press.

Feuerstein, G. (1989). *The yoga-sutra of Patanjali*. Inner Traditions International.

Figley, C. R. (2013). *Compassion fatigue: Coping with secondary traumatic stress disorder in those who treat the traumatized*. Routledge.

Firth, N., Barkham, M., Kellett, S., & Saxon, D. (2015). Therapist effects and moderators of effectiveness and efficiency in psychological wellbeing practitioners: A multilevel modelling analysis. *Behaviour Research and Therapy, 69*, 54–62. https://doi.org/10.1016/j.brat.2015.04.001

Flavell, J. H. (1979). Metacognition and cognitive monitoring: A new area of cognitive–developmental inquiry. *American Psychologist, 34*(10), 906–911. https://doi.org/10.1037/0003-066X.34.10.906

Fletcher, A. C., & Delgadillo, J. (2022). Psychotherapists' personality traits and their influence on treatment processes and outcomes: A scoping review. *Journal of Clinical Psychology, 78*(7), 1267–1287. https://doi.org/10.1002/jclp.23310

Franck, L., Molyneux, N., & Parkinson, L. (2016). Systematic review of interventions addressing social isolation and depression in aged care clients. *Quality of Life Research, 25*(6), 1395–1407. https://doi.org/10.1007/s11136-015-1197-y

Frank, J. (1961). *Persuasion and healing*. Johns Hopkins University Press.

Frank, J. D. (1987). Psychotherapy, rhetoric, and hermeneutics: Implications for practice and research. *Psychotherapy: Theory, Research, Practice, Training, 24*(3), 293–302. https://doi.org/10.1037/h0085719

Frank, J. D., & Frank, J. B. (1991). *Persuasion and healing* (3rd ed.). Johns Hopkins University Press.

Frankfurt, H. G. (2005). *On bullshit*. Princeton University Press.

Frankl, V. E. (1992). *Man's search for meaning: An introduction to logotherapy* (I. Lasch, Trans.; 4th ed.). Beacon Press. (Original work published 1959)

Freud, S. (1910). The future prospects of psychoanalytic therapy. In J. Strachey (Ed.), *The complete psychological works of Sigmund Freud* (Standard ed., pp. 139–158). Hogarth.

Fricker, M. (2007). *Epistemic injustice: Power and the ethics of knowing*. Oxford University Press.

Friedlander, M. L. (2015). Use of relational strategies to repair alliance ruptures: How responsive supervisors train responsive psychotherapists. *Psychotherapy, 52*(2), 174–179. https://doi.org/10.1037/a0037044

Fromm-Reichmann, F. (1950). *Principles of intensive psychotherapy*. University of Chicago Press.

Fuertes, J. N., & Nutt Williams, E. (2017). Client-focused psychotherapy research. *Journal of Counseling Psychology, 64*(4), 369–375. https://doi.org/10.1037/cou0000214

Fuertes, J. N., Stracuzzi, T. I., Bennett, J., Scheinholtz, J., Mislowack, A., Hersh, M., & Cheng, D. (2006). Therapist multicultural competency: A study of therapy dyads. *Psychotherapy: Theory, Research, Practice, Training, 43*(4), 480–490. https://doi.org/10.1037/0033-3204.43.4.480

Gaines, A. N., & Goldfried, M. R. (2021). Consensus in psychotherapy: Are we there yet? *Clinical Psychology: Science and Practice, 28*(3), 267–276. https://doi.org/10.1037/cps0000026

Gallagher, S. (2017). Phenomenological approaches to consciousness. In M. Velmans & S. Schneider (Eds.), *The Blackwell companion to consciousness* (2nd ed., pp. 686–696). Blackwell.

Gallagher, S., & Zahavi, D. (2020). *The phenomenological mind*. Routledge.

Gazzillo, F. (2023). Toward a more comprehensive understanding of pathogenic beliefs: Theory and clinical implications. *Journal of Contemporary Psychotherapy, 53*(3), 227–234. https://doi.org/10.1007/s10879-022-09564-5

Gendlin, E. (1981). *Focusing*. Bantam Books.

Gendlin, E. (1992). Celebrations and problems of humanistic psychology. *The Humanistic Psychologist, 20*(2–3), 447–460. https://doi.org/10.1080/08873267.1992.9986809

Gendlin, E. T. (1986). What comes after traditional psychotherapy research? *American Psychologist, 41*(2), 131–136. https://doi.org/10.1037/0003-066X.41.2.131

Gevisser, M. (2020). *The pink line: Journeys across the world's queer frontiers*. Picador.

Gilbert, P. (2020). Compassion: From its evolution to a psychotherapy. *Frontiers in Psychology, 11*, Article 586161. https://doi.org/10.3389/fpsyg.2020.586161

Gilligan, C. (1982). *In a different voice: Psychological theory and women's development*. Harvard University Press.

Giovacchini, P. L. (1989). *Countertransference: Triumphs and catastrophes*. Jason Aronson.

Gladding, S. T., & Drake Wallace, M. J. (2016). Promoting beneficial humor in counseling: A way of helping counselors help clients. *Journal of Creativity in Mental Health, 11*(1), 2–11. https://doi.org/10.1080/15401383.2015.1133361

Glasser, W. (1965). *Reality therapy*. Harper & Row.

Golubickis, M., Tan, L. B., Falben, J. K., & Macrae, C. N. (2016). The observing self: Diminishing egocentrism through brief mindfulness meditation. *European Journal of Social Psychology, 46*(4), 521–527. https://doi.org/10.1002/ejsp.2186

Goldberg, L. (2017). Therapy with former members of destructive cults. In S. Harvey, S. Steidinger, & J. A. Beckford (Eds.), *New religious movements and counselling* (pp. 63–79). Routledge.

Goldfried, M. R. (1980). Toward the delineation of therapeutic change principles. *American Psychologist, 35*(11), 991–999. https://doi.org/10.1037/0003-066X.35.11.991

Goldfried, M. R. (1995). Toward a common language for case formulation. *Journal of Psychotherapy Integration, 5*(3), 221–244. https://doi.org/10.1037/h0101272

Goldfried, M. R. (2019). Obtaining consensus in psychotherapy: What holds us back? *American Psychologist, 74*(4), 484–496. https://doi.org/10.1037/amp0000365

Goldfried, M. R., Greenberg, L. S., & Marmar, C. (1990). Individual psychotherapy: Process and outcome. *Annual Review of Psychology, 41*, 659–688. https://doi.org/10.1146/annurev.ps.41.020190.003303

Goldman, E. E., & Morrison, D. S. (1984). *Psychodrama: Experience and process*. Kendall Hunt.

Goldstein, W. N. (2013). *A primer for beginning psychotherapy*. Routledge.

Goodwin, B. J., Coyne, A. E., & Constantino, M. J. (2018). Extending the context-responsive psychotherapy integration framework to cultural processes in psychotherapy. *Psychotherapy, 55*(1), 3–8. https://doi.org/10.1037/pst0000143

Gorlin, E. I., & Békés, V. (2021). Agency via awareness: A unifying meta-process in psychotherapy. *Frontiers in Psychology, 12*, Article 698655. https://doi.org/10.3389/fpsyg.2021.698655

Goshe, S. (2019). The lurking punitive threat: The philosophy of necessity and challenges for reform. *Theoretical Criminology, 23*(1), 25–42. https://doi.org/10.1177/1362480617719450

Greenberg, J. (2019). Trauma and the metaphor of oppression. *The International Journal of Psychoanalysis, 100*(6), 1144–1153. https://doi.org/10.1080/00207578.2019.1642760

Greenberg, L. S. (1986). Change process research. *Journal of Consulting and Clinical Psychology, 54*(1), 4–9. https://doi.org/10.1037/0022-006X.54.1.4

Grencavage, L. M., & Norcross, J. C. (1990). Where are the commonalities among the therapeutic common factors? *Professional Psychology: Research and Practice, 21*(5), 372–378. https://doi.org/10.1037/0735-7028.21.5.372

Griffith, J. L., & Dsouza, A. (2012). Demoralization and hope in clinical psychiatry and psychotherapy. In R. D. Alarcon & J. B. Frank (Eds.), *The psychotherapy of hope: The legacy of persuasion and healing* (pp. 158–177). Johns Hopkins University Press.

Grossmann, I., Na, J., Varnum, M. E. W., Kitayama, S., & Nisbett, R. E. (2013). A route to well-being: Intelligence versus wise reasoning. *Journal of Experimental Psychology: General, 142*(3), 944–953. https://doi.org/10.1037/a0029560

Gupta, B. (1998). *The disinterested witness: A fragment of Advaita Vedanta phenomenology*. Northwestern University Press.

Gutierrez, D., & Czerny, A. (2018). Transtheoretical model for change. In P. Lassiter & J. Culbreth (Eds.), *Theory and practice of addiction counseling* (pp. 199–216). Sage Publications.

Hackert, B., & Weger, U. (2018). Introspection and the Würzburg school. *European Psychologist, 23*(3), 217–232. https://doi.org/10.1027/1016-9040/a000329

Hahn, R. A., & Kleinman, A. (1983). Belief as pathogen, belief as medicine: "Voodoo death" and the "placebo phenomenon" in anthropological perspective. *Medical Anthropology Quarterly, 14*(4), 3–19. https://doi.org/10.1525/maq.1983.14.4.02a00030

Haidt, J. (2024). *The anxious generation: How the great rewiring of childhood is causing an epidemic of mental illness*. Penguin.

Hamonniere, T., & Varescon, I. (2018). Metacognitive beliefs in addictive behaviours: A systematic review. *Addictive Behaviors, 85*, 51–63. https://doi.org/10.1016/j.addbeh.2018.05.018

Hanna, F. J. (1993). The transpersonal consequences of Husserl's phenomenological method. *The Humanistic Psychologist, 21*(1), 41–57. https://doi.org/10.1080/08873267.1993.9976905

Hanna, F. J. (1994). A dialectic of experience: A radical empiricist approach to conflicting theories in psychotherapy. *Psychotherapy: Theory, Research, Practice, Training, 31*(1), 124–136. https://doi.org/10.1037/0033-3204.31.1.124

Hanna, F. J. (1995). Husserl on the teachings of the Buddha. *The Humanistic Psychologist, 23*(3), 365–372. https://doi.org/10.1080/08873267.1995.9986837

Hanna, F. J. (1996). Precursors of change: Pivotal points of involvement and resistance in psychotherapy. *Journal of Psychotherapy Integration, 6*(3), 227–264. https://doi.org/10.1037/h0101102

Hanna, F. J. (1998). A transcultural view of prejudice, racism, and community feeling: The desire and striving for status. *The Journal of Individual Psychology, 54*(3), 336–345.

Hanna, F. J. (2004). Holding the family together. In L. Golden (Ed.), *Case studies in marriage and family therapy* (pp. 91–98). Merrill; Prentice-Hall.

Hanna, F. J. (2011). Freedom: Toward an integration of the counseling profession. *Counselor Education and Supervision, 50*(6), 362–385. https://doi.org/10.1002/j.1556-6978.2011.tb01921.x

Hanna, F. J., Bemak, F., & Chung, R. C. (1999). Toward a new paradigm for multicultural counseling. *Journal of Counseling and Development, 77*(2), 125–134. https://doi.org/10.1002/j.1556-6676.1999.tb02432.x

Hanna, F. J., & Black, L. L. (2007, October). *Liberation and freedom: An integration of counseling theories, social justice, and multiculturalism* [Paper presentation]. Association for Counselor Education and Supervision, Columbus, OH, United States.

Hanna, F. J., & Cardona, B. (2013). Multicultural counseling beyond the relationship: Expanding the repertoire with techniques. *Journal of Counseling and Development, 91*(3), 349–357. https://doi.org/10.1002/j.1556-6676.2013.00104.x

Hanna, F. J., Giordano, F., Dupuy, P., & Puhakka, K. (1995). Agency and transcendence: The experience of therapeutic change. *The Humanistic Psychologist, 23*(2), 139–160. https://doi.org/10.1080/08873267.1995.9986822

Hanna, F. J., & Hunt, W. P. (1999). Techniques for psychotherapy with defiant, aggressive adolescents. *Psychotherapy: Theory, Research, Practice, Training, 36*(1), 56–68. https://doi.org/10.1037/h0087842

Hanna, F. J., & Ottens, A. J. (1995). The role of wisdom in psychotherapy. *Journal of Psychotherapy Integration, 5*(3), 195–219. https://doi.org/10.1037/h0101273

Hanna, F. J., & Puhakka, K. (1991). When psychotherapy works: Pinpointing an element of change. *Psychotherapy: Theory, Research, Practice, Training, 28*(4), 598–607. https://doi.org/10.1037/0033-3204.28.4.598

Hanna, F. J., & Ritchie, M. H. (1995). Seeking the active ingredients of psychotherapeutic change: Within and outside the context of therapy. *Professional Psychology: Research and Practice, 26*(2), 176–183. https://doi.org/10.1037/0735-7028.26.2.176

Hanna, F. J., & Shank, G. (1995). The specter of metaphysics in counseling research and practice: The qualitative challenge. *Journal of Counseling and Development, 74*(1), 53–59. https://doi.org/10.1002/j.1556-6676.1995.tb01822.x

Hanna, F. J., Talley, W. B., & Guindon, M. H. (2000). The power of perception: Toward a model of cultural oppression and liberation. *Journal of Counseling and Development, 78*(4), 430–441. https://doi.org/10.1002/j.1556-6676.2000.tb01926.x

Hardy, C. (2019). Clinical sympathy: The important role of affectivity in clinical practice. *Medicine, Health Care, and Philosophy, 22*(4), 499–513. https://doi.org/10.1007/s11019-018-9872-8

Harmon-Jones, E. (Ed.). (2019). *Cognitive dissonance: Reexamining a pivotal theory in psychology* (2nd ed.). American Psychological Association. https://doi.org/10.1037/0000135-000

Harré, R. (1984). *Personal being: A theory for individual psychology.* Harvard University Press.

Harris, S. J. (1986). *Clearing the ground.* Houghton Mifflin.

Hart, C. M., Hepper, E. G., & Sedikides, C. (2018). Understanding and mitigating narcissists' low empathy. In A. D. Hermann, A. B. Brunell, & J. D. Foster (Eds.) *Handbook of trait narcissism: Key advances, research methods, and controversies* (pp. 335–343). Springer.

Hartmann, I. C. (2019). Forms of expression of a preverbal reality in child psychotherapy. *Journal of Prenatal & Perinatal Psychology & Health, 33*(4), 259–281.

Harvey, J. (2015). *Civilized oppression and moral relations: Victims, fallibility, and the moral community.* Palgrave Macmillan.

Hattie, J. A., Sharpley, C. F., & Rogers, H. J. (1984). Comparative effectiveness of professional and paraprofessional helpers. *Psychological Bulletin, 95*(3), 534–541. https://doi.org/10.1037/0033-2909.95.3.534

Hayes, J. A., Gelso, C. J., Goldberg, S., & Kivlighan, D. M. (2018). Countertransference management and effective psychotherapy: Meta-analytic findings. *Psychotherapy, 55*(4), 496–507. https://doi.org/10.1037/pst0000189

Hayes, S. C. (2005). *Get out of your mind and into your life: The new acceptance and commitment therapy.* New Harbinger Publications.

Hayes, S. C., & Linehan, M. M. (2018). Third-wave therapies. In J. O. Prochaska & J. C. Norcross (Eds.), *Systems of psychotherapy: A transtheoretical analysis* (9th ed., pp. 291–311). Oxford University Press.

Hayes, S. C., Strosahl, K. D., & Wilson, K. G. (2011). *Acceptance and commitment therapy: The process and practice of mindful change.* Guilford Press.

Heidegger, M. (1962). *Being and time.* Harper and Row. (Original work published 1927)

Hendricks, M. L., & Testa, R. J. (2012). A conceptual framework for clinical work with transgender and gender nonconforming clients: An adaptation of the minority stress model. *Professional Psychology: Research and Practice, 43*(5), 460–467. https://doi.org/10.1037/a0029597

Henriques, G. R. (2019). Toward a metaphysical empirical psychology. In T. Teo (Ed.), *Re-envisioning theoretical and philosophical psychology* (pp. 209–237). Palgrave Macmillan.

Hergenhahn, B. R. (1996). *An introduction to the history of psychology.* Wadsworth.

Herrnstein, R. J., & Boring, E. G. (Eds.). (1965). *A sourcebook in the history of psychology.* Harvard University Press.

Hibberd, F. J. (2014). The metaphysical basis of a process psychology. *Journal of Theoretical and Philosophical Psychology, 34*(3), 161–186. https://doi.org/10.1037/a0036242

Hill, C. E., Morales, K., Gerstenblith, J. A., Bansal, P., An, M., Rim, K., & Kivlighan, D. M., Jr. (2022). Therapist challenges and client responses in psychodynamic psychotherapy: An empirically supported case study. *Psychotherapy, 59*(1), 74–83. https://doi.org/10.1037/pst0000424

Hipson, W. E., Coplan, R. J., & Séguin, D. G. (2019). Active emotion regulation mediates links between shyness and social adjustment in preschool. *Social Development, 28*(4), 893–907. https://doi.org/10.1111/sode.12372

Hoener, C., Stiles, W. B., Luka, B. J., & Gordon, R. A. (2012). Client experiences of agency in therapy. *Person-Centered & Experiential Psychotherapies, 11*(1), 64–82. https://doi.org/10.1080/14779757.2011.639460

Hofmann, S. G., & Asmundson, G. J. G. (2008). Acceptance and mindfulness-based therapy: New wave or old hat? *Clinical Psychology Review, 28*(1), 1–16. https://doi.org/10.1016/j.cpr.2007.09.003

Høglend, P., & Hagtvet, K. (2019). Change mechanisms in psychotherapy: Both improved insight and improved affective awareness are necessary. *Journal of Consulting and Clinical Psychology, 87*(4), 332–344. https://doi.org/10.1037/ccp0000381

Holmes, C. (2017). *The paradox of countertransference: You and me, here and now.* Bloomsbury.

Hook, J. N., Davis, D., Owen, J., & DeBlaere, C. (2017). *Cultural humility: Engaging diverse identities in therapy.* American Psychological Association. https://doi.org/10.1037/0000037-000

Horney, K. (1987). *Final lectures.* W. W. Norton. (Original lectures given in 1952)

Howard, K. I., Kopta, S. M., Krause, M. S., & Orlinsky, D. E. (1986). The dose–effect relationship in psychotherapy. *American Psychologist, 41*(2), 159–164. https://doi.org/10.1037/0003-066X.41.2.159

Hume, D. (1978). *A treatise of human nature.* Oxford University Press. (Original work published 1739)

Husserl, E. (1970). *The crisis of European sciences and transcendental phenomenology.* Northwestern University Press. (Original work published 1936)

Husserl, E. (1982). *Ideas pertaining to a pure phenomenology and to a phenomenological philosophy: First book.* Martinus Nijhoff. (Original work published 1913)

Insel, T. R. (2022). *Healing: Our path from mental illness to mental health.* Penguin Press.

Inzlicht, M., Shenhav, A., & Olivola, C. Y. (2018). The effort paradox: Effort is both costly and valued. *Trends in Cognitive Sciences, 22*(4), 337–349. https://doi.org/10.1016/j.tics.2018.01.007

Ivey, A. E. (1995). Psychotherapy as liberation: Toward specific skills and strategies in multicultural counseling and therapy. In J. G. Ponterotto, J. M. Casas, L. A. Suzuki, & C. M. Alexander (Eds.), *Handbook of multicultural counseling* (pp. 53–72). Sage Publications.

Jacobs, D. H. (1994). Environmental failure: Oppression is the only cause of psychopathology. *Journal of Mind and Behavior, 15*(1–2), 1–18.

James, W. (1965). *Pragmatism and four essays from the meaning of truth.* New American Library. (Original work published 1909)

James, W. (1977). Does consciousness exist? In J. J. McDermott (Ed.), *The writings of William James: A comprehensive edition* (pp. 169–183). University of Chicago Press. (Original work published 1904)

James, W. (1981). *The principles of psychology.* Harvard University Press. (Original work published 1890)

Jankowski, T., & Holas, P. (2014). Metacognitive model of mindfulness. *Consciousness and Cognition, 28*, 64–80. https://doi.org/10.1016/j.concog.2014.06.005

Janosik, E. H. (1986). *Crisis counseling: A contemporary approach.* Jones & Bartlett.

Jung, C. G. (1969). *Collected works: Vol. 8. The structure and dynamics of the psyche.* Princeton University Press. (Original work published 1934)

Kajonius, P. J., & Dåderman, A. M. (2017). Conceptualizations of personality disorders with the five factor model-count and empathy traits. *International Journal of Testing, 17*(2), 141–157. https://doi.org/10.1080/15305058.2017.1279164

Kanfer, F. H., & Grimm, L. G. (1978). Freedom of choice and behavioral change. *Journal of Consulting and Clinical Psychology, 46*(5), 873–878. https://doi.org/10.1037/0022-006X.46.5.873

Kant, I. (1929). *Critique of pure reason*. St. Martin's Press. (Original work published 1787)

Karasu, T. B. (1992). *Wisdom in the practice of psychotherapy*. Basic Books.

Kazantzis, N., Dattilio, F. M., Cummins, A., & Clayton, X. (2014). Homework assignments and self-monitoring. In S. G. Hofmann, D. J. A. Dozois, W. Rief, & J. A. J. Smits (Eds.), *The Wiley handbook of cognitive behavioral therapy* (pp. 311–330). Wiley.

Kazantzis, N., & Lampropoulos, G. K. (2002). Reflecting on homework in psychotherapy: What can we conclude from research and experience? *Journal of Clinical Psychology, 58*(5), 577–585. https://doi.org/10.1002/jclp.10034

Kemp, R. (2013). Rock-bottom as an event of truth. *Existential Analysis, 24*(1), 106–116.

Kensit, D. A. (2000). Rogerian theory: A critique of the effectiveness of pure client-centred therapy. *Counselling Psychology Quarterly, 13*(4), 345–351. https://doi.org/10.1080/713658499

Kernberg, O. (1967). Borderline personality organization. *Journal of the American Psychoanalytic Association, 15*(3), 641–685. https://doi.org/10.1177/000306516701500309

Kierulff, S. (1988). Sheep in the midst of wolves: Personal-responsibility therapy with criminal personalities. *Professional Psychology: Research and Practice, 19*(4), 436–440. https://doi.org/10.1037/0735-7028.19.4.436

Kiesler, D. J. (1988). *Therapeutic metacommunication*. Consulting Psychologists Press.

Kiesler, D. J. (2017). *The process of psychotherapy: Empirical foundations and systems of analysis*. Routledge.

Kim, B. S., Ng, G. F., & Ahn, A. J. (2005). Effects of client expectation for counseling success, client-counselor worldview match, and client adherence to Asian and European American cultural values on counseling process with Asian Americans. *Journal of Counseling Psychology, 52*(1), 67–76. https://doi.org/10.1037/0022-0167.52.1.67

Kim, J. J., Brookman-Frazee, L., Gellatly, R., Stadnick, N., Barnett, M. L., & Lau, A. S. (2018). Predictors of burnout among community therapists in the sustainment phase of a system-driven implementation of multiple evidence-based practices in children's mental health. *Professional Psychology: Research and Practice, 49*(2), 131–142. https://doi.org/10.1037/pro0000182

Klein, A. C., & Wangyal, T. (2006). *Unbounded wholeness: Dzogchen, bon, and the logic of the nonconceptual*. Oxford University Press.

Klug, H. J., & Maier, G. W. (2015). Linking goal progress and subjective well-being: A meta-analysis. *Journal of Happiness Studies, 16*(1), 37–65. https://doi.org/10.1007/s10902-013-9493-0

Kocalevent, R. D., Finck, C., Pérez-Trujillo, M., Sautier, L., Zill, J., & Hinz, A. (2017). Standardization of the Beck Hopelessness Scale in the general population. *Journal of Mental Health, 26*(6), 516–522. https://doi.org/10.1080/09638237.2016.1244717

Koch, S. (1981). The nature and limits of psychological knowledge: Lessons of a century qua "science." *American Psychologist, 36*(3), 257–269. https://doi.org/10.1037/0003-066X.36.3.257

Korn, J. H., Davis, R., & Davis, S. F. (1991). Historians' and chairpersons' judgments of eminence among psychologists. *American Psychologist, 46*(7), 789–792. https://doi.org/10.1037/0003-066X.46.7.789

Korotitsch, W. J., & Nelson-Gray, R. O. (1999). An overview of self-monitoring research in assessment and treatment. *Psychological Assessment, 11*(4), 415–425. https://doi.org/10.1037/1040-3590.11.4.415

Kottler, J. A. (2022). *On being a therapist* (6th ed.). Oxford University Press.

Kramer, U., Levy, K. N., & McMain, S. (2024). *Understanding mechanisms of change in psychotherapies for personality disorders.* American Psychological Association. https://doi.org/10.1037/0000388-000

Kraus, D. R., Bentley, J. H., Alexander, P. C., Boswell, J. F., Constantino, M. J., Baxter, E. E., & Castonguay, L. G. (2016). Predicting therapist effectiveness from their own practice-based evidence. *Journal of Consulting and Clinical Psychology, 84*(6), 473–483. https://doi.org/10.1037/ccp0000083

Krebs, P., Norcross, J. C., Nicholson, J. M., & Prochaska, J. O. (2019). Stages of change. In J. C. Norcross & B. E. Wampold (Eds.), *Psychotherapy relationships that work: Evidence-based therapist responsiveness* (pp. 296–328). Oxford University Press.

Kross, E., & Ayduk, O. (2017). Self-distancing: Theory, research, and current directions. In J. M. Olsen (Ed.), *Advances in experimental social psychology* (Vol. 55, pp. 81–136). Academic Press.

Kuhn, D. (2022). Metacognition matters in many ways. *Educational Psychologist, 57*(2), 73–86. https://doi.org/10.1080/00461520.2021.1988603

Lam, K. K. L., & Zhou, M. (2022). Grit and academic achievement: A comparative cross-cultural meta-analysis. *Journal of Educational Psychology, 114*(3), 597–621. https://doi.org/10.1037/edu0000699

Lambert, M. J. (1992). Psychotherapy outcome research: Implications for integrative and eclectic therapists. In J. C. Norcross & M. R. Goldfried (Eds.), *Handbook of psychotherapy integration* (pp. 94–129). Basic Books.

Lambert, M. J., Bergin, A. E., & Collins, J. L. (1977). Therapist-induced deterioration in psychotherapy. In A. S. Gurman & A. M. Razin (Eds.), *Effective psychotherapy: A handbook of research* (pp. 452–481). Pergamon.

Larsen, D. J., & Stege, R. (2010). Hope-focused practices during early psychotherapy sessions: Part I: Implicit approaches. *Journal of Psychotherapy Integration, 20*(3), 271–292. https://doi.org/10.1037/a0020820

Laska, K. M., Gurman, A. S., & Wampold, B. E. (2014). Expanding the lens of evidence-based practice in psychotherapy: A common factors perspective. *Psychotherapy, 51*(4), 467–481. https://doi.org/10.1037/a0034332

Lavik, K. O., Veseth, M., Frøysa, H., Binder, P. E., & Moltu, C. (2018). 'Nobody else can lead your life': What adolescents need from psychotherapists in change processes. *Counselling & Psychotherapy Research, 18*(3), 262–273. https://doi.org/10.1002/capr.12166

Lazarus, A. A. (1976). *Multimodal behavior therapy.* Springer.

Lazarus, A. A. (1989a). Multimodal therapy. In R. J. Corsini & D. Wedding (Eds.), *Current psychotherapies* (4th ed., pp. 503–544). F. E. Peacock.

Lazarus, A. A. (1989b). *The practice of multimodal therapy.* Johns Hopkins University Press.

Lazarus, A. A. (1990). Can psychotherapists transcend the shackles of their training and superstitions? *Journal of Clinical Psychology, 46*(3), 351–358. https://doi.org/10.1002/1097-4679(199005)46:3%3C351::aid-jclp2270460316%3E3.0.co;2-v

Lazarus, A. A. (1993). Tailoring the therapeutic relationship, or being an authentic chameleon. *Psychotherapy: Theory, Research, Practice, Training, 30*(3), 404–407. https://doi.org/10.1037/0033-3204.30.3.404

Lazarus, A. A. (1996). The utility and futility of combining treatments in psychotherapy. *Clinical Psychology: Science and Practice, 3*(1), 59–68. https://doi.org/10.1111/j.1468-2850.1996.tb00058.x

Leahy, R. L. (2017). *Cognitive therapy techniques: A practitioner's guide.* Guilford Press.

Lee, E., Greenblatt, A., Hu, R., Johnstone, M., & Kourgiantakis, T. (2022). Developing a model of broaching and bridging in cross-cultural psychotherapy: Toward fostering epistemic and social justice. *American Journal of Orthopsychiatry, 92*(3), 322–333. https://doi.org/10.1037/ort0000611

Leschziner, V., & Brett, G. (2019). Beyond two minds: Cognitive, embodied, and evaluative processes in creativity. *Social Psychology Quarterly, 82*(4), 340–366. https://doi.org/10.1177/0190272519851791

Lester, D. (1982). Astrologers and psychics as therapists. *American Journal of Psychotherapy, 36*(1), 56–66. https://doi.org/10.1176/appi.psychotherapy.1982.36.1.56

Levitt, H. M., & Piazza-Bonin, E. (2016). Wisdom and psychotherapy: Studying expert therapists' clinical wisdom to explicate common processes. *Psychotherapy Research, 26*(1), 31–47. https://doi.org/10.1080/10503307.2014.937470

Lewin, K. (1935). *A dynamic theory of personality.* McGraw-Hill.

Lewin, K. (1936). *Principles of topological psychology.* McGraw-Hill.

Linehan, M. M. (1993). *Cognitive-behavioral treatment of borderline personality.* Guilford Press.

Liu, H., Peng, H., Song, X., Xu, C., & Zhang, M. (2022). Using AI chatbots to provide self-help depression interventions for university students: A randomized trial of effectiveness. *Internet Interventions, 27,* Article 100495. https://doi.org/10.1016/j.invent.2022.100495

Loevinger, J. (1976). *Ego development.* Jossey-Bass.

Low, A. A. (1952). *Mental health through will-training.* Willett.

Lyddon, W. J. (1989). Personal epistemology and preference for counseling. *Journal of Counseling Psychology, 36*(4), 423–429. https://doi.org/10.1037/0022-0167.36.4.423

Lyddon, W. J. (1990). First- and second-order change: Implications for rationalist and constructivist cognitive therapies. *Journal of Counseling and Development, 69*(6), 122–127. https://doi.org/10.1002/j.1556-6676.1990.tb01472.x

Lynch, T. R., Hempel, R. J., & Dunkley, C. (2015). Radically open-dialectical behavior therapy for disorders of over-control: Signaling matters. *American Journal of Psychotherapy, 69*(2), 141–162. https://doi.org/10.1176/appi.psychotherapy.2015.69.2.141

MacFarlane, P., Anderson, T., & McClintock, A. S. (2017). Empathy from the client's perspective: A grounded theory analysis. *Psychotherapy Research, 27*(2), 227–238. https://doi.org/10.1080/10503307.2015.1090038

Machado, P. P., & Beutler, L. E. (2016). Research methods and randomized clinical trials in psychotherapy. In A. J. Consoli, L. E. Beutler, & B. Bongar (Eds.), *Comprehensive textbook of psychotherapy: Theory and practice* (pp. 445–461). Oxford University Press.

Magnavita, J. J. (2006). The centrality of emotion in unifying and accelerating psychotherapy. *Journal of Clinical Psychology, 62*(5), 585–596. https://doi.org/10.1002/jclp.20250

Mahoney, M. J. (1991). *Human change processes: The scientific foundations of psychotherapy*. Basic Books.

Maibom, H. (Ed.). (2017). *The Routledge handbook of philosophy of empathy*. Taylor & Francis.

Maibom, H. (2020). *Empathy*. Routledge.

Mandela, N. (1995). *Long walk to freedom*. Abacus.

Manganaro, P. (2017). The roots of intersubjectivity—Empathy and phenomenology according to Edith Stein. In V. Lux & S. Weigel (Eds.), *Empathy: Epistemic problems and cultural-historical perspectives of a cross-disciplinary concept* (pp. 271–286). Springer.

Mann, D. (2010). *Gestalt therapy: 100 key points and techniques*. Routledge.

Marchetti, I. (2019). Hopelessness: A network analysis. *Cognitive Therapy and Research, 43*(3), 611–619. https://doi.org/10.1007/s10608-018-9981-y

Margulies, A. (1989). *The empathic imagination*. W. W. Norton.

Marquis, A., Henriques, G., Anchin, J., Critchfield, K., Harris, J., Ingram, B., Magnavita, J., & Osborn, K. (2021). Unification: The fifth pathway to psychotherapy integration. *Journal of Contemporary Psychotherapy, 51*(4), 285–294. https://doi.org/10.1007/s10879-021-09506-7

Marsh, A. A. (2018). The neuroscience of empathy. *Current Opinion in Behavioral Sciences, 19*, 110–115. https://doi.org/10.1016/j.cobeha.2017.12.016

Marshall-Lee, E. D., Hinger, C., Popovic, R., Miller Roberts, T. C., & Prempeh, L. (2020). Social justice advocacy in mental health services: Consumer, community, training, and policy perspectives. *Psychological Services, 17*(S1), 12–21. https://doi.org/10.1037/ser0000349

Martín-Baró, I. (1996). *Writings for a liberation psychology*. Harvard University Press.

Martínez-Martí, M. L., & Ruch, W. (2017). Character strengths predict resilience over and above positive affect, self-efficacy, optimism, social support, self-esteem, and life satisfaction. *The Journal of Positive Psychology, 12*(2), 110–119. https://doi.org/10.1080/17439760.2016.1163403

Masterson, J. F. (1988). *The search for the real self: Unmasking the personality disorders of our time*. Free Press.

Mayrhofer, R., Kuhbandner, C., & Lindner, C. (2021). The practice of experimental psychology: An inevitably postmodern endeavor. *Frontiers in Psychology, 11*, Article 612805. https://doi.org/10.3389/fpsyg.2020.612805

McCloskey, K. D., Cox, D. W., Ogrodniczuk, J. S., Laverdière, O., Joyce, A. S., & Kealy, D. (2021). Interpersonal problems and social dysfunction: Examining patients with avoidant and borderline personality disorder symptoms. *Journal of Clinical Psychology, 77*(1), 329–339. https://doi.org/10.1002/jclp.23033

McDowell, T., Knudson-Martin, C., & Bermudez, J. M. (2022). *Socioculturally attuned family therapy: Guidelines for equitable theory and practice*. Routledge.

McGrath, A. (2017). Dealing with dissonance: A review of cognitive dissonance reduction. *Social and Personality Psychology Compass, 11*(12), Article e12362. https://doi.org/10.1111/spc3.12362

McKay, M., Davis, M., & Fanning, P. (2021). *Thoughts and feelings: Taking control of your moods and your life*. New Harbinger.

McMullin, R. E. (1986). *Handbook of cognitive therapy techniques*. W. W. Norton.

McNeillie, N., & Rose, J. (2021). Vicarious trauma in therapists: A meta-ethnographic review. *Behavioural and Cognitive Psychotherapy, 49*(4), 1–15. https://doi.org/10.1017/s1352465820000776

McRae, L. (2013). Rehabilitating antisocial personalities: Treatment through self-governance strategies. *The Journal of Forensic Psychiatry & Psychology, 24*(1), 48–70. https://doi.org/10.1080/14789949.2012.752517

Medawar, P. B. (1984). *The limits of science*. Harper & Row.

Meichenbaum, D. B. (1977). *Cognitive-behavior modification: An integrative approach*. Plenum.

Meichenbaum, D., & Asarnow, J. (1979). Cognitive-behavioral modification and metacognitive development: Implications for the classroom. In P. C. Kendall & S. D. Hollon (Eds.), *Cognitive-behavioral interventions: Theory, research and procedures* (pp. 11–35). Academic Press.

Meichenbaum, D., & Cameron, R. (1974). The clinical potential of modifying what clients say to themselves. *Psychotherapy: Theory, Research & Practice, 11*(2), 103–117. https://doi.org/10.1037/h0086326

Merleau-Ponty, M. (1962). *The phenomenology of perception*. Humanities Press.

Merton, R. K. (1968). The Matthew effect in science. The reward and communication systems of science are considered. *Science, 159*(3810), 56–63.

Metzinger, T. (2004). *Being no one: The self-model theory of subjectivity*. MIT Press.

Meyer, I. H. (2003). Prejudice, social stress, and mental health in lesbian, gay, and bisexual populations: Conceptual issues and research evidence. *Psychological Bulletin, 129*(5), 674–697. https://doi.org/10.1037/0033-2909.129.5.674

Miller, D. (2024, January 14). *How to academy mindset: Do we have freewill? Daniel Dennettt vs. Robert Sapolsy* [Video]. Youtube. https://www.youtube.com/watch?v=aYzFH8xqhns

Miller, J. B. (1986). *Toward a new psychology of women*. Beacon Press.

Miller, W. R., & Moyers, T. B. (2021). *Effective psychotherapists*. Guilford Press.

Miller, W. R., & Rollnick, S. (2012). *Motivational interviewing: Helping people change* (2nd ed.). Guilford Press.

Mills, J. (2001). Philosophical counseling as psychotherapy: An eclectic approach. *International Journal of Philosophical Practice, 1*(1), 25–47. https://doi.org/10.5840/ijpp2001112

Mills, J. (2004). Countertransference revisited. *Psychoanalytic Review, 91*(4), 467–515. https://doi.org/10.1002/j.1556-6676.1985.tb02719.x

Moodley, R., Lo, T., & Zhu, N. (Eds.). (2017). *Asian healing traditions in counseling and psychotherapy*. Sage Publications.

Moreno, J. L. (1946). *Psychodrama: First volume*. Beacon House.

Muris, P., & Otgaar, H. (2020). The process of science: A critical evaluation of more than 15 years of research on self-compassion with the Self-Compassion Scale. *Mindfulness, 11*(6), 1469–1482. https://doi.org/10.1007/s12671-020-01363-0

Myers, J. E., & Sweeney, T. J. (2008). Wellness counseling: The evidence base for practice. *Journal of Counseling & Development, 86*(4), 482–493. https://doi.org/10.1002/j.1556-6678.2008.tb00536.x

Mylopoulos, M., & Shepherd, J. (2020). Agentive phenomenology. In U. Kriegel (Ed.), *The Oxford handbook of the philosophy of consciousness* (pp. 215–234). Oxford University Press.

Nardini, J. E. (1952). Survival factors in American prisoners of war of the Japanese. *The American Journal of Psychiatry, 109*(4), 241–248. https://doi.org/10.1176/ajp.109.4.241

Neff, K. D. (2023). Self-compassion: Theory, method, research, and intervention. *Annual Review of Psychology, 74,* 193–218. https://doi.org/10.1146/annurev-psych-032420-031047

Nelissen, R. M. (2017). The motivational properties of hope in goal striving. *Cognition and Emotion, 31*(2), 225–237. https://doi.org/10.1080/02699931.2015.1095165

Nguyen, T. (2016). *The Patanjali Yoga Sutras and its spiritual practice.* Balboa Press.

Nissen-Lie, H. A., Goldberg, S. B., Hoyt, W. T., Falkenström, F., Holmqvist, R., Nielsen, S. L., & Wampold, B. E. (2016). Are therapists uniformly effective across patient outcome domains? A study on therapist effectiveness in two different treatment contexts. *Journal of Counseling Psychology, 63*(4), 367–378. https://doi.org/10.1037/cou0000151

Norcross, J. C., & Prochaska, J. O. (1986a). Psychotherapist heal thyself: I. The psychological distress and self-change of psychologists, counselors, and laypersons. *Psychotherapy: Theory, Research, Practice, Training, 23*(1), 102–114. https://doi.org/10.1037/h0085577

Norcross, J. C., & Prochaska, J. O. (1986b). Psychotherapist heal thyself: II. The self-initiated and therapy-facilitated change of psychological distress. *Psychotherapy: Theory, Research, Practice, Training, 23*(3), 345–356. https://doi.org/10.1037/h0085622

Norman, E., & Furnes, B. (2016). The concept of "metaemotion": What is there to learn from research on metacognition? *Emotion Review, 8*(2), 187–193. https://doi.org/10.1177/1754073914552913

North, C. (1987). *Welcome, silence: My triumph over schizophrenia.* Simon & Schuster.

Northup, S. (1968). *Twelve years a slave.* Louisiana State University Press. (Original work published 1853)

Oberst, U. E., & Stewart, A. E. (2014). *Adlerian psychotherapy: An advanced approach to individual psychology.* Routledge.

O'Donohue, W. (1989). The (even) bolder model. The clinical psychologist as metaphysician–scientist–practitioner. *American Psychologist, 44*(12), 1460–1468. https://doi.org/10.1037//0003-066x.44.12.1460

Oettingen, G., & Chromik, M. P. (2017). How hope influences goal-directed behavior. In M. W. Gallagher & S. J. Lopez (Eds.), *The Oxford handbook of hope* (pp. 69–81). Oxford University Press.

Ogbe, E., Harmon, S., Van den Bergh, R., & Degomme, O. (2020). A systematic review of intimate partner violence interventions focused on improving social support and/mental health outcomes of survivors. *PLOS ONE, 15*(6), Article e0235177. https://doi.org/10.1371/journal.pone.0235177

Ogden, T. (2018). *Projective identification and psychotherapeutic technique.* Routledge.

O'Leary, E. (2021). The need for integration. In E. O'Leary & M. Murphy (Eds.), *New approaches to integration in psychotherapy* (pp. 3–11). Routledge.

Omer, H., & London, P. (1988). Metamorphosis in psychotherapy: End of the systems era. *Psychotherapy: Theory, Research, Practice, Training, 25*(2), 171–180. https://doi.org/10.1037/h0085329

Ong, A. D., Standiford, T., & Deshpande, S. (2017). Hope and stress resilience. In M. W. Gallagher & S. J. Lopez (Eds.), *The Oxford handbook of hope* (pp. 255–285). Oxford University Press.

Orlinsky, D. E., Grawe, K., & Parks, B. K. (1994). Process and outcome in psychotherapy: Noch einmal. In A. E. Bergin & S. L. Garfield (Eds.), *Handbook of psychotherapy and behavior change* (4th ed., pp. 270–376). Wiley.

Ornstein, R. (2003). *Multimind: A new way of looking at human behavior.* Macmillan.

Pagnini, F., Bercovitz, K., & Langer, E. (2016). Perceived control and mindfulness: Implications for clinical practice. *Journal of Psychotherapy Integration, 26*(2), 91–102. https://doi.org/10.1037/int0000035

Pandita, S. U. (1991). *In this very life: The liberation teachings of the Buddha.* Wisdom Publications.

Paris, J. (2017). *Psychotherapy in an age of neuroscience.* Oxford Academic Press.

Park, G., Chung, J., & Lee, S. (2023). Effect of AI chatbot emotional disclosure on user satisfaction and reuse intention for mental health counseling: A serial mediation model. *Current Psychology, 42*(32), 28663–28673. https://doi.org/10.1007/s12144-022-03932-z

Pascual-Leone, A., Greenberg, L. S., & Pascual-Leone, J. (2009). Developments in task analysis: New methods to study change. *Psychotherapy Research, 19*(4–5), 527–542. https://doi.org/10.1080/10503300902897797

Peluso, P. R., & Freund, R. (2023). Paradoxical interventions: A meta-analysis. *Psychotherapy, 60*(3), 283–294. https://doi.org/10.1037/pst0000481

Peräkylä, A. (2019). Conversation analysis and psychotherapy: Identifying transformative sequences. *Research on Language and Social Interaction, 52*(3), 257–280. https://doi.org/10.1080/08351813.2019.1631044

Pereira, J. (1976). *Hindu theology: A reader.* Image Books.

Perls, F. S. (1969). *Gestalt therapy verbatim.* Real People Press.

Perls, F. S. (1973). *The gestalt approach & eyewitness to therapy.* Science and Behavior Books.

Perls, F. S., Hefferline, R. F., & Goodman, P. (1951). *Gestalt therapy.* Dell.

Persons, J. B. (1991). Psychotherapy outcome studies do not accurately represent current models of psychotherapy: A proposed remedy. *American Psychologist, 46*(2), 99–106. https://doi.org/10.1037/0003-066X.46.2.99

Pessoa, L. (2023). The entangled brain. *Journal of Cognitive Neuroscience, 35*(3), 349–360. https://doi.org/10.1162/jocn_a_01908

Peterson, B. S. (2019). Editorial: Common factors in the art of healing. *Journal of Child Psychology and Psychiatry, 60*(9), 927–929. https://doi.org/10.1111/jcpp.13108

Peterson, D. R. (1995). The reflective educator. *American Psychologist, 50*(12), 975–983. https://doi.org/10.1037//0003-066x.50.12.975

Philips, B., & Falkenström, F. (2021). What research evidence is valid for psychotherapy research? *Frontiers in Psychiatry, 11,* Article 625380. https://doi.org/10.3389/fpsyt.2020.625380

Polster, I., & Polster, M. (1973). *Gestalt therapy integrated: Contours of theory and practice.* Vintage Books.

Pope, K. S., & Keith-Spiegel, P. (2008). A practical approach to boundaries in psychotherapy: Making decisions, bypassing blunders, and mending fences. *Journal of Clinical Psychology, 64*(5), 638–652. https://doi.org/10.1002/jclp.20477

Popper, K. (1963). *Conjectures and refutations*. Basic Books.

Powers, W. T. (1973). *Behavior: The control of perception*. Aldine.

Prochaska, J. O., DiClemente, C. C., & Norcross, J. C. (1992). In search of how people change: Applications to addictive behaviors. *American Psychologist, 47*(9), 1102–1114. https://doi.org/10.1037//0003-066x.47.9.1102

Prochaska, J. O., & Norcross, J. C. (2018). *Systems of psychotherapy: A transtheoretical analysis*. Oxford University Press.

Prochaska, J. O., Norcross, J. C., & DiClemente, C. C. (1994). *Changing for good*. Avon Books.

Puhakka, K., & Hanna, F. J. (1988). Opening the POD: A therapeutic application of Husserl's phenomenology. *Psychotherapy: Theory, Research, Practice, Training, 25*(4), 582–592. https://doi.org/10.1037/h0085385

Rahula, W. (1978). *What the Buddha taught*. Gordon-Fraser.

Rank, O. (1936). *Will therapy*. W. W. Norton.

Reber, P. J., Batterink, L. J., Thompson, K. R., & Reuveni, B. (2019). Implicit leanring: History and application. In A. Cleeremans, V. Allakhverdov, & M. Kuvaldina (Eds.), *Implicit learning: 50 years on* (pp. 16–37). Routledge.

Reggia, J. A., Katz, G., & Huang, D. W. (2016). What are the computational correlates of consciousness? *Biologically Inspired Cognitive Architectures, 17*, 101–113.

Reich, A. (1951). On countertransference. *The International Journal of Psychoanalysis, 32*, 25–31.

Reisenzein, R. (2019). Cognition and emotion: A plea for theory. *Cognition and Emotion, 33*(1), 109–118. https://doi.org/10.1080/02699931.2019.1568968

Rhodes, M. G. (2019). Metacognition. *Teaching of Psychology, 46*(2), 168–175. https://doi.org/10.1177/0098628319834381

Rholes, W. S., Michas, L., & Shroff, J. (1989). Action control as a vulnerability factor in dysphoria. *Cognitive Therapy and Research, 13*(3), 263–274. https://doi.org/10.1007/BF01173407

Richard, D. C., & Lauterbach, D. (Eds.). (2011). *Handbook of exposure therapies*. Elsevier.

Rigney, D. (2010). *The Matthew effect: How advantage begets further advantage*. Columbia University Press.

Robinson, D. N. (1990). Wisdom through the ages. In R. J. Sternberg (Ed.), *Wisdom: Its nature, origins, and development* (pp. 13–24). Cambridge University Press.

Rogers, C. R. (1951). *Client-centered therapy*. Houghton Mifflin.

Rogers, C. R. (1957). The necessary and sufficient conditions of therapeutic personality change. *Journal of Consulting Psychology, 21*(2), 95–103. https://doi.org/10.1037/h0045357

Rosengren, D. B. (2017). *Building motivational interviewing skills: A practitioner workbook*. Guilford Press.

Rowan, J. (1990). *Subpersonalities: The people inside us*. Routledge.

Ruimi, L., Hadash, Y., Zvielli, A., Amir, I., Goldstein, P., & Bernstein, A. (2018). Meta-awareness of dysregulated emotional attention. *Clinical Psychological Science, 6*(5), 658–670. https://doi.org/10.1177/2167702618776948

Russell, B. (1972). *A history of Western philosophy*. Simon & Schuster.

Russell, K. A., Swift, J. K., Penix, E. A., & Whipple, J. L. (2022). Client preferences for the personality characteristics of an ideal therapist. *Counselling Psychology Quarterly, 35*(2), 243–259. https://doi.org/10.1080/09515070.2020.1733492

Sahakian, W. S. (1976). Philosophical psychotherapy. In W. S. Sahakian (Ed.), *Psychotherapy and counseling: Techniques in intervention* (pp. 286–302). Rand McNally.

Saini, A. (2017). *Inferior: How science got women wrong—And the new research that's rewriting the story.* Beacon Press.

Sakaluk, J. K., Williams, A. J., Kilshaw, R. E., & Rhyner, K. T. (2019). Evaluating the evidential value of empirically supported psychological treatments (ESTs): A meta-scientific review. *Journal of Abnormal Psychology, 128*(6), 500–509. https://doi.org/10.1037/abn0000421

Samenow, S. E. (1998). *Straight talk about criminals.* Jason Aronson.

Samoilov, A., & Goldfried, M. R. (2000). Role of emotion in cognitive-behavior therapy. *Clinical Psychology: Science and Practice, 7*(4), 373–385. https://doi.org/10.1093/clipsy.7.4.373

Sartre, J. P. (2003). *Being and nothingness* (H. E. Barnes, Trans.). Routledge. (Original work published 1943)

Scalabrini, A., Mucci, C., Angeletti, L. L., & Northoff, G. (2020). The self and its world: A neuro-ecological and temporo-spatial account of existential fear. *Clinical Neuropsychiatry, 17*(2), 46–58. https://doi.org/10.36131/clinicalnpsych20200203

Schiepek, G., & Pincus, D. (2023). Complexity science: A framework for psychotherapy integration. *Counselling & Psychotherapy Research, 23*(4), 941–955. https://doi.org/10.1002/capr.12641

Schmid, P. F. (2019). The power of hope: Person-centered perspectives on contemporary personal and societal challenges. *Person-Centered and Experiential Psychotherapies, 18*(2), 121–138. https://doi.org/10.1080/14779757.2019.1618371

Schwartz, R. C., & Sweezy, M. (2019). *Internal family systems therapy* (2nd ed.). Guilford Press.

Segal, H. (1977). Countertransference. *International Journal of Psychoanalytic Psychotherapy, 6,* 31–37.

Seligman, M. E. P. (2006). *Learned optimism: How to change your mind and your life* (3rd ed.). Vintage Books.

Selmi, P. M., Klein, M. H., Greist, J. H., Sorrell, S. P., & Erdman, H. P. (1990). Computer-administered cognitive-behavioral therapy for depression. *The American Journal of Psychiatry, 147*(1), 51–56. https://doi.org/10.1176/ajp.147.1.51

Seow, T. X. F., Rouault, M., Gillan, C. M., & Fleming, S. M. (2021). How local and global metacognition shape mental health. *Biological Psychiatry, 90*(7), 436–446. https://doi.org/10.1016/j.biopsych.2021.05.013

Shah, P., & Mountain, D. (2007). The medical model is dead—Long live the medical model. *The British Journal of Psychiatry, 191*(5), 375–377. https://doi.org/10.1192/bjp.bp.107.037242

Shamoon, Z. A., Lappan, S., & Blow, A. J. (2017). Managing anxiety: A therapist common factor. *Contemporary Family Therapy, 39,* 43–53. https://doi.org/10.1007/s10591-016-9399-1

Shaw, M. (2015). *War and genocide: Organized killing in modern society.* Wiley.

Shoemaker, D. J. (2018). *Theories of delinquency: An examination of explanations of delinquent behavior.* Oxford University Press.

Shonin, E., & Van Gordon, W. (2016). The mechanisms of mindfulness in the treatment of mental illness and addiction. *International Journal of Mental Health and Addiction, 14*(5), 844–849. https://doi.org/10.1007/s11469-016-9653-7

Silberschatz, G. (2017). Improving the yield of psychotherapy research. *Psychotherapy Research, 27*(1), 1–13. https://doi.org/10.1080/10503307.2015.1076202

Silk, J. S., Shaw, D. S., Skuban, E. M., Oland, A. A., & Kovacs, M. (2006). Emotion regulation strategies in offspring of childhood-onset depressed mothers. *Journal of Child Psychology and Psychiatry, 47*(1), 69–78. https://doi.org/10.1111/j.1469-7610.2005.01440.x

Simard, P., Simard, V., Laverdière, O., & Descôteaux, J. (2023). The relationship between narcissism and empathy: A meta-analytic review. *Journal of Research in Personality, 102*, Article 104329. https://doi.org/10.1016/j.jrp.2022.104329

Simon, R. (1985). Take it or leave it: An interview with Carl Whitaker. *Family Therapy Networker, 9*(5), 27–37.

Simourd, D. J., Olver, M. E., & Brandenburg, B. (2016). Changing criminal attitudes among incarcerated offenders: Initial examination of a structured treatment program. *International Journal of Offender Therapy and Comparative Criminology, 60*(12), 1425–1445. https://doi.org/10.1177/0306624x15579257

Singer, B. A., & Luborsky, L. (1977). Countertransference: The status of clinical versus quantitative research. In A. S. Gurman & A. M. Razin (Eds.), *Effective psychotherapy: A handbook of research* (pp. 433–451). Pergamon.

Singer, M. T., & Lalich, J. (1996). *"Crazy" therapies: What are they? Do they work?* Jossey-Bass.

Singer, W. (2017). Conscious processing: Unity in time rather than in space. In S. Schneider & M. Velmans (Eds.), *The Blackwell companion to consciousness* (pp. 607–620). Wiley.

Skinner, B. F. (1971). *Beyond freedom and dignity.* Knopf.

Skovholt, T. (2017). *Master therapists: Exploring expertise in therapy and counseling.* Oxford University Press.

Slife, B. D. (1987). Can cognitive psychology account for metacognitive functions of mind? *Journal of Mind and Behavior, 8*(2), 195–208.

Smith, M. L., & Glass, G. V. (1977). Meta-analysis of psychotherapy outcome studies. *American Psychologist, 32*(9), 752–760. https://doi.org/10.1037/0003-066X.32.9.752

Smith, R., Lane, R. D., Nadel, L., & Moutoussis, M. (2020). A computational neuroscience perspective on the change process in psychotherapy. In R. D. Lane & L. Nadel (Eds.), *Neuroscience of enduring change* (pp. 395–432). Oxford University Press.

Smoliak, O., & Strong, T. (2018). *Therapy as discourse.* Palgrave Macmillan.

Snyder, C. R. (1994). *The psychology of hope.* Free Press.

Sperry, L. (2022). *Highly effective therapy: Effecting deep change in counseling and psychotherapy.* Routledge.

Srinivasan, T. M. (2021). Kaivalya: The ultimate freedom. *International Journal of Yoga, 14*(3), 173–174. https://doi.org/10.4103/ijoy.ijoy_123_21

Stauffer, J. (2015). *Ethical loneliness: The injustice of not being heard.* Columbia University Press.

Stefana, A. (2017). *History of countertransference: From Freud to the British object relations school.* Routledge.

Stein, D. M., & Lambert, M. J. (1995). Graduate training in psychotherapy: Are therapy outcomes enhanced? *Journal of Consulting and Clinical Psychology, 63*(2), 182–196. https://doi.org/10.1037//0022-006x.63.2.182

Sternberg, R. J. (Ed.). (1990). *Wisdom: Its nature, origins, and development.* Cambridge University Press.

Sternberg, R. J., & Glück, J. (2021). *Wisdom: The psychology of wise thoughts, words, and deeds.* Cambridge University Press.

Stevens, F. L. (2024). Revisiting the cognitive primacy hypothesis: Implications for psychotherapy. *Journal of Psychotherapy Integration, 34*(4), 450–462. https://doi.org/10.1037/int0000313

Stice, E., Shaw, H., Becker, C. B., & Rohde, P. (2008). Dissonance-based interventions for the prevention of eating disorders: Using persuasion principles to promote health. *Prevention Science, 9*(2), 114–128. https://doi.org/10.1007/s11121-008-0093-x

Strean, H. S. (1993). *Resolving counterresistances in psychotherapy.* Brunner/Maze.

Stricker, G., & Gold, J. R. (Eds.). (2013). *Comprehensive handbook of psychotherapy integration.* Springer.

Strupp, H. H. (1988). What is therapeutic change? *Journal of Cognitive Psychotherapy, 2*(2), 75–82.

Strupp, H. H. (1996). The tripartite model and the consumer reports study. *American Psychologist, 51*(10), 1017–1024. https://doi.org/10.1037//0003-066x.51.10.1017

Strupp, H. H., & Hadley, S. W. (1979). Specific versus nonspecific factors in psychotherapy. *Archives of General Psychiatry, 36*, 1125–1136.

Sue, D. W. (2010). Microaggressions, marginality, and oppression: An introduction. In D. W. Sue (Ed.), *Microaggressions and marginality: Manifestation, dynamics and impact* (pp. 3–22). Wiley.

Sue, D. W., Sue, D., Neville, H. A., & Smith, L. (2022). *Counseling the culturally diverse: Theory and practice.* Wiley.

Sultanoff, S. M. (2013). Integrating humor into psychotherapy: Research, theory, and the necessary conditions for the presence of therapeutic humor in helping relationships. *The Humanistic Psychologist, 41*(4), 388–399. https://doi.org/10.1080/08873267.2013.796953

Swift, J. K., Owen, J., & Miller, S. D. (2023). Client factors. In S. D. Miller, D. Chow, S. Malins, & M. A. Hubble (Eds.), *The field guide to better results: Evidence-based exercises to improve therapeutic effectiveness* (pp. 47–78). American Psychological Association. https://doi.org/10.1037/0000358-004

Ta, V., Griffith, C., Boatfield, C., Wang, X., Civitello, M., Bader, H., DeCero, C., & Loggarakis, A. (2020). User experiences of social support from companion chatbots in everyday contexts: Thematic analysis. *Journal of Medical Internet Research, 22*(3), Article e16235. https://doi.org/10.2196/16235

Tapper, K. (2018). Mindfulness and craving: Effects and mechanisms. *Clinical Psychology Review, 59*, 101–117. https://doi.org/10.1016/j.cpr.2017.11.003

Teater, M., & Ludgate, J. (2014). *Overcoming compassion fatigue: A practical resilience workbook.* PESI Publishing & Media.

Tedeschi, R. G., & Moore, B. A. (2021). Posttraumatic growth as an integrative therapeutic philosophy. *Journal of Psychotherapy Integration, 31*(2), 180–194. https://doi.org/10.1037/int0000250

Teyber, E., & Teyber, F. M. (2014). Working with the process dimension in relational therapies: Guidelines for clinical training. *Psychotherapy*, *51*(3), 334–341. https://doi.org/10.1037/a0036579

Theise, N. D., & Kafatos, M. C. (2016). Fundamental awareness: A framework for integrating science, philosophy and metaphysics. *Communicative & Integrative Biology*, *9*(3), Article e1155010. https://doi.org/10.1080/19420889.2016.1155010

Tirch, D., Silberstein, L. R., & Kolts, R. L. (2015). *Buddhist psychology and cognitive-behavioral therapy: A clinician's guide*. Guilford Press.

Totton, N. (2018). Power in the therapeutic relationship. In R. Tweedy (Ed.), *The political self* (pp. 29–42). Routledge.

Townshend, C. (1987). The necessity of political violence: A review article. *Comparative Studies in Society and History*, *29*(2), 314–319. https://doi.org/10.1017/S0010417500014523

Travers-Hill, E., Dunn, B. D., Hoppitt, L., Hitchcock, C., & Dalgleish, T. (2017). Beneficial effects of training in self-distancing and perspective broadening for people with a history of recurrent depression. *Behaviour Research and Therapy*, *95*, 19–28. https://doi.org/10.1016/j.brat.2017.05.008

Ucar, G. K., Hasta, D., & Malatyali, M. K. (2019). The mediating role of perceived control and hopelessness in the relation between personal belief in a just world and life satisfaction. *Personality and Individual Differences*, *143*, 68–73. https://doi.org/10.1016/j.paid.2019.02.021

Vafaie, N., & Kober, H. (2022). Association of drug cues and craving with drug use and relapse: A systematic review and meta-analysis. *JAMA Psychiatry*, *79*(7), 641–650. https://doi.org/10.1001/jamapsychiatry.2022.1240

Vago, D. R., Farb, N., & Spreng, R. N. (2022). Clarifying internally-directed cognition: A commentary on the attention to thoughts model. *Psychological Inquiry*, *33*(4), 261–272. https://doi.org/10.1080/1047840X.2022.2141005

Vahdani, R., & Phillips, M. (2021). Existential–Jungian analysis: Reconciling the personal and archetypal realms in the consulting room. *Journal of Humanistic Psychology*, *61*(5), 806–827. https://doi.org/10.1177/0022167819880039

Vallejo, Z., & Amara, H. (2009). Adaptation of mindfulness-based stress reduction program for addiction relapse prevention. *The Humanistic Psychologist*, *37*(2), 192–206. https://doi.org/10.1080/08873260902892287

van der Kolk, B. A. (2014). *The body keeps the score: Brain, mind, and body in the healing of trauma*. Viking.

van Ede, F., & Nobre, A. C. (2021). Toward a neurobiology of internal selective attention. *Trends in Neurosciences*, *44*(7), 513–515. https://doi.org/10.1016/j.tins.2021.04.010

van Inwagen, P. (2024). *The abstract and the concrete: Further essays in ontology*. Oxford University Press.

Van Kaam, A. (1966). *Existential foundations of psychology*. Duquesne University Press.

Van Wagoner, S. L., Gelso, C. L., Hayes, J. A., & Diemer, R. A. (1991). Countertransference and the reputedly excellent therapist. *Psychotherapy: Theory, Research, Practice, Training*, *28*(3), 411–421. https://doi.org/10.1037/0033-3204.28.3.411

Vargas, S. M., Huey, S. J., Jr., & Miranda, J. (2020). A critical review of current evidence on multiple types of discrimination and mental health. *American Journal of Orthopsychiatry*, *90*(3), 374–390. https://doi.org/10.1037/ort0000441

Vickery, P. J., Hanna, F. J., & Wilkinson, B. D. (2023). Techniques in the freedom-from oppression model: An integrative existential-cognitive therapy. *The Journal of Humanistic Counseling, 62*(3), 173–186. https://doi.org/10.1002/johc.12205

Wachtel, P. L. (1977). *Psychoanalysis and behavior therapy: Toward an integration*. Basic Books.

Wachtel, P. L. (2018). Pathways to progress for integrative psychotherapy: Perspectives on practice and research. *Journal of Psychotherapy Integration, 28*(2), 202–212. https://doi.org/10.1037/int0000089

Walrond-Skinner, S. (1986). *Dictionary of psychotherapy*. Routledge; Kegan Paul.

Walsh, L. M., Roddy, M. K., Scott, K., Lewis, C. C., & Jensen-Doss, A. (2019). A meta-analysis of the effect of therapist experience on outcomes for clients with internalizing disorders. *Psychotherapy Research, 29*(7), 846–859. https://doi.org/10.1080/10503307.2018.1469802

Wampold, B. E. (2001). *The great psychotherapy debate: Models, methods, and findings*. Routledge.

Wampold, B. E., & Flückiger, C. (2023). The alliance in mental health care: Conceptualization, evidence and clinical applications. *World Psychiatry, 22*(1), 25–41. https://doi.org/10.1002/wps.21035

Wampold, B. E. & Imel, Z. E. (2015). *The great psychotherapy debate: The evidence for what makes psychotherapy work* (2nd ed.). Routledge.

Wampold, B. E., & Ulvenes, P. G. (2019). Integration of common factors and specific ingredients. In J. C. Norcross & M. R. Goldfried (Eds.), *Handbook of psychotherapy integration* (pp. 69–87). Oxford University Press.

Wang, M., Zhang, L. J., & Hamilton, R. (2023). Developing the Metacognitive Awareness of Grit Scale for a better understanding of learners of English as a foreign language. *Frontiers in Psychology, 14*, Article 1141214. https://doi.org/10.3389/fpsyg.2023.1141214

Wang, Y., Chung, M. C., Wang, N., Yu, X., & Kenardy, J. (2021). Social support and posttraumatic stress disorder: A meta-analysis of longitudinal studies. *Clinical Psychology Review, 85*, Article 101998. https://doi.org/10.1016/j.cpr.2021.101998

Warth, M., Zöller, J., Köhler, F., Aguilar-Raab, C., Kessler, J., & Ditzen, B. (2020). Psychosocial interventions for pain management in advanced cancer patients: A systematic review and meta-analysis. *Current Oncology Reports, 22*(1), Article 3. https://doi.org/10.1007/s11912-020-0870-7

Watkins, M. (2002). Seeding liberation: A dialogue between depth psychology and liberation psychology. In D. Slattery & L. Corbett (Eds.), *Depth psychology: Meditations in the field* (pp. 204–225). Daimon Verlag.

Watson, L. B., DeBlaere, C., Langrehr, K. J., Zelaya, D. G., & Flores, M. J. (2016). The influence of multiple oppressions on women of color's experiences with insidious trauma. *Journal of Counseling Psychology, 63*(6), 656–667. https://doi.org/10.1037/cou0000165

Watts, R. E., & Bluvshtein, M. (2020). Adler's theory and therapy as a river: A brief discussion of the profound influence of Alfred Adler. *Journal of Individual Psychology, 76*(1), 99–109. https://doi.org/10.1353/jip.2020.0021

Watzlawick, P., Weakland, J. H., & Fisch, R. (1974). *Change: Principles of problem formation and problem resolution*. W. W. Norton.

Weinberger, J., & Eig, A. (1999). Expectancies: The ignored common factor in psychotherapy. In I. Kirsch (Ed.), *How expectancies shape experience* (pp. 357–382). American Psychological Association. https://doi.org/10.1037/10332-015

Weiner, M. F. (1982). *The therapeutic impasse*. Free Press.

Weintraub, J., Nolan, K. P., & Sachdev, A. R. (2023). The cognitive control model of work-related flow. *Frontiers in Psychology, 14*, Article 1174152. https://doi.org/10.3389/fpsyg.2023.1174152

Weiss, P. (1958). Common sense and beyond. In S. Hook (Ed.), *Determinism and freedom: In the age of modern science* (pp. 211–224). Collier Books.

Wells, A. (2007). Cognition about cognition: Metacognitive therapy and change in generalized anxiety disorder and social phobia. *Cognitive and Behavioral Practice, 14*(1), 18–25. https://doi.org/10.1016/j.cbpra.2006.01.005

Whitaker, C. (1976). The hindrance of theory in clinical work. In P. D. Guerin (Ed.), *Family therapy: Theory and practice* (pp. 154–164). Gardner Press.

Whitaker, C. (1989). *Midnight musings of a family therapist*. W. W. Norton.

Whitehead, A. N. (1925). *Science and the modern world*. Free Press.

Whitehead, A. N. (1938). *Modes of thought*. Capricorn Books.

Wilken, B., & Miyamoto, Y. (2018). Dialectical emotions. In J. Spencer-Rodgers & K. Peng (Eds.), *The psychological and cultural foundations of East Asian cognition: Contradiction, change, and holism* (pp. 509–546). Oxford University Press.

Wilkinson, B. D. (2019). A refined and further defined argument on the limits of neuroscience in counseling: Response to Field, Luke, and Beeson and Miller. *The Journal of Humanistic Counseling, 58*(2), 119–134. https://doi.org/10.1002/johc.12101

Wilkinson, B. D. (2023). Understanding experiential awareness in humanistic-phenomenological counseling. *The Journal of Humanistic Counseling, 62*(2), 145–159. https://doi.org/10.1002/johc.12196

Wilkinson, B. D., & Hanna, F. J. (2018). Using the precursors model of change to facilitate engagement practices in family counseling. *The Family Journal, 26*(3), 306–314. https://doi.org/10.1177/1066480718795502

Wilkinson, B. D., & Wilkinson, K. A. (2024). The ecological-enactive approach to embodiment in humanistic psychotherapy. *The Humanistic Psychologist*. Advance online publication. https://doi.org/10.1037/hum0000349

Winnicott, D. W. (2018). Ego distortion in terms of true and false self. In L. Caldwell (Ed.), *The person who is me* (pp. 7–22). Routledge. (Original work published 1960)

Wolpe, J. (1958). *Psychotherapy by reciprocal inhibition*. Stanford University Press.

Woods, A., Solomonov, N., Liles, B., Guillod, A., Kales, H. C., & Sirey, J. A. (2021). Perceived social support and interpersonal functioning as predictors of treatment response among depressed older adults. *The American Journal of Geriatric Psychiatry, 29*(8), 843–852. https://doi.org/10.1016/j.jagp.2020.12.021

Yaden, D. B., Johnson, M. W., Griffiths, R. R., Doss, M. K., Garcia-Romeu, A., Nayak, S., Gukasyan, N., Mathur, B. N., & Barrett, F. S. (2021). Psychedelics and consciousness: Distinctions, demarcations, and opportunities. *The International Journal of Neuropsychopharmacology, 24*(8), 615–623. https://doi.org/10.1093/ijnp/pyab026

Yadlin-Gadot, S. (2016). *Truth matters: Theory and practice in psychoanalysis*. Brill.

Yalom, I. D. (1980). *Existential psychotherapy*. Basic Books.

Yalom, I. D. (1989). *Love's executioner and other tales of psychotherapy*. HarperCollins.

Yalom, I. D. (1995). *Theory and practice of group psychotherapy*. Basic Books.

Yang, Y., & Hayes, J. A. (2020). Causes and consequences of burnout among mental health professionals: A practice-oriented review of recent empirical literature. *Psychotherapy, 57*(3), 426–436. https://doi.org/10.1037/pst0000317

Zahavi, D. (2014). Empathy and other-directed intentionality. *Topoi, 33*(1), 129–142. https://doi.org/10.1007/s11245-013-9197-4

Zahavi, D. (2017). *Husserl's legacy: Phenomenology, metaphysics, and transcendental philosophy.* Oxford University Press.

Zahavi, D. (2018). Brain, mind, world: Predictive coding, neo-Kantianism, and transcendental idealism. *Husserl Studies, 34*(1), 47–61. https://doi.org/10.1007/s10743-017-9218-z

Zerubavel, N., & Messman-Moore, T. L. (2015). Staying present: Incorporating mindfulness into therapy for dissociation. *Mindfulness, 6*(2), 303–314. https://doi.org/10.1007/s12671-013-0261-3

Zilcha-Mano, S. (2021). Toward personalized psychotherapy: The importance of the trait-like/state-like distinction for understanding therapeutic change. *American Psychologist, 76*(3), 516–528. https://doi.org/10.1037/amp0000629

Zvi-Beiman, S., & Shahar, G. (2015). Psychotherapy integration. In R. Cautin & S. Lilienfeld (Eds.), *The encyclopedia of clinical psychology* (pp. 1–6). Wiley.

INDEX

paradox, use of, 122
role-plays of others, 120
as savoir faire, 115–116
self-monitoring, 121
significant moments of change involving, 109–110
situation, defined, 116
techniques for cultivating, 113–125
unaware person, example of, 114–115

B

Bad breath metaphor, 114
Bandura, A., 95
Bateson, G., 57
Beck, A. T., 107, 114
Beck Hopelessness Scale, 94
Being and Time (Heidegger), 146
Benign stereotyping, 247
Bettelheim, B., 90
Bibliotherapy, 31–32, 36
Black Lives Matter movement, 241
Blaming others, 160–161
Blind spots metaphor, 113
Body odor metaphor, 114
Boundaries setting, 65
Brodley, B. T., 117
Burnout, 216, 227–228, 230, 255

C

Cannon, W. B., 90
Caring, 63–64
prioritizing, 226–227
Cautela, J. R., 124
Cautionary note, 189
Change deficits, 20, 35
CHANGES assessment
case examples, 216–221
across diagnoses, 208
empirical validation of, 198–199
examples of, 204–207
form, 198, 199–202
with groups and families, 207–208
James case, 219–221
Joy case, 205–206
Kurt case, 217–218
Nancy case, 218–219
rating for, 197–208
Ricky case, 206–207
scoring of, 202–204
therapist interference, 211–216
Tommy case, 204–205
CHANGES Assessment for Businesses and Corporations, 275–279
CHANGES model, 4. *See also* Therapeutic change
advantages of, 273–274

assessing individual, team, and organizational change, 275–279
future applications of, 274–275
to metatheoretical framework, 279–286
technological freedom and, 285–286
unique aspects of, 6–9
Chatbots, 36, 184
Civilized oppression, 241
Cleansing metaphor, 154
Client-specific factors, 16–17
Clinical markers
awareness, 110–111
confronting, 76–77
effort, 172–173
grit, 150–151
hope, 92–93
necessity, 129–130
social support, 186–187
Cognitive behavioral therapy, 24, 26, 42, 107, 171, 267
Cognitive dissonance, 138–141
asking questions, 138–139
Jason case, 139–141
role of, 128–129
spitting in the client's soupis technique, 139, 141
Compartmentalizing, 112
Compassion, 63–64, 233–234
Compassion fatigue, 227
Concentration-based techniques, 87
Concentric-circle technique, 68, 190–191
Concretized confronting, 85–87
Confidence, 92
Conflicted client, 174–175
Confrontation, 116–118
avoiding, 229
with compassion and empathy, 233–234
with impatience, 229
Confronting the problem, 5, 18, 276–277
absence of, 77–78
ancient approaches to, 72–73
clinical markers of, 76–77
concentration-based techniques, 87
concretized, 85–87
cutting to essence of, 71–72
deficit in, 212
defined, 69
hesitancy to confront, 79
holding problem steady, 70
idea of change itself, 79
impatience, 229
leading to therapeutic change, 70–75
metaphor of strength, 78–79
miracle question, 88
mirroring, 85
onion peeler, 83–84
power of problem, removing, 74–75
reality testing, 73

recognizing, 76–77
representational, 85–87
significant moments of change involving, 75–76
simplicity and complexity, 73
smaller problem space, 74
and systematic desensitization, 71
techniques for enhancing, 78–88
vaccine effect of, 75
in vivo, 80–83
Confusion, building tolerance of, 125
Consciousness-raising strategy, 31–32, 107–108
Contagion, hope as, 100–101
Contexts, contrasting, 122–123
Control
  effort, 169–170
  Grit, 161–162
  necessity, 142
  of thoughts and images, 169–170
Countertransference, 209–210, 211
Courtesy, 54–55
Cravings
  influencing, 270
  management, 269
  mindfully riding, 269–270
  techniques for reducing, 269–270
Creative narratives, 102–103
Crenshaw, K., 246
Crisis, 9, 91, 94, 121
  defined, 37
Cross-purposes, 141–142

D

Decentering, 107
Decision making, 180
Defensiveness, 145, 230
Degree of change, 9–10
Degrees of conscious awareness, 106
Diagnostic and Statistical Manual of Mental Disorders, 39, 208, 266
Dialectical thinking, 31, 231
Difficult clients, 15–34, 52, 210–211
  antisocial clients, 64
  autonomy and freedom, respecting and encouraging, 62–63
  back off, option of telling to, 57
  at basis of techniques, 27–28
  at basis of theory, 22–27
  being courteous, 54–55
  being persuasive, 55–56
  boundaries setting, 65
  change as skill, 28–29
  chunks, addressing problems in, 64
  client's meaning system, 60–61
  compassion and caring, displaying, 63–64
  concentric circle technique, 68

defense systems, bringing down, 62
defined, 20
emotional state matching, 65–66
empathy, increasing therapist capacity for, 59–60
framing techniques, 28
hesitancy, expecting, 64–65
"I Behind The Eye", 67
Joy case, 40, 205–206
Kathy case, 42–43
making, 35–48
matching therapist with, 67
metacognitive aspects of change, 29–31
metalogue, attending to, 57–58
perspicacity, as wisdom characteristic, 67
positive qualities, validating, 56–57
precursors of change, 17–19, 21–22, 33
problem, redefining, 61–62
realigning psychotherapy theories around change, 24–26
reflecting meanings before feelings, 58–59
relationship with, 54–68
requesting permission from, 54–55
Ricky case, 40–41, 206–207
as teachers, 236–237
theories for clients, 26–27
therapeutic change and client-specific factors, 16–17
therapeutic modalities, 68
therapeutic window, opening, 66
Tommy case, 39–40, 204–205
transtheoretical model and motivational interviewing, 31–33
uncooperativeness as protection of freedom, 63
value of model for therapy with, 20–22
"what's-in-it-for-me?" question, 63
Difficult therapists, 210–211
Difficulty. *See also* Grit, or the willingness to experience anxiety or difficulty
  implicit learning and maladaptive beliefs, 41–43
  Kurt case, 38, 217–218
  and resistance as self-protection, 36–41
  roots of, 41–43
  therapist variables influencing therapeutic success, 43–47
  training to be difficult by therapists, 37–39
  training wisdom out of therapist, 46–47
  wisdom and wise therapist, 44–46
Disappointment, 94
Discouragement, 94, 215, 235
Disequilibrium, 37
Disgusting, 235
Doubling, 265
Douglass, F., 249

freedom-from, 282, 284
freedom-to, 282, 284–285
freedom-with, 282–283, 285
modes of, 281–283, 284
respecting and encouraging, 62–63
as teleological approach to integration,
    283–285
uncooperativeness as protection of, 63
Freedom-from-oppression model (FOM), 250
Freedom of choice, 176
Freud, S., 20, 107, 209
Freud, Sigmund, 3
Fromm-Reichmann, F., 210

G

Gendlin, E., 3, 6, 67, 87, 119
Genuineness, 46, 51, 53, 66
Gestalt therapy, 26, 28, 83, 87, 120, 262
Glass, G. V., 23
Glasser, W., 168
Goal, clarification of, 176–177
Goldfried, M. R., 22
Graduated tasks, assigning, 177
Graduate training, 43, 44, 46
Grand reframe of addictive behaviors,
    255–259
Grit, or the willingness to experience anxiety
    or difficulty, 5, 18, 30, 278
    absence of, 151–152
    anxiety accompanying change, 146
    clinical markers of, 150–151
    control or freedom challenge, 161–162
    deficit in, 215
    defined, 145
    internal dialogue avoiding anxiety,
        155–157
    leading to change, 147–149
    maladaptive beliefs about, 164–165
    metaphors, 152–155
    ownership taking and blame stopping,
        160–161
    paradox, use of, 157–160
    person owning problem, 147
    philosophical roots of, 146–147
    recognizing, 150–151
    self-monitoring, 162–164
    significant moments of change
        involving, 149
    techniques for establishing, 152–165
Group therapy, 8, 68, 103, 125, 192–193,
    207–208, 266
Guts metaphor, 154–155

H

Hadley, S. W., 43
Hanna, F. J., 4, 266
Harris, Sydney J., 5

Harvey, J., 241
Heidegger, M., 26, 72, 146–147, 250
Hermeneutical injustice, 242
Hesitance, 64–65
    to confronting, 79
Hooking and unhooking approach, 227
Hope for change, 5, 18, 277
    absence of, 93–94
    clinical markers of, 92–93
    clues to presence of, 92
    as contagion, 100–101
    converting threats into challenges,
        98–100
    creative narratives, 102–103
    deficit in, 213
    defined, 89
    empowerment strategies, 97
    hopelessness, reflecting, 97–98
    and humor, 93
    Jamesian Device, 96–97
    leading to therapeutic change, 90–91
    maladaptive beliefs, examining, 103–104
    moments of change involving, 91–92
    negative behaviors, reframing, 98
    negative role models and, 95–96
    recognizing, 92–93
    relating and rewriting, 102–103
    sense of worthiness and, 101–102
    techniques for building, 94–104
    telling stories of recovery, 103
Hopelessness, 91, 94, 97–98, 235
Horney, K., 216, 232
Hostility, with equanimity and humor,
    234–235
House cleaning metaphor, 176
Human being, as active agent, 8–9
Human Change Processes (Mahoney), 37
Hume, D., 25, 169
Humor, 93, 234–235
Husserl, E., 26, 71–72, 83, 107

I

Idea of making changes, 79
Implicit learning, 41–42
Implicit oppression, 241–242
Individual therapy, 68
Inductive reasoning process, 58
Integrative existential-cognitive therapy.
    See Existential-cognitive therapy
Intelligence, 44, 46
Intentional unawareness, handling,
    123–124
Intentions, mapping, 179–180
Interpersonal input, 125
Interpersonal savvy, role of, 7–8
In vivo confronting, 80
    Marvin case, 80–81
    Rusty case, 81–83

ABOUT THE AUTHORS

Brett D. Wilkinson, PhD, LMHC, is an associate professor in the Department of Counseling and Graduate Education at Purdue University Fort Wayne (PFW). He serves as editor-in-chief of the *Journal of Humanistic Counseling* and founding director of the PFW Institute for Counseling Research. His research examines therapeutic change mechanisms, experiential-humanistic interventions, and cognitive complexity development. He is also author of the textbook *Educational Psychology for Learners*, now in its third edition. He has 15 years of therapy experience working with adolescents, adults, couples, and families in community agencies and private practice and provides consulting services on the CHANGES model, reflective supervision practices, and experiential interventions.

Fred J. Hanna, PhD, is a professor and codesigner of the PhD program in Counseling at Adler University in Chicago. He is also a senior faculty associate at Johns Hopkins University, where he taught graduate counseling courses for 25 years, including 11 years full time, leaving as a full professor. Fred has authored or coauthored over 70 peer-reviewed and professional publications. An award-winning teacher, he has also delivered well over 500 presentations at conferences, seminars, trainings, and workshops across America. Fred was the recipient of the 2019 Humanistic Impact Award, a national award granted by the Association for Humanistic Counseling. He also received the Adler University Social Justice Award for 2020. Fred has served as a consultant and trainer to the medical, mental health, corrections, business, and education communities, including at such places as the Johns Hopkins School of Medicine Department of Psychiatry; the Fort Peck Sioux Reservation in Montana; the Department of Psychiatry at Yale University; and a wide variety of school systems, community agencies, prisons, and criminal justice settings from coast to coast. His research interests have focused on developing the CHANGES model as well as developing, publishing, and presenting many evidence-based, innovative psychotherapy techniques and strategies designed for application in the areas of client motivation, therapy resistance, addictions, diversity and multiculturalism, oppression, liberation, trauma, spirituality, criminality, defiant adolescents, personal development, and difficult personalities. He is also an accomplished world traveler, having explored many remote areas in Asia over a period of 2 years.